Drugs of Abuse

FORENSIC

SCIENCE AND MEDICINE

Steven B. Karch, MD, SERIES EDITOR

DRUGS OF ABUSE: *BODY FLUID TESTING*
edited by **Raphael C. Wong and Harley Y. Tse,** *2005*

A PHYSICIAN'S GUIDE TO CLINICAL FORENSIC MEDICINE: *SECOND EDITION*
edited by **Margaret M. Stark,** *2005*

FORENSIC MEDICINE OF THE LOWER EXTREMITY: *HUMAN IDENTIFICATION AND TRAUMA ANALYSIS OF THE THIGH, LEG, AND FOOT,* by **Jeremy Rich, Dorothy E. Dean, and Robert H. Powers,** *2005*

FORENSIC AND CLINICAL APPLICATIONS OF SOLID PHASE EXTRACTION, by **Michael J. Telepchak, Thomas F. August, and Glynn Chaney,** *2004*

HANDBOOK OF DRUG INTERACTIONS: *A CLINICAL AND FORENSIC GUIDE,* edited by **Ashraf Mozayani and Lionel P. Raymon,** *2004*

DIETARY SUPPLEMENTS: *TOXICOLOGY AND CLINICAL PHARMACOLOGY,* edited by **Melanie Johns Cupp and Timothy S. Tracy,** *2003*

BUPRENOPHINE THERAPY OF OPIATE ADDICTION, edited by **Pascal Kintz and Pierre Marquet,** *2002*

BENZODIAZEPINES AND GHB: *DETECTION AND PHARMACOLOGY,* edited by **Salvatore J. Salamone,** *2002*

ON-SITE DRUG TESTING, edited by **Amanda J. Jenkins and Bruce A. Goldberger,** *2001*

BRAIN IMAGING IN SUBSTANCE ABUSE: *RESEARCH, CLINICAL, AND FORENSIC APPLICATIONS,* edited by **Marc J. Kaufman,** *2001*

TOXICOLOGY AND CLINICAL PHARMACOLOGY OF HERBAL PRODUCTS,
edited by **Melanie Johns Cupp,** *2000*

CRIMINAL POISONING: *INVESTIGATIONAL GUIDE FOR LAW ENFORCEMENT, TOXICOLOGISTS, FORENSIC SCIENTISTS, AND ATTORNEYS,*
by **John H. Trestrail, III,** *2000*

A PHYSICIAN'S GUIDE TO CLINICAL FORENSIC MEDICINE,
edited by **Margaret M. Stark,** *2000*

Drugs of Abuse

Body Fluid Testing

Edited by

Raphael C. Wong, MS, MBA

Branan Medical Corporation, Irvine, CA

Harley Y. Tse, PhD, MBA

Department of Immunology and Microbiology,
Wayne State University School of Medicine,
Detroit, MI

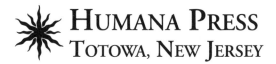
HUMANA PRESS
TOTOWA, NEW JERSEY

© 2005 Humana Press Inc.
999 Riverview Drive, Suite 208
Totowa, New Jersey 07512
www.humanapress.com

This publication is printed on acid-free paper. ∞

ANSI Z39.48-1984 (American Standards Institute) Permanence of Paper for Printed Library Materials.

Production Editor: Tracy Catanese

Cover design by Patricia F. Cleary

For additional copies, pricing for bulk purchases, and/or information about other Humana titles, contact Humana at the above address or at any of the following numbers: Tel: 973-256-1699; Fax: 973-256-8341; E-mail: orders@humanapr.com, or visit our Website at www.humanapress.com

Printed in the United States of America. 10 9 8 7 6 5 4 3 2 1

e-ISBN: 1-59259-951-6

Library of Congress Cataloging in Publication Data

Drugs of abuse : body fluid testing / edited by Raphael C. Wong, Harley Y. Tse.
    p. cm. -- (Forensic science and medicine)
  Includes bibliographical references and index.
  ISBN 1-58829-435-8 (alk. paper)
  1. Drugs of abuse--Analysis. 2. Forensic pharmacology. 3. Body fluids--Analysis. I. Wong, Raphael C.
II. Tse, Harley Y. III. Series.
  RA1160.D785 2005
  614'.1--dc22
                                                                        2005000317

Preface

Although not exactly a common topic for social conversations, drug testing directly and indirectly touches the lives of many people. Circumstances surrounding employment, traffic accidents, sports, and perhaps encounters with law enforcement inevitably involve some facets of drug testing. During the past two decades, drug testing has been greatly facilitated by the development of lateral flow immunoassays that simplify the testing procedures and make test results available in a timely fashion. Urine has been the biological specimen of choice for testing. However, recent technological advances have now made it possible to use alternative body fluids for this purpose. Subsequently, the field of drug testing has flourished as a science. It is with this view in mind that the present volume, *Drugs of Abuse: Body Fluid Testing*, is written. It is intended to be both informative and timely. Its audience includes not only professionals and scientists, but also cursory readers interested in understanding the societal impact as well as the limitations of drug testing.

Drugs of Abuse: Body Fluid Testing begins with a historical recounting of events that have led to the establishment of federal regulatory policies specifically pertaining to drug testing. This is followed by a broad description of the various body fluid specimens suitable for use in testing for illicit drugs. These two initial chapters are both informative and interesting to read. The next three chapters are designed for the technically minded. Chapter 3 presents a comprehensive review of all commonly used analytical technologies and their utilities in drug testing, both in laboratory-based and on-site settings. Chapters 4 and 5 then provide rather detailed accounts of the structural as well as manufacturing aspects of on-site testing devices based on lateral flow immunoassays. Because the use of urine as a testing matrix has been exhaustively discussed over the years in numerous publications, we have chosen in this volume to avoid repetition and concentrate on the use of other body fluids, such as saliva and sweat, and hair. The advantages as well as the pitfalls of using these specimens are the subject matter of Chapters 6–11. Of the alternative biological specimens, oral fluid has the best potential of succeeding urine as the next matrix of choice for drug detection. Therefore, four popular saliva testing devices are selected for discussion. Following this section is Chapter 12, the author of which adopts the viewpoint that drug testing is, in practice, information transfer and argues that, to comply with privacy and accuracy issues, the processes of drug testing should be automated with as little human intervention as possible. On the application of drug testing in the legal system, Chapter 13 describes what occurs within the drug court system with intriguing statistics. Finally, any discussion on drug testing cannot be complete without an appreciation of the current status of sample adulteration. Two chapters are devoted to this purpose. Because drug addiction is not just a problem confined to the United States, the next two chapters of this volume bring the reader up to date on how the European Union deals with this problem. A large-scale roadside drug-testing program (ROSITA) was undertaken, the results of which would benefit not just the European Union, but also countries worldwide. Thus, this book covers a wide spectrum of issues related to body fluid testing of drugs of abuse, and is written by experts in their respective fields. The subject matter should appeal to a wide variety of readers.

Raphael C. Wong
Harley Y. Tse

Contents

Preface v
Contributors ix

CHAPTER 1   Historical Aspects of Drugs-of-Abuse Testing
             in the United States
             Lawrence A. Reynolds *1*

CHAPTER 2   Specimens for Drugs-of-Abuse Testing
             Leo J. Kadehjian *11*

CHAPTER 3   Drug-Testing Technologies and Applications
             Jane S-C. Tsai and Grace L. Lin *29*

CHAPTER 4   The Use of Nitrocellulose Membranes
             in Lateral-Flow Assays
             Michael A. Mansfield *71*

CHAPTER 5   Antibody–Label Conjugates in Lateral-Flow Assays
             Paul Christopher, Nikki Robinson, and Michael K. Shaw *87*

CHAPTER 6   Lateral-Flow Assays: *Assembly and Automation*
             David Carlberg *99*

CHAPTER 7   Oral-Fluid Drug Testing Using the Intercept® Device
             R. Sam Niedbala and Keith W. Kardos *115*

CHAPTER 8   Dräger DrugTest®: *Test for Illegal Drugs
             in Oral-Fluid Samples*
             Stefan Steinmeyer, Rainer Polzius, and Andreas Manns *133*

vii

CHAPTER 9   On-Site Oral-Fluid Drug Testing by Oratect®
Raphael C. Wong *145*

CHAPTER 10   Saliva and Sweat Testing With Drugwipe®: *A Review*
Franz Aberl and Robert VanDine *161*

CHAPTER 11   Hair Analysis in Drugs-of-Abuse Testing
Michael I. Schaffer and Virginia A. Hill *177*

CHAPTER 12   Instrumented Urine Point-of-Collection Testing
Using the eScreen® System
Murray Lappe *201*

CHAPTER 13   Adulteration of Drugs-of-Abuse Specimens
Amitava Dasgupta *215*

CHAPTER 14   Adulteration Detection by Intect® 7
Raphael C. Wong and Harley Y. Tse *233*

CHAPTER 15   Drug Testing and the Criminal Justice System:
A Marriage Made in Court
John N. Marr *247*

CHAPTER 16   Drug-of-Abuse Testing: *The European Perspective*
Alex Yil Fai Wong *259*

CHAPTER 17   The Results of the Roadside Drug Testing
Assessment Project
Alain Verstraete *271*

CHAPTER 18   Trends in Drug Testing: *Concluding Remarks*
Raphael C. Wong *293*

Index *297*

Contributors

FRANZ ABERL • *Securetec Detektions-Systeme AG, Ottobrunn, Germany*

DAVE CARLBERG • *Kinematic Automation Inc., Twain Harte, CA*

PAUL CHRISTOPHER • *British BioCell International, Cardiff, Wales, UK*

AMITAVA DASGUPTA • *Department of Pathology and Laboratory Medicine, University of Texas-Houston Medical School, Houston, TX*

VIRGINIA A. HILL • *Psychemedics Corporation, Culver City, CA*

LEO J. KADEHJIAN • *Biomedical Consulting, Palo Alto, CA*

KEITH W. KARDOS • *OraSure Technologies Inc., Bethlehem, PA*

MURRAY LAPPE • *eScreen Inc., Beverly Hills, CA*

GRACE L. LIN • *Roche Diagnostics, Indianapolis, IA*

ANDREAS MANNS • *Dräger Safety AG & Co. KGaA, Lübeck, Germany*

MICHAEL A. MANSFIELD • *Millipore Corporation, Danvers, MA*

JOHN N. MARR • *Johnson City, TN*

R. SAM NIEDBALA • *Chemistry Department, Lehigh University, Bethlehem, PA*

RAINER POLZIUS • *Drägerwerk AG, Lübeck, Germany*

LAWRENCE A. REYNOLDS • *LAR Consulting, San Jose, CA*

NIKKI ROBINSON • *British BioCell International, Cardiff, Wales, UK*

MICHAEL I. SCHAFFER • *Psychemedics Corporation, Culver City, CA*

MICHAEL K. SHAW • *Department of Immunology and Microbiology, Wayne State University School of Medicine, Detroit, MI*

STEFAN STEINMEYER • *Dräger Safety AG & Co. KGaA, Lübeck, Germany*

JANE S-C. TSAI • *R&D, Roche Diagnostics, Indianapolis, IN*

HARLEY Y. TSE • *Department of Immunology and Microbiology, Wayne State University School of Medicine, Detroit, MI*

ALEX YIL FAI WONG • *Frost & Sullivan, London, UK*

RAPHAEL C. WONG • *Branan Medical Corporation, Irvine, CA*

ROBERT VANDINE • *Secutetec Contraband Detection & Identification Inc., South Williamsport, PA*

ALAIN VERSTRAETE • *Clinical Biology Laboratory, Ghent University Hospital, Gent, Belgium*

Chapter 1

Historical Aspects of Drugs-of-Abuse Testing in the United States

Lawrence A. Reynolds

SUMMARY

This chapter examines the early history of testing for abused drugs, starting in Vietnam, and traces its growth and expanded applications in the workplace, criminal justice, and schools. It also examines the role played by drug abuse-related accidents on the USS *Nimitz* and Amtrak in shaping the field of drug testing. Standardization and process have been applied to this field of analysis through government regulation of mandated testing for government employees. The chapter examines the collection process, laboratory testing, review of test results, and the role of third-party administrators for workplace testing. These methods have also been applied to testing for the private sector. Standards for testing have also been influenced by a combination of technological advances that allow more accurate and useful test results, and government regulations that help ensure the reliability of the testing process.

1. INTRODUCTION

This chapter examines the early history of drug testing in body fluids, from the first military applications to regulated workplace testing and in the private sector of today. The manner in which federal rules and regulations have shaped the process is also reviewed.

From: *Forensic Science and Medicine: Drugs of Abuse: Body Fluid Testing*
Edited by R. C. Wong and H. Y. Tse © Humana Press Inc., Totowa, NJ

2. THE BEGINNING

Drug abuse has been part of our society for centuries, but the technology to test body fluids for drugs has only been available for less than 50 yr. Testing for illicit drugs first began in Vietnam *(1)*. In the late 1960s, an unusually large number of soldiers began returning home from Southeast Asia as heroin addicts. Identifying these GIs proved difficult. The unpopularity of the Vietnam War was already a public relations disaster for the Nixon administration, and sending our soldiers home as heroin addicts was another war tragedy that the Administration did not want. White House staffers began to look for tools that could be used to rapidly screen thousands of GIs before they returned to the United States. The search ended in 1970, when SYVA Company, a small research organization located in Palo Alto, California, developed a rapid test system capable of detecting opiates in urine. The system used an innovative homogeneous methodology based on the tumbling action of free radicals in solution. This technology was known commercially as free radical assay technique (FRAT) *(2)*. The test was conducted by using an electron spin resonance spectrometer to measure the action of the free radicals. The equipment to conduct this test was somewhat cumbersome, but it was quickly deployed to Vietnam and became an effective screening tool. The FRAT technology had a short but successful commercial life and was replaced 2 yr later by a more robust technology from SYVA known as enzyme-multiplied immunoassay technique (EMIT) *(3)*. This new system utilized an enzymatic reaction that was measured on a simple spectrophotometer. EMIT became the gold standard for the next generation of successful drug-testing methodologies. Other screening technologies followed from Roche, Abbott, and Microgenics. Each of these new technologies further refined the screening tools to identify drug users by testing their body fluids. These technologies will be discussed in more detail in Chapter 3.

3. GROWTH OF DRUG TESTING

By the mid-1970s, the field of drug testing had begun to take root, as many young Americans, both military and civilian, experimented with illegal drugs such as marijuana (tetrahydrocannabinol, or THC), lysergic acid diethylamide (LSD), and cocaine. Most urine testing for illicit drugs was being done either by forensic laboratories or in methadone treatment programs. In these programs, patients undergoing methadone substitution therapy for heroin addiction were monitored for illicit drug use and compliance with the methadone therapy *(4)*. A modest amount of drug testing was being conducted in the workplace by innovative companies that recognized the productivity value of promoting a drug-free work environment.

Then on May 26, 1981, an event occurred that had tremendous reper-cussions on the drug-testing industry *(5)*. There was a serious and deadly crash involving fighter aircraft on the carrier USS *Nimitz*, in the Atlantic Fleet. Fourteen servicemen died, 48 were injured, and $150 million in damage was sustained. Results from the crash investigation revealed that some of the crewmen involved had drugs in their system at the time of the accident. As a result of this incident, the Navy adopted a zero-tolerance drug policy that would ensure that it would be the first drug-free branch of the armed forces. The Navy was committed to ensure that a similar disaster would not occur again. All new recruits were subjected to screening; enlisted personnel and officers were subjected to "for cause" testing. The Navy urine-testing program became the model used by other branches of the US mili-tary and was later adopted by the armies and navies of several other NATO members.

Throughout the 1980s, urine drug testing continued to grow in the civil-ian world as well, with many Fortune 500 companies adopting the policies of, and the procedures for, a drug-free workplace. Some unions adopted these poli-cies as well and undertook testing programs for their members. Drug testing, however, was not applied to government employees until another major deadly event occurred. At noon on January 4, 1987, Amtrak's Colonial passenger train headed out of Washington's Union Station. An hour later, disaster struck in Chase, Maryland, when the Amtrak Colonial collided with a locomotive oper-ated by Conrail engineer Ricky Gates *(6)*. An investigation by the National Transportation Safety Board revealed that Gates and his brakeman had THC in their urine and plasma, ignored the warning signals, and drove the locomotive into the path of the oncoming Amtrak train. This incident alone raised the awareness in both the private and public sectors of the importance of a drug-free workplace in industries like transportation that could endanger the public safety. As a result of both public and private pressures and by an executive order in September 1988, the National Institute on Drug Abuse (NIDA), a department within the US Department of Health and Human Services (HHS), published the first "Mandatory Guidelines for Federal Workplace Drug Testing Programs." The Department of Transportation was the first government agency to adopt the guidelines.

4. REGULATION OF DRUG TESTING

4.1. Federal Regulations

Before the NIDA published its mandatory guidelines in 1988, the only government regulation for drug testing was that the equipment and reagents used had to meet the Food and Drug Administration's (FDA) standards of an in vitro diagnostic medical device. Commercial suppliers of drug-testing products were required to submit test results that demonstrated to the FDA that the performance of the medical device was consistent with the product performance claims. If the results were satisfactory, the FDA would grant approval, known as a 510(k), which allowed the commercial sale of the product. Standards for sample collection, screening levels, and confirmation were, in many cases, left up to the discretion of the laboratory and/or the manufacturer. Each manufacturer of immunoassays had its own cutoffs for drug or metabolite assays and its own interpretations for measuring cross-reactivity to metabolites or interfering substances. In many cases, their claims and interpretations were written in ways to present their tests as comparable with competitive drug-testing products. With the issuance of the mandatory guidelines, everything changed. Drug testing in both the public and private sectors now had a standard to follow. NIDA, which later became The Substance Abuse and Mental Health Services Administration (SAMHSA), developed and implemented substance-abuse programs for the workplace that continue today. The first draft of the mandatory guidelines addressed the following important topics:

- Dilution and adulteration;
- Specimen collection and handling procedures;
- Training and qualifications of personnel;
- Screening levels;
- Confirmation testing and certifying test results;
- Laboratory certification.

Since 1988, the mandatory guidelines have been revised several times to incorporate technological advancements and process revisions. They became the *de facto* standard for all workplace drug-testing programs, including private industry. The regulations were revised and re-issued on August 1, 2001. That version of the mandatory guidelines incorporates many of the technological advancements that have been made in testing for illicit drugs. They address drug screening of urine as well as alternate matrix samples, such as oral fluid, sweat, and hair. They also address regulations and procedures for on-site testing, called point-of-collection testing (POCT). These standards were developed by SAMHSA's Drug Testing Advisory Board (DTAB). To develop standards for the products that represent the next generation in drug testing, this forum utilized input from industry representatives, laboratory professionals, and academics. A complete summary of the mandatory guidelines can be found on SAMHSA's web site: http://workplace.samhsa.gov/resourcecenter.

Meanwhile, the FDA has continued to review and issue 510(k) approvals for new assays, applications for tests of new equipment, and tests utilizing alternative matrices. In addition, the FDA has also begun to address standards for validation of on-site test devices. They have issued guidelines for validation and evaluation of POCT devices. These guidelines have not yet been issued, but are being followed for some new POCT devices. More information can be found at www.FDA.gov.

4.2. State Regulations

Of the 50 states, 31 have also adopted some type of employment drug-testing statute or regulation. These laws address which industries are required to test, what kinds of samples are allowed, and where the actual testing is done—e.g., laboratory or on-site. There are 14 states with voluntary laws that will qualify an employer for a discount on its workers' compensation premiums and/or a legal shield against litigation of drug testing that is conducted in accordance with the law. Additional states currently have laws under consideration that address workplace drug testing.

4.3. Determination of Cutoff Concentrations and Confirmations

Prior to the mandatory guidelines, the cutoffs for screening tests were established by each manufacturer supplying the immunoassay kit, and the confirmation level was determined by the sensitivity of the equipment and methodology used by the reference lab to confirm the nonnegative or positive sample. To publish the mandatory guidelines with established cutoffs for the initial or screening test and to set confirmation levels that ensure that true negatives will be identified and discarded and true positives will be identified and confirmed as positive was a formidable challenge for SAMHSA. Today, this problem becomes even more challenging, because levels were needed for oral fluid, hair, and sweat, as well as urine.

Although no system is perfect and absolute, the objective is to set the initial screening threshold at a level that will identify 95–98% of the true negatives as negative, but to also place it at a level that will pick up 100% of the true positives. Setting the appropriate cutoff level is further complicated when the immunoassay detects a primary metabolite with greater sensitivity than the parent drug. Finally, consideration is given to the differences in sensitivity found in commercially available technologies. The validation of the screening cutoff is usually done through several iterations of blind proficiency samples. Setting the confirmation cutoff is somewhat easier because it involves a chemical separation and measurement of the targeted drug or metabolite. It still means identifying the lower threshold or sensitivity level of the confirmatory method that will ensure that greater than 95% of all screened nonnegatives will be confirmed as positive. The cutoff values for screening and confirmation, in some cases, have to be set for the parent drug, as well as the drug's metabolite. Understanding the pharmacology of each drug's metabolism is key to setting the optimum screening and confirmation cutoffs. The cutoff concentrations for the initial and confirmation test can be found in Section 3.3 of the mandatory guidelines.

5. Drug Testing of Body Fluids in the 21st Century

Although the exact size of the drug-testing market in the United States is not known, most industry experts estimate it to be over 120 million tests annually and increasing. This estimate includes criminal justice, workplace testing, emergency medicine, and the newest area of drug testing—schools.

5.1. Criminal Justice

The largest segment of the drug-testing market, criminal justice, is divided into five areas: (1) drug courts, (2) corrections (probation/parole), (3) drug treatment programs, (4) driving under the influence of drugs (DUID), and (5) correctional facilities. Of the five areas, the largest volume of testing occurs in drug courts, drug treatment programs, and corrections.

5.1.1. Drug Courts

Drug courts are the fastest growing area of the criminal justice market. The drug court system (*see* Chapter 15) has 1093 courts nationally and will continue to grow with the addition of dozens of new courts each year *(7)*. Each program participant is tested monthly, and in some cases weekly, for illicit drugs. In each drug court, the judge usually sets the policies for drug testing (i.e., determining which test will be used, how positive results will be administered, and whether positive screening results will be confirmed). In most courts the positives are not confirmed.

5.1.2. Corrections

It is estimated that 4.8 million adults are under supervision of the courts for either probation or parole reasons *(8)*. The National Survey on Drug Use and Health reported that 28% of these adults reported illicit drug usage in 2002. Sample collection and testing is usually conducted during periodic visits with the parole or probation officers. Because most of these programs are funded by the state or county, budgetary resources are limited for testing. Many parole officers would prefer to use on-site test devices because immediate results are more effective if they need to take the individual into custody. For budgetary reasons, they are forced either to send samples to laboratories for screening (because these lab results are, in most cases, less expensive than using the on-site test device) or, when funds are no longer available, to simply discard the sample. It should also be noted that, in many cases, nonnegative test results may not be confirmed and are treated as positives by the probation or parole program.

5.1.3. Drug Treatment Programs

The drug treatment programs have not changed much since their inception in the 1970s. They continue to dispense methadone, provide counseling, and conduct periodic drug testing. Testing is done weekly. Because the turnaround time for results is not critical, samples are usually sent to reference labs for screening. Confirmation of nonnegative results is usually done; however, there are few punitive results for a positive other than a loss of methadone take-home privileges, unless the methadone patient is assigned to the program by the criminal justice system. In this case, their freedom or rights may be revoked by the courts.

5.2. Workplace

The second largest but most developed segment of the drug-testing market is workplace testing. According to HHS, there are estimated to be 16.6 million illicit drug users over 18 yr of age; of these adults, 12.4 million (74.6%) were employed either full or part time *(8)*. Over half of these employed adults work full time. Currently, 67% of all major US corporations have drug-testing policies. Industry experts have estimated that approx 40 million workplace drug tests are conducted annually. Drug testing in the workplace is divided into two areas: (1) government-mandated drug testing and (2) nonregulated employers or private sector. Of the total, approx 7 million tests are government-mandated tests. The remaining 33 million tests in the private sector are primarily pre-employment tests of new hires to assess their use of illicit drugs. The volume of pre-employment testing is usually found to be in direct correlation with the health of the economy; during a soft economic period, the amount of pre-employment testing will decline as a result of decreased hiring by employers.

5.2.1. Workplace Testing Process

The typical process for a drug screen starts with the employer, who is either operating in a regulated industry, such as transportation, or has made a corporate commitment to provide a drug-free work environment for its employees. The demand for drug-free policies is driven by two key factors: (1) the cost and liability of an unsafe workplace, and (2) federally mandated drug testing of employees in certain safety-sensitive jobs—most notably, the transportation and nuclear industries. Demand in this segment will continue to grow as a result of increased awareness, program effectiveness measures, and policy in government segments.

There are five primary types of drug tests performed in the workplace:

1. Pre-employment
2. Random selection
3. Post-accident
4. Reasonable suspicion/cause
5. Return to duty/follow-up

5.2.2. Collection

All drug tests start with the collection of the sample. For regulated testing programs, the collector must be certified by HHS. The type of specimen collected is determined by the type of test being requested (e.g., a hair sample can be collected only for pre-employment, random selection, or return to duty/follow-up purposes). A minimum quantity must be collected in a manner as outlined by the mandatory guidelines. The sample also may be tested on-site with an appropriate FDA-approved test device, or it may be packaged in an approved sealed shipping container along with the necessary chain-of-custody documents and forwarded to an HHS-certified laboratory for testing. Although most testing programs dictate that urine samples must be collected and sent to an approved lab for screening and confirmation, the emergence of alternate test matrices devices have allowed employers to utilize tools that are less invasive to the privacy of their employees, such as oral fluid. The availability of POCT devices allows the employer to better utilize the employee's time by conducting the drug test on-site, thus minimizing time away from the job by the employee, and possibly the supervisor. A complete description of the collection procedure used to collect each type of specimen can be found in the HHS Specimen Collection Handbook for Federal Workplace Drug Testing Programs. The handbook can be found at www.SAMHSA.gov.

5.2.3. Laboratory

Each HHS-certified laboratory has to meet the standards of the National Laboratory Certification Program (NLCP). To meet these qualifications, the laboratory must pass three consecutive proficiency sample tests, pass an on-site inspection, undergo maintenance inspections twice a year, and continue to pass proficiency sample tests each quarter. When the employee's sample arrives at the laboratory, an initial immunoassay test is conducted to determine the true negatives. In addition, specimen validity (adulteration) tests are conducted on all samples to validate the integrity of the sample. Tests may include creatinine, specific gravity, pH, oxidizing agents, and surfactants. Samples testing nonnegative for parent or drug metabolites are retested for confirmation using a procedure that combines chromatographic separation methods with mass spectrometric identification (gas chromatography–mass spectrometry [GC-MS]; *see* Chapter 3).

5.2.4. The Medical Review Officer

Before confirmed positive results can be reported to the employer, the results must be reviewed by a medical review officer (MRO). A certified MRO must be a licensed physician with training in the collection, chain of custody, interpretation of test results, and federal workplace regulations policies. After complete review of the collection process, drug testing, and adulteration test results, the MRO will report his or her findings to the employer. Only with the MRO review are the results certified as positive for the drug in question.

5.2.5. The Third-Party Administrator

In many cases there is another party involved in the drug-testing process. This individual or organization is known as a third-party administrator (TPA). The employer may contract with the TPA to manage the entire drug-testing process. TPAs can arrange for the collection, shipment to a certified laboratory, and review by an MRO. If on-site tests are requested, they often provide the collector and test materials for the on-site test. In some cases, the TPA may also provide MRO and laboratory services as well.

5.3. Emergency Medicine

The emergency testing field is relatively small and currently estimated at 2.5 million tests annually. In this kind of situation, speed and proximity of obtaining results for the tests are of prime importance. Urine or blood samples are usually collected at the emergency center and the testing is done in a clinical laboratory. The objective of testing in this area is focused on determining what class of drugs has been ingested and approximately what quantities are present. With these results, an effective antidotal treatment can be formulated. Confirmation of test results is not done in most cases.

5.4. Schools

The emerging arena for drug testing is found in public and private schools. In June 2002, the US Supreme Court ruled that random drug tests could be conducted on all middle and high school students participating in competitive extracurricular activities *(9)*. A national survey titled Monitoring the Future estimated in 2001 that more than half of all students had used illicit drugs by the time they had finished high school *(10)*. Testing in this new field has been slow to develop. With opposition coming from the American Civil Liberties Union (ACLU) and parents, school authorities have been cautious in the development of programs to stem drug abuse in schools. School districts that have instituted drug testing have carefully written policies and procedures that ensure close communication with parents and follow many of the procedures outlined in SAMHSA's mandatory guidelines for the workplace.

6. CONCLUSIONS

The field of testing for illicit drugs in body fluids is a dynamic industry. The standard for testing has been shaped by a combination of technological advances, government regulations, and social values. The field has changed dramatically over the past 30 yr and will undoubtedly continue to evolve in the next 30 yr with new analytical technologies and refined government regulations.

REFERENCES

1. Lewis JH. Drug detection and its role in law enforcement. Trends & Issues in Crime and Criminal Justice 2001;205:2.
2. Leute RK, Ullman EF, and Goldstein A. Special immunoassay of opiates in urine and saliva. J Amer Med Assoc 1972;211:1231–1234.
3. Schneider RS, Lundquist P, Wong ET, Rubenstein KE, and Ullman EF. Homogeneous immunoassay for opiates in urine. Clin Chem 1973;19:821–825.
4. Dole VP, Kim WK, and Eglitis I. Detection of narcotic drugs, tranquilizers, amphetamines, and barbiturates in urine. J Amer Med Assoc 1966;198:349–352.
5. Gilmore GJ. DoD winning 30-year war against drugs in the ranks. DefenseLINK. American Forces Press Service, October 19, 2000.
6. Marshall S. High-speed collision. Firehouse Magazine, April 1987.
7. OJP Drug Court Clearinghouse and Technology Assistance Project, May 27, 2004.
8. The National Survey on Drug Use and Health. Office of Applied Studies, Department of Health and Human Services, 2002.
9. Board of Education of Independent School District No. 92 of Pottawatomie County vs. Earls.
10. Johnson LD, O'Malley PM, and Bachman JG. Monitoring the Future—National Results on Adolescent Drug Use: Overview of Key Findings. NIH Publication No. 03-5374 2002; p. 5.

Chapter 2

Specimens for Drugs-of-Abuse Testing

Leo J. Kadehjian

SUMMARY

A wide variety of body fluid specimens have been utilized for analysis for the presence of drugs of abuse. Urine has been and remains the most widely used body fluid specimen for routine testing for drugs of abuse, but several alternative specimens are establishing their place as suitable for drug testing. Hair, sweat, and oral fluid have reached a sufficient level of scientific credibility to be considered for use in the federally regulated workplace drug-testing programs. Each specimen provides different information about time and extent of use and likelihood of impairment. Some of these specimens (e.g., urine and oral fluid) can even be analyzed with simple on-site, noninstrumented testing devices, as well as through standard laboratory methods. These drug-testing tools, as objective pieces of information identifying drug use, have proven highly useful in addressing our society's ongoing substance abuse challenges. This chapter reviews the use of these various body fluid specimens for drugs-of-abuse testing, addressing the balances between ease of specimen collection and handling, the ease and accuracy of analytical methods, the capability for sound interpretation of results, and, ultimately, legal defensibility.

1. INTRODUCTION

Drug abuse remains a significant public health issue worldwide. Although major advances have been made in our understanding of the neurobiology of addiction and the pharmacology of abused drugs, society still has few tools to

From: *Forensic Science and Medicine: Drugs of Abuse: Body Fluid Testing*
Edited by R. C. Wong and H. Y. Tse © Humana Press Inc., Totowa, NJ

effectively address drug abuse and addiction. However, drug testing has proven to be one of the key objective tools to at least identify those who have used and abused drugs of abuse. Furthermore, drug testing, with appropriate responses and sanctions for positive test results, has deterred drug use. These tests have demonstrated their utility in a wide variety of clinical and nonclinical settings, including emergency toxicology, perinatal testing, criminal justice, the workplace, schools, and drugged driving.

Urine is the most widely used specimen for such routine drugs-of-abuse testing, but several "alternative" specimens are establishing their place as suitable for drug testing *(1–3)*. Hair, sweat, and oral fluid (*see* Chapters 7–11) have reached a sufficient level of scientific credibility to be considered for use in the federally regulated workplace drug-testing programs under the Substance Abuse and Mental Health Services Administration (SAMHSA) *(4)*. Each of these specimens offers a different balance among ease of specimen collection and handling, ease and accuracy of analytical methods, capability for sound interpretation of results, and legal defensibility. Legal defensibility is important because tests for drugs of abuse are often utilized in a variety of criminal, civil, and administrative adversarial proceedings.

All of these specimens lend themselves to accurate analysis of drug and/or metabolite levels through conventional scientific techniques, i.e., immunoassays and chromatographic methods such as high-performance liquid chromatography (HPLC), gas chromatography (GC), and gas chromatography–mass spectrometry (GC-MS; *see* Chapter 3). However, some specimens are clearly easier to analyze than others, with simple noninstrumented, on-site devices having been developed for urine and oral fluid. Furthermore, the analyte(s) in question varies between specimens, with the parent drug being predominant in some specimens (hair, sweat, oral fluid) whereas more polar metabolites are predominant in others (urine). Finally, issues of specimen collection, handling, transport, and stability also vary. Of importance are concerns about handling of biological specimens and the relative risks of exposure to, and transmission of, infectious agents. In 1991, the Occupational Safety and Health Administration (OSHA) published the Bloodborne Pathogen Standards at 29 CFR 1910.1030 (and subsequent OSHA Standards Interpretation and Compliance letters), which address the handling and infection risks of various biological specimens *(5)*.

This chapter addresses the various body specimens that have been routinely utilized to identify use and abuse of drugs.

2. BLOOD

Blood is widely regarded as the specimen offering the best correlation between drug levels and likely dosing and likely concomitant pharmacological, cognitive, and psychomotor effects. There have been many controlled dosing studies examining blood levels of drugs and concomitant effects. However, owing to ethical concerns, not all abused drugs have been subjected to such controlled dosing studies. Drug levels found in blood are often quite low (ng/mL) and often short-lived. The analysis of drugs in blood is time-consuming, generally requiring extraction procedures before further analyses can be performed. There have been several publications addressing the application of urine immunoassays to the analysis of blood specimens, after appropriate extraction protocols *(6,7)*.

Although blood is widely used for drug testing in clinical and emergency toxicology settings, especially for alcohol, the invasiveness of the collection of blood specimens does not lend itself to routine testing in other nonclinical contexts, such as in workplace-, student-, and corrections-testing environments. Furthermore, there is much greater risk of transmission of infectious disease through handling of blood specimens than with many other routinely tested specimens for drugs-of-abuse testing. Accordingly, blood will not be further considered in this review.

3. URINE

3.1. Urine Specimens

By far, urine is the most widely used specimen for drugs-of-abuse testing. It offers the advantages of large specimen volume and relatively high drug concentrations, because of the approx 100-fold concentrating effect of the kidneys (each minute, approx 125 mL of blood plasma is filtered in the kidneys by the glomeruli and concentrated to approx 1 mL of urine). There is an extensive body of literature addressing the detection of drugs and their metabolites in urine specimens, and much is known about the pharmacokinetics of drug and metabolite elimination in urine. There are several well-established guidelines and laboratory certification programs, most notably those originally established by the National Institute on Drug Abuse (NIDA) in 1988 for federally regulated workplace drug-testing programs. These guidelines, called the NIDA Guidelines, are now overseen by SAMHSA *(8)*. These guidelines address testing for five drugs of abuse: cannabinoids (marijuana), cocaine metabolites, opiates, amphetamines, and phencyclidine (PCP). These workplace drug-testing guidelines are widely regarded as the "gold standard" in urine drug testing. As of March 2005, there were 49 laboratories (including 2 in Canada) certified under this program to perform such federally regulated workplace drug testing.

Urine is 95% water, with sodium chloride and urea in about equal amounts as the main dissolved substances, and with much smaller amounts of a wide variety of other constituents. Urine is attractive as a specimen because it can be conveniently provided as a normal waste product in relatively large volumes. Typical urine production rates are about 1 mL/min during waking hours, so collection of a specimen of sufficient volume for both initial screening by immunoassay as well as any subsequent confirmation testing is generally not problematic. Furthermore, the large specimen volume allows the option of splitting the specimen into two portions at the time of collection for assurance of proper chain of custody and specimen integrity in the event of adversarial challenges to the test results. Drugs and their metabolites are reasonably stable in urine when specimens are refrigerated or frozen. As far as specimen handling is concerned, urine is generally not considered infectious unless visibly contaminated with blood *(5)*.

3.2. Urine Analysis

Urine is relatively easy to collect and analyze. There are a wide variety of immunoassays available for detection of most common drugs of abuse and/or their metabolites in urine. Furthermore, in part because of the relatively high drug and/or metabolite concentrations in urine, simple noninstrumented, on-site immunoassays have been developed and are widely used in a variety of settings. There are numerous versions of these simple-to-use, noninstrumented immunoassays (i.e., visually read dipsticks, cassettes, cups) which allow the ready on-site testing of urine specimens outside of a formal laboratory. Some of these devices have even been cleared by the US Food and Drug Administration (FDA) for at-home use. Studies of the performance of these noninstrumented, on-site devices have demonstrated impressive performance for some devices at levels comparable to bench-top laboratory analyzers, even when performed by those without any formal laboratory experience *(9,10)*.

3.3. Urine Issues

In spite of the well-established place of urine as a specimen for drug testing, its use is not without its challenges. One issue is the potential invasion of privacy involved in specimen collection. Unlike within the criminal justice testing programs (pretrial, probation, prisons, drug courts, and so on) (*see* Chapter 15), most workplace and other drug-testing programs do not allow direct observation of specimen collection, except under special circumstances. Without direct observation, the opportunity for specimen adulteration and substitution exists (*see* Chapters 13 and 14). To respond to such efforts to thwart the integrity of the testing, specimen collection and laboratory guidelines have been developed to minimize the opportunities for such tampering. Furthermore, laboratory procedures to detect such efforts have been established. Adulteration is generally easily detected and is difficult at best when collection is performed under direct observation, as in criminal justice contexts. Although there are many adulterants available, there are also many simple test strips as well as laboratory methods to detect such adulterants.

Specimen dilution (in vivo), however, is a much greater challenge, as it is fairly easy to drink sufficient excess fluids prior to specimen donation and dilute one's urine by a factor of up to 10 or even more, thereby minimizing the chance of testing positive at conventional screening cut-offs. Although there are established criteria for what constitutes an excessively dilute specimen (e.g., creatinine less than 20 mg/dL and specific gravity less than 1.003), these regulatory criteria are undergoing scrutiny to ensure that false accusations of intentional efforts at dilution are not made.

Another limitation to the utility of urine specimens in drug testing is the relative difficulty in correlating urine drug and/or metabolite levels with likely dosing and likelihood of impairment. Granted, the correlation between urine drug levels and time and extent of drug use and likelihood of impairment is weak. Unfortunately, some toxicologists claim that urine drug levels should *never* be interpreted, but this clearly is an extreme and incorrect position. In some situations, urine levels may clearly be commensurate with the claims of the user or not, and as such can be highly useful. Furthermore, very high urine levels can clearly demonstrate recent and significant use, whereas low drug levels are much more difficult to interpret. But to deny any value in urine drug levels for interpretation is incorrect.

4. ORAL FLUID

4.1. Oral Fluid Specimens

The alternative specimen receiving the most recent interest appears to be saliva or, more appropriately, oral fluid *(11-15)*. Although *saliva* has been the commonly used term to describe fluid specimens from the oral cavity, this fluid, as collected by current simple swabbing or absorbent pad devices, is really a complex mixture of several different oral fluids, including saliva. Accordingly, the broader term *oral fluid* is preferred. Oral fluid represents a mixture of not only the saliva from the three oral salivary glands (parotid, submandibular, and submaxillary), but other oral fluids as well (e.g., gingival crevicular fluid).

The first experiments to measure biological analytes in saliva were performed in the mid-19th century. Further experiments in the 1930s demonstrated the role of lipid solubility and ionizability in the partitioning of solutes into saliva. Oral fluid has been used for a wide variety of analytes, including steroids, hormones, enzymes, antibodies, DNA typing, therapeutic drugs, and drugs of abuse. From the earliest days of immunoassay development for drug testing in the early 1970s, saliva has been considered a suitable specimen. In fact, one of the first papers published on the use of homogeneous immunoassays for the detection of drugs (a spin immunoassay developed by Syva Company, called free radical assay technique [FRAT], a forerunner of the now well-established enzyme-multiplied immunoassay technique [EMIT] assay), specified in the title the use of both urine and saliva for morphine testing *(16)*.

The key advantage of oral fluid for drugs-of-abuse testing is the ease of specimen collection, without invoking privacy or gender concerns. Oral fluid for drug testing offers great promise for roadside driving-under-the-influence scenarios, which prove prohibitive for the collection of a urine specimen (*see* Chapters 8 and 17). Furthermore, there is the potential for immediate test results with on-site, noninstrumented immunoassays already developed. In addition, there has been the promise that saliva drug levels may correlate better with blood levels than urine, thereby allowing for better assessment of the level of likely impairment. Unfortunately, a close review of the literature indicates that although oral-fluid levels may correlate better with blood levels than urine drug levels, the correlation is not so strong that a clear relationship with impairment exists. Finally, the possibility of specimen adulteration appears to be minimal. Some limitations are the very low specimen volume and the low analyte levels. Although oral fluid as a specimen for drugs-of-abuse testing is receiving active research interest, oral fluid has been widely studied for use in therapeutic drug monitoring *(17)*.

Ethanol was apparently first reported in saliva in 1875. Saliva ethanol levels have been shown to demonstrate excellent correlation with blood alcohol levels, with a saliva/blood ratio close to 1; this is why saliva as a specimen for initial alcohol testing is authorized under the Department of Transportation (DOT) program as well as under several state driving statutes *(18–20)*. The DOT regulations detail saliva collection and testing procedures. In conjunction with the DOT rulemaking, the National Highway Traffic and Safety Administration (NHTSA) included performance evaluations of nonevidential alcohol-screening devices for saliva for use in the DOT testing program. Those devices fulfilling NHTSA's criteria are listed in their Conforming Products List (CPL), periodically published in the Federal Register *(20)*. In addition, there is ongoing review by SAMHSA's Division of Workplace Testing of the use of saliva for federally regulated workplace testing for other drugs of abuse as well *(4)*. There is also a program in Europe called Roadside Testing Assessment (ROSITA), which examines a variety of specimens and technologies for their suitability in roadside testing, with much attention paid to saliva *(21)*.

Saliva is effectively an ultrafiltrate of blood. All of the organic compounds present in plasma have been detected in saliva, albeit in trace amounts for some analytes. Saliva is about 98% water, with a specific gravity of 1.00–1.02. Saliva contains both electrolytes (primarily Na, K, Cl, and HCO_3) and proteins, and its osmolality is less than or equal to that of plasma. The electrolyte concentrations and pH are markedly dependent upon saliva flow rate. Accordingly, stimulating saliva flow for speed of specimen collection can alter the partitioning of drugs between blood and oral fluid and thus affect the saliva:blood ratio. The protein concentration in saliva is less than 1% of that in plasma. However, saliva has proven a suitable specimen for forensic DNA analysis as well as antibody testing for human immunodeficiency virus (HIV).

Typical daily saliva secretion is 500–1500 mL—average 0.6 mL/min (range 0.1–1.8; during sleep, 0.05 mL/min). Production rates for stimulated saliva have been reported to average about 2 mL/min but have reached as high as 7 mL/min. Saliva pH is typically 6.7 (5.6–7.9, flow rate dependent), vs 7.4 for plasma.

The mechanism by which drugs are found in saliva is passive diffusion, although there are examples of active secretion (e.g., lithium). The major factors affecting drug entry into saliva are lipid solubility and degree of ionization at saliva pH.

Unfortunately, oral fluid has not proven very sensitive for detection of cannabis use, as it appears that cannabinoids are not secreted from the blood into oral fluid. Rather, it is only from contamination of the oral cavity after smoking or oral ingestion of cannabis that cannabinoids may be detected in oral fluid. Accordingly, detection of cannabis use is likely only for several hours after use *(22,23)*. However, this may prove beneficial in testing programs where the goal is to demonstrate a likelihood of impairment. If an appropriate threshold cut-off is established, then a positive result in oral fluid would clearly represent use within the past few hours, with demonstrated cognitive and psychomotor deficits.

4.2. Oral Fluid Analysis

Analysis of oral fluid for drugs is relatively straightforward. However, there are limitations in repeat and multiple confirmation tests as a result of low specimen volumes. Both on-site and laboratory-based methods have been developed *(24,25)*.

Specimens may be collected through a variety of techniques, although simple expectoration (spitting) into plastic (polypropylene) tubes (either stimulated or unstimulated) or absorption of oral fluid with an absorbent material (foam pad, cotton fiber wad) are the most common. Spitting causes a saliva secretion rate of approx 0.5 mL/min. The flow of saliva can be stimulated through a variety of techniques, such as chewing paraffin, or through the use of chemical stimulants, such as citric acid or sour candy drops. Of course, the use of any foreign material to stimulate saliva must be carefully considered so that the specimen is not altered or contaminated in a way that might limit subsequent analyses or interpretations. Chewing paraffin will cause secretion rates of 1–3 mL/min, but paraffin may absorb highly lipophilic compounds, causing a reduction in measured saliva levels. Citric acid candies are potent stimulators, leading to secretion rates of 5–10 mL/min. Stimulated saliva appears to have a fairly narrow pH range (approx 7.4) relative to the broader range for unstimulated saliva. Again, the variability in pH may be important for the saliva/plasma ratios of weakly basic or weakly acidic compounds. The pH of saliva increases from approx 6.2 to 7.4 as the secretion rate increases. It is generally approx pH 7 for stimulated saliva, whereas unstimulated saliva shows a greater pH variation. This variation in saliva pH resulting from variations in secretion rates can have a significant impact on the saliva/plasma ratio for certain drugs, depending on their pKa.

Generally, a specimen is collected with an absorbent pad placed in the mouth for a few minutes. After the pad is saturated with oral fluid or a specific amount has been absorbed, the pad is placed in a tube of buffer for shipment to the laboratory. On-site methods may similarly collect the specimen with an absorbent pad from which the specimen is applied to a noninstrumented or instrumented immunoassay device. There is even a device that aspirates a specimen directly into a bench-top analyzer. However, drug levels in oral fluid are generally much lower than those found in urine specimens, except when there is direct contamination of the oral cavity.

Specimen handling is relatively straightforward. Saliva has been shown to be source of infectious microorganisms, and appropriate precautions should be taken in the handling of oral fluid *(5)*. Court cases have addressed the relative infectivity of saliva when one subject has been bitten by another.

4.3. Oral Fluid Issues

One promise of oral fluid testing is a supposed better correlation with blood levels and, accordingly, impairment. Unfortunately, a detailed review of the literature indicates that although oral fluid levels generally correlate better with blood levels than, for example, urine, the correlation is not so close as to allow a strong prediction of blood levels. This is especially so shortly after drug use by oral ingestion, smoking, or nasal insufflations, when contamination of the oral cavity by drug can lead to dramatically elevated drug levels, much greater than corresponding blood levels, at least for several hours. Another issue is that oral fluid testing is relatively insensitive for the detection of cannabis use, as it appears that cannabinoids are not secreted from the blood into oral fluid. Rather, detection of cannabis use is possible only as long as there is contamination of the oral cavity with cannabinoids. This period of detection is much shorter than the several days for detection of cannabinoids in urine. However, by choosing an appropriate cut-off, one can insure that a positive cannabis result in oral fluid can occur only within a few hours of use, and thus provides a clear indication of likely impairment.

5. HAIR

5.1. Hair Specimens

It has been demonstrated that a very wide variety of ingested drugs and/or their metabolites may be found in hair specimens. Hair specimens from ancient mummies have been demonstrated to contain cocaine. Several famous deceased persons have also had their hair analyzed for drug exposure (Napoleon Bonaparte, Ludwig van Beethoven, William Butler Yeats) *(26,27)*.

Hair testing has gained interest because of its ability to provide a history of drug use, dependent on the length of hair tested (*see* Chapter 11). Unlike other conventional biological specimens used for drug testing with detection times measured in days, drugs have been demonstrated to remain in hair for extended periods of time: years, decades, and even longer. Current hair-testing protocols examine segments of hair representing about 3 mo of growth (head hair typically grows approx 1 cm/mo). That drug residues may be detected in hair over extended periods of time has been amply demonstrated in a large number of published studies. Hair specimens examined include not only head hair, but also beard hair, axillary hair, body hair, and even pubic hair. Furthermore, even neonatal hair has been analyzed to demonstrate possible prenatal drug exposure *(28)*.

There have been numerous national and international scientific meetings specifically addressing hair testing, with the establishment of a few professional societies dedicated to hair testing. In 1990, there was a small conference addressing this new technology convened in Washington, DC, by the Society of Forensic Toxicology, the National Institute on Drug Abuse, and the National Institute of Justice. Although most attendees were critical of hair testing, subsequent research has demonstrated its utility. The first international meeting addressing hair testing was held in Genoa in 1992 *(29)*; an international workshop was held in 1994 in Strasbourg *(30)*; a joint The International Association of Forensic Toxicologists (TIAFT)/Society of Forensic Toxicologists (SOFT) meeting was held in 1994 in Tampa with a special session dedicated to hair testing; another international meeting held in 1995 in Abu Dhabi; and the first European meeting held in Genoa in 1996 *(31)*. The proceedings of several of these meetings have been published as full issues of the journal *Forensic Science International*. Since then, hair-testing science and technology has been extensively addressed at numerous forensic science and toxicology meetings. A large body of experimental and epidemiological scientific data has been published *(32–36)*.

The mechanism of drug incorporation in hair has been found to be not as simple as originally proposed. It was thought that drugs within the blood capillaries bathing the follicle were transferred into the growing hair shaft and effectively locked in place. However, it has been shown that such a simple mechanism does not account for all the experimental observations. It has been demonstrated that drugs can also enter the hair shaft via sweat and sebum. Also, environmental contamination of the hair has been demonstrated. One question is whether hair analysis can differentiate between drugs in hair from actual drug use as opposed to environmental exposure (*see* Chapter 11).

5.2. Hair Analysis

Hair analysis is performed by cutting a segment of hair from close to the scalp, generally representing about three months' growth. Hair typically grows approx 1 cm/mo, although there are inter-individual differences in hair-growth rates. The cut hair specimen is washed to remove potential external contamination and then digested. The digest solution is tested by immunoassay and GC-MS. In addition, some laboratories also test the initial wash solutions for an assessment of the possibility of environmental contamination and its likely contribution to the subsequent test results.

Unlike the multitude of laboratories offering urine drug-testing services, there are only a few laboratories offering hair-testing services. There are currently no formal hair-testing laboratory regulations or guidelines, although there are a few professional societies as well as some proficiency-testing programs *(37)*. However, hair testing is on the list of alternative specimens proposed for federally regulated workplace testing, with some laboratory and testing standards established, at least in draft form *(4)*.

5.3. Hair Issues

The main issues facing hair testing are (1) distinguishing environmental exposure/contamination of the hair from drug incorporation in the hair shaft from use and (2) addressing the possibility of hair-color bias. Both of these issues have been reasonably well investigated but still appear to remain subjects of controversy *(38)*.

Hair-testing laboratories claim that they can distinguish between actual drug use and contaminating environmental exposure by a comparison of the levels of drugs that might be found in the preliminary wash solutions and the level of drugs found in the actual hair digest. If there are high levels of drugs in the wash solutions relative to those found in the digest, external contamination is considered likely. However, there appears to remain some controversy surrounding these claims.

It has been well demonstrated that drugs bind to hair differentially, dependent upon the physicochemical properties of the drug in question and those of the hair. It is known that many drugs bind preferentially to dark-pigmented hair over fair-colored hair, leading some to make claims of a hair-color bias in hair testing, unfairly identifying those with heavily pigmented hair over those with fair hair. Some have even called this a racial bias *(39–42)*.

Another issue is the possibility of specimen adulteration *(43–45)*. It has been demonstrated that hair color plays a significant role in binding of drugs to hair and that bleaching or other treatments can dramatically reduce the amount of drug found in hair. In addition, there are shampoos being sold on the Internet claiming that they can rid the hair of drugs *(43)*. It seems clear that the opportunity to thwart hair testing through such chemical treatments exists. Of course, drug users could also shave their heads and even other body hair to prevent testers from obtaining an incriminating specimen.

Some claim that by segmental analysis of the hair shaft, a time profile of drug use may be obtained, although others challenge the scientific validity of such segmental analysis *(46–48)*. Some experimental studies have challenged the simple view that drugs are neatly deposited along the hair shaft from the blood capillaries bathing the hair follicle, and remain in place as the hair shaft grows to provide a timeline of drug use. It has been demonstrated that this model of drug deposition and incorporation into hair is too simplistic and that drugs may be incorporated into and onto the hair shaft by a variety of mechanisms, including sweat and sebum excretion.

There have been numerous court challenges to the admissibility, probative value, and interpretation of hair drug tests. On balance, it now appears that hair testing has been generally accepted by the courts *(49)*.

Another issue to consider when using hair testing in the workplace setting is that by examining *prior* drug use where there may not be *current* drug use, any sanctions may run afoul of the Americans with Disabilities Act. This act precludes employers from discriminating against otherwise qualified applicants or employees based on *prior* drug use, as long as they are not *currently* using drugs. Whether a positive hair test that looks back 3 mo in time represents *current* use appears not to have been conclusively decided in the courts.

6. SWEAT

6.1. Sweat Specimens

Drugs of abuse and their metabolites have long been known to be excreted in sweat. Quinine was detected in sweat in 1844, morphine in 1942, and amphetamines in 1972. The development and patenting of a sweat patch collection device by PharmChem Laboratories (Haltom City, TX) in the 1990s has allowed for the ready detection of drug use over a period of approx 1 wk of patch wear *(50–54)*. The sweat patch is a simple Band-Aid®-like device consisting of a small 3 × 5 cm absorbent cellulose pad covered by a gas-permeable polyurethane membrane that allows water vapor to pass through while trapping in the absorbent pad any drugs and/or their metabolites excreted in sweat. The patch is held in place on the torso or arm by a special Band-Aid-like adhesive layer surrounding and covering the cellulose collection pad. After a wear period of approx 1 wk, the analysis of the sweat patch is relatively straightforward—drugs are eluted from the collection pad and the extract subsequently analyzed by immunoassay and GC-MS.

The criminal justice community has shown great interest in sweat-patch testing for drugs of abuse. The patch offers the primary advantage of constantly monitoring for any drug use over a period of approx 1 wk, obviating the need for multiple urinalyses to effectively monitor for any drug use over that period. The patch cannot be removed or tampered with without it being apparent to a trained technician. There has also been interest in the use of the sweat patch for federally regulated workplace drug-testing applications *(4)*. However, given the invasion-of-privacy implications of an employer monitoring the off-duty behavior of an employee, the sweat patch would likely be used only as a last-chance agreement between an employee and employer after a prior failed drug test or other evidence of workplace drug use.

Sweat arises from both eccrine and apocrine sweat glands. The eccrine sweat glands are found on most parts of the body, whereas apocrine sweat glands are found primarily in the axillary, inguinal, and perineal areas. The apocrine sweat glands open directly onto the hair follicle and are less well studied and understood than eccrine sweat glands. Eccrine sweat-gland density varies widely, from 60/cm^2 on the back to 600/cm^2 on the sole of the foot. Glandular sweat production is approx 1–5 nL/min/gland. Insensible sweat amounts to 400–700 mL/d. Sweat is 99% water, originally isotonic with plasma, but water re-absorption makes it hypotonic. Sweat pH when resting is 5.8, but exercise increases sweat pH to 6.1–6.4.

6.2. Sweat Analysis

The patch is applied to the torso or arm after precleaning the skin with alcohol wipes. The cleaning is designed to not only remove any possible surface contaminants but also to ensure an effective seal of the adhesive. The patch is worn for about a week, absorbing sweat and any drug and metabolites present in that sweat. The patch absorbs approx 300 µL of sweat each day, or approx 2 mL/wk. After approx 1 wk, the patch is removed and sent to Pharm-Chem Laboratories for elution and analysis by immunoassay and GC-MS. Elution is performed using an aqueous methanol/acetate buffer. Cut-off levels for reporting a positive result are on the order of 25 ng/patch. The Administrative Office of the US Federal Courts has also administratively required that to report positive test results for cocaine or methamphetamine, their respective metabolites must also be present at their limits of detection.

6.3. Sweat Issues

The patch has been demonstrated to be sensitive and accurate, although its use has not been without challenges. There have been claims that the patch may be contaminated from exposure to drugs, both from the environment and from residual levels of drug in the skin from prior use *(55,56)*. It has been demonstrated that under certain laboratory conditions, drugs applied in certain pH solutions to the outside of the patch can migrate through the polyurethane outer membrane into the underlying collection pad when the underlying pad is also soaked with certain pH buffers. However, these laboratory experimental conditions are not likely to occur in a real-world setting. In addition, it has been demonstrated that when alcohol-precleaned skin is doped with drug in solution, the preplacement cleaning procedure does not remove all of the drugs from the skin and can generate a positive test result. Again, these conditions are not likely to occur in a real-world setting. Although at least one federal court has recognized the possibility for such external contamination, these contamination challenges have been effectively rebutted in several subsequent cases. Further research would be welcome to define more accurately whether the patch may be prone to the possibility of contamination under more real-world drug-exposure conditions.

7. OTHER SPECIMENS

A wide variety of additional body specimens have been analyzed for drugs of abuse. These are not widely used, but a few will be addressed briefly.

7.1. Meconium

Meconium is a newborn's first stool. It is formed over the last trimester of pregnancy, and thus can represent exposure to drugs over 16–20 wk prepartum. Meconium is collected from the neonate's diaper and extracted with solvents. The extract is then analyzed by conventional immunoassay and GC-MS techniques *(57)*.

7.2. Breast Milk

Drugs and alcohol have also been detected in mother's breast milk, with implications for healthcare concerns about neonatal exposure. It has been demonstrated that alcohol is eliminated in breast milk, and that newborns can detect the flavor of alcohol in breast milk and actually suck harder but obtain less milk as a result of alcohol's inhibition of prolactin secretion, thereby inhibiting milk release. More dramatically, methamphetamine and cocaine have been found in mother's breast milk and linked to adverse neonatal health effects *(58,59)*.

7.3. Vernix Caseosa

Vernix caseosa is a white deposit of sebum and desquamated cells covering the skin of neonates and has been analyzed for evidence of prenatal cocaine exposure *(60)*.

7.4. Semen

Semen has been demonstrated to have measurable levels of drug after drug use. It is occasionally proposed as a basis to explain positive drug tests as a result of exposure to drugs through sexual relations. However, the absolute amount of drug present in semen is very low and could not account for significant exposure *(61)*.

7.5. Nails

Drugs are found in nails, as they are in hair. Nails have been used to detect drugs in both adults and neonates *(62–65)*.

7.6. Vitreous Humor

Vitreous humor is the gel that fills the eye. It is obtained at autopsy and analyzed for drugs *(66)*.

8. CONCLUSIONS

A wide variety of body fluid specimens have been analyzed for the presence of drugs of abuse. The analytical methods are sound and well developed. Each specimen provides different information about time and extent of use and likelihood of impairment. However, the interpretation of test results from each of these types of specimen offers its own challenges. Formal regulatory criteria have been established for several of these specimens, and case law addressing their admissibility and probative value has been developed for some. These drug-testing tools, as an objective piece of information identifying drug use, have proven highly useful in addressing the ongoing challenge of substance abuse.

REFERENCES

1. Cone EJ. Legal, workplace, and treatment drug testing with alternate biological matrices on a global scale. Forensic Sci Int 2001;121:7–15.
2. Caplan, YH and Goldberger, BA. Alternative specimens for workplace drug testing. J Anal Toxicol 2001;25(5):396–399.
3. Guidelines for Testing Drugs Under International Control in Hair, Sweat, and Saliva. United Nations Office for Drug Control and Crime Prevention, United Nations Publications, New York, NY, 2001.
4. Mandatory Guidelines for Federal Workplace Drug Testing Programs. SAMHSA, Notice of Proposed Revisions, 69 FR 19673-19732, April 13, 2004. www.work place.samhsa.gov
5. Occupational Exposure to Bloodborne Pathogens. Final Rule. December 6, 1991. 56 FR 64004–64182. www.osha.gov/SLTC/bloodbornepathogens/index.html
6. Moeller MR and Kraemer T. Drugs of abuse monitoring in blood for control of driving under the influence of drugs. Ther Drug Monit 2002;24(2):210–221.
7. Moeller MR, Steinmeyer S, and Kraemer T. Determination of drugs of abuse in blood. J Chromatogr B Biomed Sci Appl 1998;713(1):91–109.
8. workplace.samhsa.gov.
9. Kadehjian L. Performance of five non-instrumented urine drug-testing devices with challenging near-cutoff specimens. J Anal Tox 2001;25(8):670–679.
10. Willette R and Kadehjian L. Drugs-of-abuse test devices: a review, in On-Site Drug Testing (Jenkins AJ and Goldberger BA, eds), Humana Press, Totowa, NJ: 2002; pp. 219–252.
11. Cone EJ, Presley L, Lehrer M, et al. Oral fluid testing for drugs of abuse: positive prevalence rates by Intercept immunoassay screening and GC-MS-MS confirmation and suggested cutoff concentrations. J Anal Toxicol 2002;26(8): 541–546.
12. Samyn N, Verstraete A, van Haeren C, and Kintz P. Analysis of drugs of abuse in saliva. Forensic Sci Rev 1999;11:1–19.
13. Höld KM, de Boer D, Zuidema J, and Maes AA. Saliva as an analytical tool in toxicology, Int. J. Drug Testing, 1996, 1, 1–34. www.criminolgy.fsu.edu/journal/ hold.html.
14. Schramm W, Smith RH, Craig PA, and Kidwell DA. Drugs of abuse in saliva: a review. J Anal Toxicol 1992;16(1):1–9.
15. Spiehler V, Baldwin D, and Hand C. Analysis of drugs of abuse in saliva, in On-Site Drug Testing (Jenkins AJ and Goldberger BA, eds). Humana, Totowa, NJ: 2002; pp. 95–109.
16. Leute R, Ullman EF, and Goldstein A. Spin immunoassay of opiate narcotics in urine and saliva. JAMA 1972;221(11):1231–1234.
17. Drobitch RK and Svensson CK. Therapeutic drug monitoring in saliva. An update. Clin. Pharmacokinet. 1992;23(5):365–379.
18. Dubowski K. Analysis of ethanol in saliva, in On-Site Drug Testing (Jenkins, AJ and Goldberger BA, eds). Humana, Totowa, NJ: 2002; pp. 77–93.
19. Department of Transportation. Procedures for Transportation Workplace Drug and Alcohol Testing; Final Rule, 69 FR 79461, December 19, 2000.

20. Department of Transportation, National Highway Traffic Safety Administration. Highway Safety Programs; Conforming Products List of Screening Devices To Measure Alcohol in Bodily Fluids, 66 FR 22639, May 4, 2001.
21. www.rosita.org/
22. Niedbala RS, Kardos KW, Fritch DF, et al. Detection of marijuana use by oral fluid and urine analysis following single-dose administration of smoked and oral marijuana. J Anal Toxicol 2001;25(5):289–303.
23. Yacoubian GS, Wish ED, and Perez DM. A comparison of saliva testing to urinalysis in an arrestee population. J Psychoactive Drugs 2001;33(3):289–294.
24. Walsh JM, Flege R, Crouch DJ, Cangianelli L, and Baudys J. An evaluation of rapid point-of-collection oral fluid drug-testing devices, J Anal Toxicol 2003; 27:429–439.
25. Barrett C, Good C, and Moore C. Comparison of point-of-collection screening of drugs of abuse in oral fluid with a laboratory-based urine screen. Forensic Sci Int 2001;122:163–166.
26. Baez H, Castro MM, Benavente MA, et al. Drugs in prehistory: chemical analysis of ancient human hair. Forensic Sci Int 2000;108(3):173–179.
27. Cartmell LW, Aufderhide A, and Weems C. Cocaine metabolites in pre-Columbian mummy hair. J Okla State Med Assoc 1991;84(1):11–12.
28. Graham K, Koren G, Klein J, Schneiderman J, and Greenwald M. Determination of gestational cocaine exposure by hair analysis. JAMA 1989;262(23):3328–3330.
29. Proceedings published in Forensic Sci. Int. 63, 1993; 1–315.
30. Proceedings published in Forensic Sci. Int. 70 (1–3), 1995; 1–222.
31. Proceedings published in Forensic Sci. Int. 84(1–3), 1997; 1–312.
32. Cairns T, Kippenbereger DJ, and Gordon AM. Hair analysis for detection of drugs of abuse, in Handbook of Analytical Therapeutic Drug Monitoring and Toxicology (Wong SHY and Sunshine I, eds), CRC, Boca Raton, FL: 1997; pp. 237–251.
33. Sachs H. History of hair analysis. Forensic Sci Int 1997;84:7–16.
34. Kintz P (ed). Drug Testing in Hair. CRC, Boca Raton, FL: 1996.
35. Cone EJ. Mechanisms of drug incorporation into hair. Ther Drug Monit 1996; 18(4):438–443.
36. Kidwell DA and Blank DL. Hair analysis: techniques and potential problems. In Recent Developments in Therapeutic Drug Monitoring and Clinical Toxicology (Sunshine I, ed), Marcel Dekker, New York, NY: 1992; pp. 555–563.
37. Sniegoski LT and Welch MJ. Interlaboratory studies on the analysis of hair for drugs of abuse: results from the fourth exercise. J Anal Toxicol 1996;20(4): 242–247.
38. Wennig R. Potential problems with the interpretation of hair analysis results. Forensic Sci Int 2000;107:5–12.
39. Mieczkowski T and Newel R. An analysis of the racial bias controversy in the use of hair assays, in Drug Testing Technology. Assessment of Field Applications (Mieczkowski T, ed), CRC, Boca Raton, FL: 1999; pp. 313–348.
40. Henderson GL, Harkey MR, Zhou C, Jones RT, and Jacob P 3rd. Incorporation of isotopically labeled cocaine into human hair: race as a factor. J Anal Toxicol 1998; 22(2):156–165.

41. Joseph RE Jr, Su TP, and Cone EJ. In vitro binding studies of drugs to hair: influence of melanin and lipids on cocaine binding to Caucasoid and Africoid hair. J Anal Toxicol 1996;20(6):338–344.

42. Gygi SP, Joseph RE Jr, Cone EJ, Wilkins DG, and Rollins DE. Incorporation of codeine and metabolites into hair. Role of pigmentation. Drug Metab Dispos 1996; 24(4):495–501.

43. Rohrich J, Zorntlein S, Potsch L, Skopp G, and Becker J. Effect of the shampoo Ultra Clean on drug concentrations in human hair. Int J Legal Med 2000;113(2): 102–106.

44. Potsch L and Skopp G. Stability of opiates in hair fibers after exposure to cosmetic treatment. Forensic Sci Int 1996;81(2–3):95–102.

45. Cirimele V, Kintz P, and Mangin P. Drug concentrations in human hair after bleaching. J Anal Toxicol 1995;19:331–332.

46. Pragst F, Rothe M, Spiegel K, and Sporkert F. Illegal and therapeutic drug concentrations in hair segments—a timetable of drug exposure? Forensic Sci Rev 1998;10:81–111.

47. Henderson GL, Harkey MR, Zhou C, Jones RT, and Jacob P. 3rd. Incorporation of isotopically labeled cocaine and metabolites into human hair: 1. dose-response relationships. J Anal Toxicol 1996;20(1):1–12.

48. Strano-Rossi S, Bermejo-Barrera A, and Chiarotti M. Segmental hair analysis for cocaine and heroin abuse determination. Forensic Sci Int 1995;70(1–3):211–216.

49. Huestis M. Judicial acceptance of hair tests for substances of abuse in the United States: scientific, forensic, and ethical aspects. Ther Drug Monit 1996;18:456–459.

50. Sunshine I and Sutliff JP. Sweat it out, in Handbook of Analytical Therapeutic Drug Monitoring and Toxicology (Wong SHY and Sunshine I, eds). CRC Press, Boca Raton, FL: 1997; pp. 253–264.

51. Kidwell DA, Holland JC, and Athanaselis S. Testing for drugs of abuse in saliva and sweat. J Chrom B 1998;713:111–135.

52. Baer J and Booher J. The patch: a new alternative for drug testing in the criminal justice system. Fed Probation 1994;58 (2):29–33.

53. Fay J, Fogerson R, Schoendorfer D, Niedbala RS, and Spiehler V. Detection of methamphetamine in sweat by EIA and GC-MS. J Anal Toxicol 1996;20(6): 398–403.

54. Winhusen TM, Somoza EC, Singal B, Kim S, Horn PS, and Rotrosen J. Measuring outcome in cocaine clinical trials: a comparison of sweat patches with urine toxicology and participant self-report. Addiction 2003;98(3):317–324.

55. Kidwell DA, Kidwell JD, Shinohara F, et al. Comparison of daily urine, sweat, and skin swabs among cocaine users. Forensic Sci Int 2003;133(1–2):63–78.

56. Kidwell DA and Smith FP. Susceptibility of PharmChek drugs of abuse patch to environmental contamination. Forensic Sci Int 2001;116(2–3):89–106.

57. Kadehjian L. Drug testing of meconium: determination of prenatal drug exposure, in Handbook of Analytical Therapeutic Drug Monitoring and Toxicology (Wong SHY and Sunshine I, eds). CRC Press, Boca Raton, FL: 1997; pp. 265–279.

58. Winecker RE, Goldberger BA, Tebbett IR, et al. Detection of cocaine and its metabolites in breast milk. J Forensic Sci 2001;46(5):1221–1223.

59. Dickson PH, Lind A, Studts P, Nipper HC, Makoid M, and Therkildsen D. The routine analysis of breast milk for drugs of abuse in a clinical toxicology laboratory. J Forensic Sci 1994;39(1):207–214.
60. Moore C, Dempsey D, Deitermann D, Lewis D, and Leikin J. Fetal cocaine exposure: analysis of vernix caseosa. J Anal Toxicol 1996;20:509–511.
61. Pichini S, Zuccaro P, and Pacifici R. Drugs in semen. Clin Pharmacokin 1994; 26(5):356–373.
62. Palmieri A, Pichini S, Pacifici S, Zuccaro P, and Lopez A. Drugs in nails. Physiology, pharmacokinetics and forensic toxicology. Clin Pharmacokin 2000;38(2): 95–110.
63. Lemos NP, Anderson RA, Valentini R, Tagliaro F, and Scott RT. Analysis of morphine by RIA and HPLC in fingernail clippings obtained from heroin users. J Forensic Sci 2000;45(2):407–412.
64. Engelhart D, Lavins ES, and Sutheimer CA. Detection of drugs in nails. J Anal Toxicol 1998;22:314–318.
65. Skopp G and Potsch L. A case report on drug screening of nail clippings to detect prenatal drug exposure. Ther Drug Monitor 1997;19:386–389.
66. Bost RO. Analytical toxicology of vitreous humor, in Handbook of Analytical Therapeutic Drug Monitoring and Toxicology (Wong SHY and Sunshine I, eds). CRC Press, Boca Raton, FL: 1997; pp. 281–302.

Chapter 3

Drug-Testing Technologies and Applications

Jane S-C. Tsai and Grace L. Lin

SUMMARY

Over the past few decades, a remarkable gamut of increasingly sophisticated technologies has been employed for the development of drug-testing applications. Recent advancements in analytical instrumentation and computer technologies have further expanded the capabilities and dimensions for drug testing and toxicological analysis. Technologies of different chemical principles can be used sequentially or in combination to accomplish the specific goals and requirements of the drug analysis programs. Ligand-binding assays such as immunoassays are commonly used for screening. Separation techniques such as chromatography or electrophoresis, as well as their coupling with powerful detectors such as mass spectrometry, can be effectively used for confirmatory testing of preliminary positive results or systematic analysis of generally unknown toxic compounds. Each of these technology categories can be further broken down into multiple selections for instrumentations and methodologies. This chapter presents a general overview of the commonly used analytical technologies and their utilities in drug testing. The analytical technologies afford a powerful means toward the detection, identification, and quantification of the presence of abused drugs in biological specimens. However, the overall interpretation of analytical results ought to take into consideration the reasons for testing and the performance characteristics of the applied technologies.

1. INTRODUCTION

"Drugs-of-abuse testing" is a simple term but comprises diverse fields of drug testing, with manifold medico-legal and socioeconomic implications.

From: *Forensic Science and Medicine: Drugs of Abuse: Body Fluid Testing*
Edited by R. C. Wong and H. Y. Tse © Humana Press Inc., Totowa, NJ

Although the objectives of drug testing are mainly the detection, identification, and/or deterrence of substance abuse or misuse, the processes and regulations related to this topic may vary among different drug-testing sectors. The scopes of different drug-testing applications can vary, depending on the types of specimen tested, the regulations for testing procedures and programs, the drug-use prevalence in the population tested, the desired menu of drugs for analysis, the choice of testing technologies, and the interpretation and reporting of testing results. Depending on the goals and requirements of the drug-testing programs, technologies of different chemical principles can be employed sequentially or in combination to accomplish the detection, identification, and quantification of the drugs present in a biological specimen.

In general, the choice of analytical drug-testing technologies can be grouped into three major categories of general analytical techniques. Each of the three categories listed below can be further broken down into multiple selections for instrumentations and methodologies.

1. Assays that are based on molecular recognition and ligand binding, with immunoassays being the most popular techniques for drugs-of-abuse screening. Depending on the circumstances and requirements of testing, both instrumented immunoassays for laboratory testing and noninstrumented immunoassays for point-of-collection testing (POCT) are widely employed as initial tests for drugs of abuse (1–17).

2. Separation methodologies, such as various chromatographic or electrophoresis techniques, which physically separate the analyte(s) of interests from the other sample components. Examples include gas chromatography (GC), high-performance liquid chromatography (HPLC), thin-layer chromatography (TLC), capillary electrophoresis (CE), and capillary electrochromatography. A variety of detection methods are available for each of the separation techniques (18–34).

3. Mass spectrometry (MS), which identifies, quantifies, and/or elucidates the structure of substances in diverse types of sample matrix. The mass spectrometer is one of the most powerful detectors for various separation techniques, and is used for the majority of the "hyphenated" or "coupled" techniques. For example, GC-MS has become an integral part of forensic toxicology and abused drug confirmation. Notable progress has been made in the development of the interface for LC-MS and CE-MS in recent years. Comprehensive two-dimensional gas chromatography (GC × GC) with MS has recently been applied for drug screening and confirmation. Moreover, the advances in tandem MS (MS-MS) or multi-stage MS provide additional dimensions in the analysis of minute concentrations of compounds in various biological matrices (35–64).

To date, the most common drug-testing practices are based on a two-tier approach of initial immunoassay screening followed by confirmatory testing of preliminary positive screen results. Various separation methodologies or GC-MS in scan mode have also been employed as initial drug-screening tools. The hyphenated techniques are effective tools for confirmatory testing of presumptive positive results or for systematic analysis of generally unknown compounds. In the field of behavioral toxicology, the initial steps of drug recognition examination involve a series of physiological evaluations, including psychomotor tests and the examination of the eye *(65–67)*. Nevertheless, the evaluation often culminates in the collection of biological specimens for chemical analysis.

This chapter presents a general overview of drugs-of-abuse testing and analytical drug-testing technologies. The applications and general considerations of drugs-of-abuse testing are discussed first, because the analytical results are often interpreted in the context of the drug-testing applications. Then the principles of each of the technologies are compendiously reviewed, and the more commonly used drug-testing techniques are discussed. In addition to the abundance of methodology choices, there are myriad existing literature sources on all aspects of the technologies. Therefore, the aim of this chapter is to provide a synopsis of the technologies and their utilities in drugs-of-abuse testing.

2. THE ESSENCE OF DRUGS-OF-ABUSE TESTING

To understand the principles underlying the array of drug-testing technologies, some basic knowledge is required in terms of the drug metabolism and the intent of the particular drug-testing program. The route and method of drug administration, drug dose, and drug metabolism are closely related to the presence and amounts of the drug and/or its metabolites in the testing specimen at the time of specimen collection.

Over the past several decades, significant efforts have been devoted to the research of drug pharmacokinetics (i.e., the process by which a drug is absorbed, distributed, metabolized, and eliminated by the body), pharmacodynamics (i.e., the mechanism of drug action and effect on the body), as well as toxicological and epidemiological investigations. Advances have also been made in understanding the intra-individual and inter-individual variabilities of drug metabolism and excretion.

It should always be noted that the actual testing of abused drugs in any given biological specimen is only one component of a specific drug-testing program or application. There are legal, legislative, social, forensic, and/or medical elements of drug testing. Modern analytical technologies allow the pursuit of detecting and measuring the identified analyte(s) in a biological specimen with proper accuracy and precision. The interpretation and judgment of analytical measurement results, however, is not a straightforward process. There is bountiful active research in these fields, and reports from a wide spectrum of investigations will continue to be published. Nevertheless, the collective knowledge from all aspects of related scientific studies has provided the essential foundations for the design, execution, quality assurance, and outcome interpretation of chemical drug analysis.

2.1. The Applications of Drugs-of-Abuse Testing

The applications of drugs-of-abuse testing touch all walks of life in society. The highest volume of drugs-of-abuse testing comes from workplace drug testing (WDT). In the United States, programs for federal workplace drug testing are regulated by the Substance Abuse and Mental Health Services Administration (SAMHSA) of the US Department of Health and Human Services (HHS). In general, drug-testing programs regulated by the US Mandatory Guidelines (68) have established systems of protocols applicable to the testing of large numbers of urine specimens for the presence of five classes of drugs. These drugs (and their respective target analytes for confirmation) are as follows: amphetamines (amphetamine and methamphetamine), cannabinoids (11-nor-Δ^9-tetrahydrocannabinol-9-carboxylic acid, abbreviated as THC-COOH), cocaine metabolites (benzoylecgonine), opiates (morphine and codeine), and phencyclidine (PCP). The proposed new guidelines (69) will allow federal drug-testing programs the option to incorporate the testing of these drug classes in alternative specimens (oral fluid, sweat, or hair). Furthermore, the confirmation techniques will be expanded to couple the use of GC or LC with MS or MS-MS.

Additional classes of abused or misused drugs have also been tested in various societal sectors or clinical drug-testing programs worldwide (70–102). The main examples include benzodiazepines, barbiturates, lysergic acid diethylamide (LSD) and/or metabolite (2-oxo-3-hydroxy-LSD), methadone and/or metabolite (2-ethylidene-1,5-dimethyl-3,3-diphenylpyrrolidine, EDDP), methaqualone, propoxyphene, tricyclic antidepressants (TCA), and so on. The testing of the amphetamines group has recently been expanded to include designer drugs, especially 3,4-methylenedioxymethamphetamine (MDMA), as specific assay target analytes. Several studies were conducted for the detection of certain benzodiazepines, especially flunitrazepam. There is also growing interest in testing additional target classes of opioids and certain synthetic analgesics, such as buprenorphine and metabolites, 6-monoacetylmorphine (6-MAM or 6-AM), oxycodone, fentanyl, and so on. An expanded menu and more flexible drug-testing options are often desirable for clinical and medicolegal assessment, including clinical forensic medicine and emergency department drug testing. Different classes of drugs of abuse may provoke various signs of mental disorder, and testing for the presence of suspected drugs can help psychiatric clinics to differentiate between endogenous and drug-induced mental illness. For drug-dependence treatment or detoxification centers, the "objective evidence" of compliance monitoring is via regular drug testing of individuals with prescribed medication. Periodic drug testing is also used to ensure continued abstinence during rehabilitation. Similarly, scheduled testing can be used to check on previous drug offenders on parole and probation. Drugs-of-abuse testing is also frequently employed in the criminal justice system to identify drug offenders and to deter the abuse of drugs.

Drugs-of-abuse testing is mostly considered "forensic testing" because of its legal consequences and the high probability of legal challenges. Urine specimens are sufficient for most drug-testing applications; however, the analysis of the urine alone for drugs is insufficient for various forensic toxicology investigations. Interest in drug testing in alternative specimens, such as oral fluid/saliva, sweat, hair, as well as meconium for neonate exposure, has markedly increased over the past few years *(103–117)* (*see* Chapters 8, 10, and 11). In human-performance toxicological evaluations, blood is generally considered a suitable specimen for impairment investigation *(50,51)*. Nevertheless, interest in effective and timely drug testing for traffic safety has led to a number of projects that have evaluated the utility of various onsite urine- and saliva-testing devices for roadside drug testing *(17,118–122)* (*see* Chapter 17). Antemortem or postmortem forensic toxicology further requires the development of an assortment of tests for comprehensive screening of drugs in a variety of specimen types. A number of analytical techniques have been developed and evaluated for the systematic toxicological analysis (STA) of "generally unknown" toxic compounds *(18,20–22,46,55–60)*. The availability of reliable methods for the STA of drugs and poisons is important for laboratories involved in clinical and forensic toxicology investigations. In general, two or more assays are required for laboratories wishing to cover a reasonably comprehensive range of drugs of toxicological significance.

2.2. General Considerations and Guidelines

Regardless of their applications in identifying or excluding the abuse of drugs, most testing technologies need a defined or declared threshold concentration in order to distinguish a positive from a negative result. Conventionally, the threshold decision can be made based on either the assay limit of detection or a pre-defined, higher concentration that takes into account special requirements for the analysis. The limit of detection and limit of quantification usually are important for forensic purposes. For most drugs-of-abuse testing programs, however, "administrative cutoffs" have been chosen that are sufficiently above the assay limit of detection but still low enough to allow the detection of drug use within a reasonable time frame.

The SAMHSA regulation authorizes rapid initial testing within a framework of extensive quality control and specifies defined rules if confirmation is required. This allows the administrative cutoffs to be used for comparison across different assay technologies. Likewise, a number of countries, organizations, and professional societies have developed guidelines and recommended cutoff levels for drugs-of-abuse testing. The European guidelines for WDT *(123)* allow individual countries to operate within the requirements of national customs and legislation. For most regulated testing, a sample containing drugs below a specified cutoff concentration, or no drug at all, is reported as negative on the initial test and usually not further tested. A positive screen result is considered "presumptive positive"; thus, adequate confirmation is required in the majority of forensic testing, mandated workplace drug testing, and recommended in clinical testing.

Prior to the use of an analytical technique for the purpose of drug testing, a battery of analytical performance specifications and characteristics must be established, validated, and verified. The basic performance evaluation criteria include precision (i.e., intra-run, inter-run, and total precision), analytical sensitivity or lower limit of detection, accuracy by comparison studies to "gold" standards, method comparison to predicate systems/reference devices, and specificity (cross-reactivity profile). The performance evaluations for most immunoassays also include near cut-off performance, accuracy by analytical recovery studies, robustness against potential interference and adulteration substances, and a variety of stability studies. Immunoassays for abused-drug testing can be performed in either qualitative or semi-quantitative mode but are not considered quantitative. For technologies used for quantitative analysis, linearity, selectivity, resolution, and/or limit of quantification are also assessed. In addition, the implementation of proper quality-assurance programs is critical for testing programs or laboratories to produce accurate, reliable, and defensible results.

For most diagnostic testing, the generally accepted definition of "true negative" is a negative test result for a disease or condition in a subject in whom the disease or condition is absent. Likewise, "true positive" (TP) is a positive test result when the disease or condition is present in a subject. In comparison, the criteria for a "true-negative" (TN) drugs-of-abuse testing result also include the presence of drug concentration below that of both the screen and confirmation cutoff concentrations. Therefore, the presence of a drug concentration below the screen cutoff yet above the confirmation cutoff concentration is considered a "false-negative" (FN) result. By the same token, the presence of drug concentration above the screen cutoff yet below the confirmation cutoff is considered a "false-positive" (FP) result. These are important considerations for result interpretation and analysis of comparative evaluations of drugs-of-abuse testing.

A number of factors can impact the evaluations of sensitivity (TP/[TP + FN] × 100%), specificity (TN/[TN + FP] × 100%), and efficiency ([TP + TN]/

[TP + TN + FP + FN] × 100%) of a drug immunoassay, because such calculations are related to the comparison of the results of the screening techniques to those of the confirmation techniques. The prevalence of drug use in the studied population will also affect the calculated sensitivity and specificity. Because measurement uncertainties and inter-assay variations exist for all analytical methodologies, the comparison of screening and confirmation results for near-cutoff samples can vary from one study to another. In addition, it has been well published that immunoassay sensitivity, specificity, and predictive values, and hence the drug detection rate and detection time, can all be affected by the manipulation of the cutoff concentrations used for drug testing *(124–131)*.

3. MOLECULAR-RECOGNITION- AND LIGAND-BINDING-BASED ASSAYS

Assay technologies that rely on specific molecular recognition of analytes by high-affinity binding partners have played pivotal roles in diverse areas of biomedical and chemical analyses. The most versatile binding partners are the antibody molecules that are widely utilized in immunoassays for the detection of the analyte of interest (i.e., antigen) in a variety of sample matrices. Other binding partners used for drug testing include the specific drug receptor for various formats of receptor assay *(132–135)*. Depending on the type of specimen used, the specific molecular binding allows for the direct detection of the target analyte(s) in the specimen with minimal or no sample pretreatment. In general, urine samples do not require pretreatment, although enzymatic hydrolysis with glucuronidase can be applied to enhance the detection of certain drug classes *(4)*. Immunochemical assays can be developed to possess adequate sensitivity and specificity for the target class of drugs or drug metabolites. Once the reagents are developed and optimized, immunoassays are simple to use and allow relatively fast screening of a large number of samples. The availability of various commercial kits and instruments further facilitates the versatility of immunoassays in meeting the specific needs of drug-testing fields.

3.1. Immunoassays

Immunoassays for drug screening have been designed to efficiently detect the presence of the target class or classes of drugs above the defined threshold in a biological specimen. Consequently, immunoassays as a screening technique remain the most cost-effective way to rule out drug presence in the majority of samples submitted for routine drugs-of-abuse testing. The discriminatory power of the antibody binding site bestows the assay specificity; however, all ligand-binding-based assays can exhibit cross-reactivity with congeners, or sometimes with surprisingly unrelated structures *(136,137)*. Hence, a screened positive result is considered preliminary or presumptive positive.

The majority of immunoassays for drug screening are based on the competition of free drug molecules in the specimen and drug derivatives in the assay reagents for binding to a pre-optimized amount of antibody molecules in the reagent kit. A label is attached to one of the binding partners to serve as an indicator for monitoring and reporting the outcome of the competitive immunoreaction. The labels possess a measurable property that confers the analytical characteristics to meet the performance requirements of the specific assay. In practice, the apparent drug concentration in a specimen is determined by comparing the amount of this measured property in a sample to that of reference standards containing known concentrations of the target analyte.

Generally, there are two configurations of competitive immunoassays. A "heterogeneous" immunoassay requires the physical separation of free, labeled binding partner (antigen or antibody) from the labels that are bound in an immune complex in order to measure the quantity of labels. A "homogeneous" immunoassay can detect the analyte-induced signal change of the label characteristics without any separation steps. Both types of immunoassays are important for drugs-of-abuse screening. There are a variety of immunoassay techniques that are applicable to drug testing. The nomenclature of these techniques is based on the type of specific assay label used and the reaction principle of each of these immunoassays. Table 1 provides a summary of the technologies, assay labels, and reaction principles of these immunoassays.

3.1.1. Heterogeneous Competitive Immunoassay Techniques

Radioimmunoassay (RIA) *(1–3,5,7,138)* is a technique of saturation analysis that consists of three major components: a label for antigen (with ^{3}H, ^{131}I, or ^{125}I), a saturable compartment (specific antibody), and a separation step. The radiolabeled drug derivative binds to the antibody and forms a complex that is subsequently separated from the unbound labels. Solid phases that allow the removal of the unbound label in the supernatant (e.g., coated-tube technique) and second antibody binding to precipitate the ^{125}I-drug-antibody complex (e.g., double-antibody approach) are the most frequently used separation methods for drug RIA. After washing, the radioactivity of the labeled-drug-antibody complex can be measured in counts per minute (CPM). A dose-response curve can be constructed using the calculated radioactivity value vs analyte concentration for each of the calibrators. A standard curve can also be plotted using logit B/B_0 (B/B_0 = CPM of the test sample/CPM of the zero control) vs the natural logarithm (i.e., $\log_e$) of the drug concentrations. The concentration of drug in the sample is inversely proportional to the calculated radioactivity value.

Enzyme-linked immunosorbent assays (ELISAs) *(6,11,12,14,139)* are by far the most versatile techniques for diverse fields of biochemical, toxicological,

Table 1

Commonly Used Competitive Immunoassays for Instrumented Drugs-of-Abuse Screening

Nomenclature of immunoassay technology (abbreviation)	Enzyme-multiplied immunoassay technique (EMIT)	Fluorescence polarization immunoassay (FPIA)	Kinetic interaction of microparticles in solution (KIMS)	Cloned enzyme donor immunoassay (CEDIA)	Radioimmunoassay (RIA)	Enzyme-linked immunosorbent assay (ELISA)
Assay labels and reaction indicator	G6P-DH enzyme oxidizes G-6-P and reduces NAD. The generation of NADH is measured by absorbance rate change at 340 nm.	Excited Fluorophore (fluorescein) emits light at a second wavelength (fluorescence). A filter mechanism is used to determine the polarization of the emitted light (mP)	Microparticle-labeled reagent reacts with the binding-partner and promotes the aggregation reaction The proceeding of the reaction results in the kinetic absorbance increase with time.	The association of the ED and EA fragments forms active enzyme β-Galactosidase that hydrolyzes CPRG. The generation of CPR is measured by the absorbance rate change at 570 nm.	^{125}I-drug binds with antibody to form a radio-labeled drug-antibody complex. The radioactivity of the ^{125}I-drug-antibody complex can be measured (CPM)	Enzyme (HRP)-drug conjugate binds to immobilized antibody. The HRP conversion of TMB to a colored product is measured by absorbance at 450 nm
Major reagent composition (excluding the bulk agents, stabilizer, and preservative, etc.)	1. Antibody, G-6-P, and NAD. 2. Drug-G6P-DH conjugate	1. Antibody 2. Pretreatment solution 3. Drug-fluorescein tracer 4. Wash solution	*Gen I KIMS* 1. Antibody, diluent 2. Drug microparticles *Gen II KIMS* 1. Drug-polymer 2. Antibody-microparticles	1. EA reagent + EA reconstitute buffer and antibody 2. Drug-ED conjugate + ED reconstitute buffer, and CPRG	*Coated tube RIA* 1. Antibody-coated tube 2. ^{125}I-drug reagent *Second Ab RIA* 1. Antibody reagent 2. ^{125}I-drug reagent 3. Second antibody with polyethylene glycol	1. Antibody-coated wells in microtiter plates or strips 2. Drug-labeled enzyme reagent 3. Substrate reagent 4. Stop solution

NAD, nicotinamide adenine dinucleotide; ED, enzyme donor; EA, enzyme acceptor; CPRG, chlorophenol red b-d-galactopyranoside; HRP, horseradish peroxidase; OD, optical density; CPM, counts per minute; TMB, tetramethylbenzidine.

and medical analysis. Customized ELISA can be developed for drug testing in forensic and clinical toxicology laboratories. Approximately a dozen commercial ELISA kits are available for testing a spectrum of forensic matrices, such as urine, blood, serum, oral fluid, sweat, meconium, bile, vitreous humor, and tissue extracts. Competitive ELISAs for drug testing rely on competition between enzyme-labeled drug derivatives and free drug in the sample for binding to solid-phase (micro-well strips or plates) immobilized capture antibody. The competition of free drug for binding to the surface-coated antibody inhibits the binding of drug-enzyme conjugate and results in reduced enzymatic activity. An optical density (OD_{450}) value or color intensity can be used to qualitatively interpret a negative or a presumptive positive result. From the calibration curve, drug concentration is inversely related to the amount of signal generated.

3.1.2. Homogeneous Competitive Immunoassay Techniques

The homogeneous immunoassays are relatively easier to perform and can be readily adapted to screening large numbers of samples using automatic analyzers. The progress of immunoassay reagent development has been complemented by the advancement of sophisticated laboratory-automation instruments and data-management systems. After sample loading, an analyzer can screen a large number of samples per hour with minimal laboratory personnel intervention. However, application parameters have to be developed for specifically optimized reagent-instrument interfaces. Some of the reagents are used with applications validated by the laboratories (i.e., user-defined tests). Examples of applications development include the scheme and mode of pipetting, the sample and reagent volume ratio, the reaction modes and kinetics, the reading window and choice of measuring points, the calibration models and curve assessment, and the result determination and report.

Enzyme-multiplied immunoassay technique (EMIT) *(1–4,7,16,140–143, 147)* is based on the modulation of enzymatic activities by the binding of antibody to the enzyme-labeled drug derivative. Among the enzymes investigated, the most popular choice is glucose-6-phosphate dehydrogenase (G6PDH), which oxidizes glucose-6-phosphate to form glucuronolactone-6-phosphate. The reaction is coupled with the reduction of the cofactor nicotinamide adenine dinucleotide (NAD) to NADH, which can be monitored spectrophotometrically with absorbance at a maximum wavelength of 340 nm. In the presence of free drugs in the specimen, the competition for antibody binding results in a higher amount of free enzyme. Thus the enzyme is less inhibited when the concentration of free drugs is increased.

Cloned enzyme donor immunoassay (CEDIA) *(3,16,144–147)* is based on the complementation of two inactive polypeptide fragments to form an active enzyme. The enzyme acceptor (EA) and the enzyme donor (ED) can spontaneously associate in solution to form the active enzyme, i.e., recombinant microbial β-galactosidase. The catalytic activity of the enzyme on the substrate chlorophenol red β-D-galactopyranoside (CPRG) can be monitored spectrophotometrically with absorbance at the maximum wavelength (approx 570 nm). The absorbance rate change is measured as a function of time (mA/min). The antibody binding to the drug derivative–ED conjugate in the reaction cuvet prevents the formation of an active enzyme. The presence of drug in the specimen competes for antibody binding and hence allows the free drug–ED conjugate to reassociate with the EA. Therefore, the concentration of drugs in the sample is proportional to the enzymatic activity detected.

Fluorescence polarization immunoassay (FPIA) *(2–4,16,143,148)* is a technique that utilizes the properties of fluorescent molecules for biomedical analysis. Excitation of fluorophores in solution leads to selective absorption of light by appropriately oriented molecules. Polarized emission of these molecules occurs when their rate of rotation is low relative to the rate of fluorescent emission. Fluorescein-labeled drug derivatives (i.e., tracer for the immunoassay) rotate rapidly before light emission occurs, resulting in depolarization of the emitted light. When the tracer is bound to a macromolecule, the rotation is slowed and the fluorescence remains polarized. FPIA utilizes a known amount of tracer that competes with the free drug in the specimen for antibody binding. Increasing the concentration of drug in the specimen that binds to antibody leads to a greater amount of unbound tracer, which contributes to depolarization of the emitted light. Hence, the drug concentration is inversely related to the degree of polarization, which is measured in milliPolarization (mP) units.

There are two formats of kinetic interaction of microparticles in solution (KIMS) *(1–4,7,16,149–152)* techniques for drug immunoassays. Generation I KIMS (Abuscreen OnLine) is based on the competition between microparticle-labeled drug derivative and the free drugs in the specimen for antibody binding in solution. The binding of antibody and microparticle-bound drug conjugates leads to the formation of particle aggregates that scatter transmitted light. Generation II KIMS (ONLINE II) contain polymer-conjugated drug derivatives and microparticle-labeled antibodies. The interaction of the soluble conjugates and antibody on the microparticles promotes particle lattice formation. As the aggregation reaction proceeds, there is a kinetic increase in absorbance values. Any drug in the sample competes for antibody binding and inhibits particle aggregation; thus, drug concentration is inversely related to the absorbance change.

3.1.3. Competitive Immunoassay Techniques With Combined Labels

Enzyme immunoassay can be combined with other labels for drug analysis in either heterogeneous or homogeneous format *(153–155)*. For example, substrate-labeled fluorescence immunoassay combines the use of the enzyme β-galactosidase and a fluorogenic substrate. Microparticle enzyme immunoassay combines the use of antibody-coated microparticles and alkaline phosphatase enzyme-labeled drugs. The enzymes can hydrolyze a fluorogenic substrate, and the rate of fluorescence generation can be measured with a fluorometer. Enzyme-enhanced chemiluminescence immunoassay (IMMULITE) utilizes alkaline phosphatase (ALP) as the enzyme label and 1,2-dioxetane as the chemiluminescent substrate. The substrate is destabilized by ALP, leading to an unstable dioxetane intermediate that can emit light upon decay back to the ground state. The IMMULITE instrument employs a proprietary tube that contains polystyrene beads as the solid phase to capture antibody. The tube allows for the separation of reaction components through high-speed spin about the longitudinal axis for decanting and washing. When the chemiluminescent substrate is added to the tube, the light emission is read with a photon counter, and this reading is then converted to analyte concentration by an external computer.

Immunoassays can also be combined with various flow-injection or chromatographic techniques to develop a flow immunosensor assay or a multianalyte capillary electrophoretic immunoassay *(156)*. More recently, a number of immunosensor-based or biochip-based *(157–159)* competitive immunoassays have been designed or investigated for their applications in drug testing.

3.1.4. Point-of-Collection Drugs-of-Abuse Testing

The immediacy of a drugs-of-abuse test result, especially the result that rules out drug presence at the point of collection (POCT or "on-site"), is desirable for certain drug-testing programs *(7–10)*. The availability of POCT can benefit programs that require a faster personnel decision-making process, an immediate safety or compliance assessment, or an aid in clinical management. The implementation of POCT has included three areas:

1. The performance of instrument-based immunoassays at on-site initial screening-only testing facilities;
2. On-site sample processing for further laboratory analysis;
3. The utilization of single-use, disposable POCT devices.

Early versions of on-site drug testing were mostly based on the microparticle agglutination-inhibition methods in the 1970s. The techniques had been further developed for single-unit, visually read, homogeneous immunoassay devices such as Abuscreen OnTrak *(160)*.

The use of paper chromatography (PC) for drugs-of-abuse screening was explored in the 1980s, but the initial products suffered from a number of performance issues. Enzyme was the initial choice for membrane-based assays but was later replaced by colored microparticles, which allow the visualization of results without the need of additional substrate reagents. Similarly to the evolution of other immunoassay technologies that were first developed for larger molecules or polypeptides, the application of these technologies to competitive assays for small molecules typically required further development. The visually read, lateral-flow immunochromatography that was first available for sandwich immunoassays in the late 1980s was further developed for drug testing in the 1990s and has since become the most popular technique for drug POCT *(161–167)*.

The two basic formats of lateral-flow test strip for drug testing include the colloidal gold-based test strip configuration and a colored latex-enhanced immunochromatography. Both formats depend on the competition of free drugs in the sample with the immobilized drug-derivative conjugate on the result zone for binding to antibody on the colored particles. In the absence of drugs, antibody binds to the immobilized drug derivative, and hence a colored band is visible in the result zone. The presence of free drugs inhibits such binding; thus, no color is visible on the strip. The techniques were developed for urinalysis and more recently have also been used in the production of alternative specimen POCT.

The ascend multimmunoassay technique (such as Biosite Triage) *(7,10, 168)* depends on competitive binding of drugs in the sample with colloidal gold-labeled drug derivatives for antibody binding sites. After a 10-min incubation, the mixture is transferred to a strip of membrane onto which several specific antibodies are immobilized in discrete lines. In the absence of drugs, all the colloidal gold-labeled drugs are bound by their specific antibodies and cannot bind to the immobilized antibodies. Therefore, no color band is formed. The presence of drugs in the sample reduces the amount of antibody binding to the gold-labeled drugs, and hence the free gold-labeled drugs can bind to the membrane-immobilized antibodies and form a visible band.

Table 2 shows a summary of POCT techniques used for drugs-of-abuse testing. All of the ready-to-use devices have been pre-calibrated during manufacturing, and therefore on-board calibration or multilevel cutoff flexibility does not apply. There have been concerns about near-cutoff result reading; however, these assays in routine use are generally considered comparable to the performance with conventional immunoassays in most drug-screening settings that demand a rapid turnaround. In recent years, there has been a remarkable proliferation in the varieties of onsite drug-testing products as well as a significantly increased number of distributors for such tests. Because no specialized high-cost analyzers are required, the market for POCT has a lower entry barrier and is highly dynamic.

3.2. Receptor Assays

Many drugs exert their action through an interaction with one or more receptor types or subtypes in vivo. Theoretically, a receptor assay (RA) permits

Table 2
Examples of Competitive Immunoassays for Point-of-Collection Drugs-of-Abuse Screening

Nomenclature of immunoassay technology (Abbreviation)	Latex agglutination-inhibition (LAI)	Membrane enzyme immunoassay (EIA)	Ascend multiimmunoassay (AMIA)	Colored latex-based lateral flow immunochromatography	Gold sol-based lateral flow immunochromatography	Gold-labeled optically read rapid immunoassay (GLORIA)
Assay labels	Latex microparticles	Enzyme-HRP	Gold sol nanoparticles	Colored latex micro/nanoparticles	Gold sol nanoparticles	Gold sol nanoparticles
Reagents and solid phase	Three dropper bottles Drug conjugate on microparticles; antibody reagent; buffer [Slide with capillary tracks]	Enzyme-drug conjugate Positive and negative control solutions, antibody immobilized in the reaction site of membrane	Three lyophilized pellets: Drug conjugates on Gold sol; antibodies; buffer Wash solution bottle [antibody immobilized in membrane strip]	Antibody-latex dried on latex pad Drug conjugate immobilized in membrane strip	Antibody-Gold sol dried on gold conjugate pad Drug conjugate immobilized in membrane strip	Antibody on Gold sol Antibody in membrane Drug conjugate in pad
Assay procedure	1. Pipette sample to the mixing well on assay slide. 2. Add one drop each of the antibody reagent, reaction buffer, and latex reagent. 3. Stir and start the run.	1. Pipette sample to the wells on assay card. 2. Apply positive and negative controls to respective wells. 3. Add one drop of enzyme to all wells. 4. Wash 5. Apply substrate to all wells.	1. Pipette sample to the Reaction cup 2. Incubate for 10 min 3. Transfer the reaction mixture from the cup to the detection area 4. Allow the mixture to soak through 5. Wash, allow soaking through	Introduce sample to sample-receiving pad (method is device-dependent)	Introduce sample to sample-receiving pad (method is device-dependent)	Dip the test strip into the sample and then drain for 3–5 s
Result reading time	Read results when complete (about 4 min)	Read results in 3 min	Read results within 5 min of completion	Read results when test is valid (about 3–5 min)	Read results when test is valid (mostly 5–10 min)	Read results when test is complete (about 2 min)

HRP, horseradish peroxidase.

the simultaneous measurement of the molecules that bind to the receptor, providing a total estimate of all pharmacologically active forms of the drugs (i.e., parent drug and active metabolites). RAs have also been proposed as a tool for systematic toxicological analysis because they can be applied toward the detection of an entire pharmacological class of drugs *(132)*.

The RA technique makes use of the property of the analyte to competitively replace a labeled ligand from the same receptor binding site. The amount of labeled ligand replaced is a measure of the amount and the affinity of the analyte. Even though RAs do not exploit the physicochemical properties of the analyte, the result may offer information regarding the biological or pharmacological activity of the analyte by distinguishing the compounds on the basis of their specific binding reactions rather than specific molecular structure recognition. It should be noted, however, that drug binding to the cell receptor may have agonist or antagonist properties, so the activity can be either positive or negative for similar concentrations of related drugs. RA techniques such as the radio-receptor assay (RRA) have been used in various investigations of benzo-diazepines *(132,133)*. In general, results from RRA have been reported to be equal to or better than immunoassays and to correlate well with chromatographic methods. A few nonisotopic RAs have been developed for benzo-diazepines. Other nonisotopic labels such as fluorescence have been proposed as an alternative to RRAs for benzodiazepines assay in biological systems and to screen new benzodiazepine-like compounds from nature *(134)*.

4. SEPARATION METHODOLOGIES FOR DRUGS-OF-ABUSE TESTING

Analytical identification and quantification of the analyte of interest require the physical separation of the analyte from the mixture of sample components. The most important separation methodologies for drugs-of-abuse testing are the chromatographic technologies, although electrophoresis techniques have also been developed for drug analysis.

4.1. The Chromatographic Techniques: PC, TLC, GC, and HPLC

As defined by the International Union of Pure and Applied Chemistry (IUPAC) Compendium of Chemical Terminology *(169)*, *chromatography* is a physical method of separation in which the components to be separated are distributed between two phases, one of which is stationary (stationary phase) while the other (the mobile phase) moves in a definite direction. There are more than 20 types of chromatographic technologies, at least four of which have been applied to drug analysis. Liquid–liquid (partition) chromatography and PC were experimented with in the 1940s, and gas–liquid chromatography

(GLC) and TLC (planar chromatography) were further developed in the 1950s and 1960s. Currently, TLC such as Toxi-Lab is still in use for drug testing. Further advances in recent years in both gas and liquid chromatographies and their interfaces with mass spectrometry have further facilitated the progression of drug analysis technologies. The "hyphenated techniques" of chromatography and MS now are indispensable tools of drugs-of-abuse confirmatory testing and forensic analysis. Impressive congeries of publications and comprehensive reviews have been published for GC, LC, and especially for their hyphenated techniques. A wealth of specific technical details has been published for the analysis of a wide spectrum of drug classes. The goal for the following sections is to present an overview of these technologies, and we will not specifically describe details for their manifold applications.

4.1.1. Thin-Layer Chromatography

In planar chromatography, the stationary phase is a thin layer of absorbent material coated on a glass or metal plate (in TLC) *(170–172)*, or impregnated in a sheet of cellulose or fiberglass material (in PC). To run TLC, the sample is applied as a small spot near the lower edge of the plate and the plate is placed in a solvent chamber. As the solvent rises in the stationary phase, the components in the sample move up the plate at different rates and are separated into different spots. Visualization of the separated components on the plates can be performed under ultraviolet (UV) light and fluorescence. The plates can also be sprayed with various staining reagents to produce color spots. The distance a component migrates from its point of application is calculated as the R_f value. The corrected R_f values are dependent on chemical characteristics and can be used as identification parameters to determine the presumptive presence of a substance. TLC is relatively inexpensive for screening a variety of substances but has relatively higher and variable detection limits. TLC is labor intensive; a prototype Toxi-Prep system developed to automate the process of sample extraction, washing, and elution onto a chromatogram was shown to achieve an overall labor reduction for extraction and spotting of approx 40% *(172)*. A modified TLC technique, high-performance TLC (HPTLC), employs smaller sorbent particles and thicker stationary phase to achieve a better and more efficient separation in a shorter time and with less consumption of solvents *(173–175)*.

4.1.2. Gas Chromatography

GC is commonly used for the separation of thermally stable, volatile compounds. GC separates components of a mixture into its constituent components by forcing the gaseous mixture and carrier gas through a column of stationary phase and then measuring specific spectral peaks for each component of the vaporized sample. Each peak size, measured from baseline to apex, is proportional to the amount of the corresponding substance in the sample. Retention time is the time elapsed between injection and elution from a column of a single component of the separated mixture. The principle of the separation lies in the partitioning of sample components with different retention times, which depends on the chemical and physical characteristics of the analyte molecules. A substance with little or no affinity for the stationary phase of the column will elute rapidly, while a substance with high affinity for the stationary phase will be impeded and therefore slower to elute.

The general design of a GC instrument incorporates (1) a sample injection port (i.e., injector), (2) a mobile phase supply (i.e., carrier gas) and flow control apparatus, (3) a column to perform chromatographic separation between mobile and stationary phases, (4) a detector, and (5) a system to collect and process data (i.e., computer).

4.1.2.1. Preparation of Samples and Internal Standards

Sample preparations such as hydrolysis, extraction, and derivatization have to be carried out prior to sample injection for GC analysis. Depending on the type of specimen used, sample pretreatment such as protein precipitation may also be required. The hydrolysis step *(176–178)* is used to cleave the conjugate, and may involve fast acid hydrolysis or relatively gentle enzymatic hydrolysis. Alkaline hydrolysis is mostly used for the cleavage of ester conjugates. Scores of studies have been published, reporting specific sample preparation methods that demonstrate enhancement of extraction efficiency *(179–185)* and improvement of GC-MS analyses. In short, the most commonly used extraction techniques are liquid–liquid extraction (LLE), solid-phase extraction (SPE), and solid-phase microextraction (SPME). A wide variety of solvents and solid-phase materials have been developed, and large selections of commercial columns are also available. The choice of solid-phase cartridges, such as those based on hydrophobic, polar, ionic, or mixed mode of retention mechanisms, is based on both the chemical properties of the analyte(s) and the sample matrix. The development of direct extractive alkylation *(186–188,190)* under alkaline conditions allows the simultaneous extraction and derivatization of acidic compounds. In addition, antibodies have been used for an immunoaffinity extraction procedure that allowed the simultaneous analysis of Δ9-THC and its major metabolites in urine, plasma, and meconium by GC-MS *(106)*.

Derivatization chemistry *(189–191)* is employed to convey volatility to nonvolatile compounds and to permit analysis of polar compounds not directly amenable to GC and/or MS analysis. On the other hand, for compounds that have excess volatility, derivatization can be designed to yield less volatile compounds, to minimize losses during the procedure, and to help separate the GC sample peaks from the solvent front. In addition, derivatization can be utilized to yield a more heat-stable compound and hence improve chromatographic performance and peak shape. Analytical derivatization techniques can be developed to improve chromatographic separation of a closely related compound. Moreover, appropriate derivatization can be utilized to improve the detecting power of certain detectors. An excellent comprehensively review was published by Segura et al. *(191)*. In brief, the common derivatization methods for GC include (1) silylation (to give, e.g., trimethylsilyl [TMS] derivatives, commonly using *N,O*-bis[trimethylsilyl]trifluoroacetamide [BFSTFA] as the derivatizing agent, or *tert*-butyldimethylsilyl [TBDMS] derivatives); (2) acylation (to give acetyl; pentafluoropropionyl [PFP]; heptafluorobutyryl [HFB]; or trifluoroacetyl [TFA], using, e.g., *N*-methyl-bis[trifluoroacetamide] [MBTFA] derivatives); (3) alkylation (to give, e.g., methyl or hexafluoroisopropylidene [HFIP] derivatives); and (4) the formation of cyclic or diastereomeric derivatives. In addition, chiral derivatization reagents such as fluoroacyl-prolyl chloride, *S*-(-)-heptafluorobutyryl-prolyl chloride, and *S*-(-)-trifluoroacetyl-prolyl chloride can be used to distinguish enantiomers when using a non-chiral chromatographic column.

Internal standards *(192,193)* are required to avoid or minimize possible errors during the extraction and derivatization processes. Internal standards are also used to ensure correct chromatographic behavior and quantitation as well as to help in structural elucidation. In GC-MS applications, deuterated internal standards are often used. However, a variety of compounds have been selected as internal standards because such compounds usually have similar structure and possess chromatographic behavior and retention times similar to those of the target analyte.

4.1.2.2. Injector and Carrier Gas-Mobile Phase

The analyte(s) must be in the gas phase for GC separation, and a variety of sample introduction systems have been developed to vaporize liquid samples. In conventional GC with packed columns, samples are injected via an on-line injector using the syringe/septum arrangement or direct connected loop injector. In capillary column GC, the isothermal split or splitless injector system is typically used. The splitless mode of injection is designed for a diluted sample so that most of the sample injected is directed into the column. Temperature-programmable injection ports can be used in either the split or splitless mode to allow the separation of solvent-removal and analyte vaporization, hence improving analyte detection. In addition, cold direct injection and cold on-column injection have been developed to minimize discrimination against higher boiling-point components by the injector.

Upon injection into the GC inlet port, a small amount of sample is vaporized immediately by the high-temperature conditions, which are maintained throughout the GC process by the enclosing oven. An inert carrier gas then transfers the vaporized sample onto the column with minimal band broadening, where it undergoes chromatographic separation. The selection of carrier gas (usually helium, hydrogen, or nitrogen) is influenced by several factors, such as the column type, detector, and the laboratory operation considerations. A constant gas flow from the mobile phase supply is sustained by monitoring flow meters and pressure gages.

4.1.2.3. Columns: Stationary Phase and Temperature Control

The necessity for high temperatures to volatilize drugs for GC requires a special stationary phase that is stable and nonvolatile under the operational conditions. There are two types of stationary phases; the nonselective type separates analytes by molecular size and shape, whereas the selective type separates analyte according to the selective retention of certain groups. There are two major types of GC columns: packed columns and capillary columns (i.e., wall-coated open tubular [WCOT] column).

A multitude of GC columns are available for selection from a variety of commercial suppliers. Many of the supplier catalogs, literature, or application notes provide information on stationary-phase materials and their compatibility with solvent, the amount of polarity, the recommended operating temperature range, and other related information. After the injected sample is directed into the column and carried by the mobile gas phase, the various components of the sample will partition according to the vapor pressure and solubility of each component in the stationary phase of the column. A lower vapor pressure, corresponding to a higher boiling point, will cause the compound to remain longer in the stationary phase and hence elute slower. A compound that is more soluble in the stationary phase will also produce a longer retention time.

4.1.2.4. Detectors and Computer

Ideally, the separated sample components are introduced one at a time into a detector. The choice of a GC detector from the wide variety available is made according to its particular utility and analytical performance requirements. Examples of detectors include MS, flame ionization detector (FID), electron capture detector (ECD), thermal conductivity detector (TCD), atomic emission detector (AED), and many others. MS and FID are universal detectors that may be used for the detection of many volatile organic compounds, although both detectors will also destroy the sample. Because of its ability to provide detailed structural information, MS is the most widely used detector in forensic toxicology. ECD and AED display selectivity in detector response; ECD is often used in the analysis of halogenated compounds, whereas AED is preferred for certain elements such as carbon, sulfur, nitrogen, and phosphorous. TCD is concentration-dependent, whereas FID is mass-flow-rate-dependent.

Following detection, the spectral output is recorded and displayed visually by computer. The computer provides both system-control and data-processing functions. The data are stored and used to calculate analyte concentration from the area or height of each of the chromatographic peaks, to construct calibration curves, to calculate conversion factors from internal or external calibration, and to generate a report.

4.1.3. Liquid Chromatography

For drug analysis, liquid chromatography (LC) is used for the separation of nonvolatile compounds. Separation by LC is based on the distribution of the solutes between a liquid mobile phase and a stationary phase. The most widely used LC technique for drug analysis is HPLC. HPLC utilizes particles of small diameter as the stationary phase support to increase column efficiency. Because the pressure drop is related to the square of the particle diameter, relatively high pressure is needed to pump liquid mobile phase through the column. Similarly to GC, a wide variety of HPLC columns and systems are available from a number of vendors.

Akin to GC, the general design of an LC instrument incorporates (1) an injector, (2) a mobile phase supply (solvent reservoir) and pumps to force the mobile phase through the system, (3) a column to perform chromatographic separation between mobile and stationary phases, (4) a detector, and (5) a system to collect and process data (computer).

Sample preparation for LC also includes the appropriate protein precipitation, hydrolysis, and LLE or SPE; however, the majority of analytes do not require analytical derivatization for LC analysis. The most frequently used injector for LC is the fixed-loop injector. The injector can be used at high pressure and can be programmed in an automatic system. A number of high-precision, microprocessor-controlled autosamplers are available from various vendors. Degassed solvent from the solvent reservoir is pumped into the system using a mode selected for the purpose of the particular LC analysis (e.g., isocratic or gradient mode). To protect the analytical column, either a precolumn (placed between the pump and the injector) or a guard column (located between the injector and the LC column) is commonly used. As with GC, there are a wide range of commercial LC columns offered from a number of suppliers. However, stereoselective HPLC can be optimized for the determination of the individual enantiomers *(194,195)*.

The commonly used detectors for LC include UV spectrophotometers, such as diode array detectors (DAD), fluorometers, refractometers, and electrochemical detectors. Detectors that can simultaneously monitor column effluent at a range of wavelengths using multiple diodes or rotating filter disks are useful as drug screening methods. As with GC, the most powerful detector for

LC is MS. However, in comparison with GC-MS, more sophisticated interfaces must be developed for LC-MS. The introduction of two atmospheric pressure ionization (API) interfaces—electrospray ionization (ESI) and atmospheric pressure chemical ionization (APCI)—has facilitated the major evolution of LC-MS. In the past year, the importance of LC-MS, especially LC-MS-MS, has dramatically increased in diverse biochemical applications, from proteomics to clinical and forensic toxicology. Improvements made to the interfaces of LC and MS include the nebulization of the liquid phase, the removal of the bulk solvent, the dissociation of solvent-analyte clusters, and ionization techniques. Commonly used ionization techniques for the coupling of chromatography and MS will be further discussed under Subheading 5.2.

A number of limitations associated with LC-MS have been investigated, including its susceptibility to matrix effect and ion-suppression effect *(196–199)*. Dams et al. *(198)* evaluated the matrix effect resulting from the combination of bio-fluid, sample preparation technique, and ionization type. The authors concluded that matrix components interfered at different times and to a varying extent throughout the study. The residual matrix components were higher in plasma than those in oral fluid, whereas oral fluid has more matrix interferences than urine.

4.2. The Electrophoretic Techniques: CE, HPCE, CZE, MECC, CITP

CE is based on the principle of electrophoresis in a capillary format that separates compounds based on the combined properties of their electrophoretic mobility, isoelectric point, partitioning, molecular size, and so on *(29–34)*. Over the past decade, CE and high-performance CE (HPCE) have emerged as effective and promising separation techniques as a result of its high separation efficiency, minimal sample preparation, negligible sample and solvent consumption, and broad analytical spectrum. Instrumentation for CE utilizing fused silica capillaries has been developed and evaluated for diverse applications in biomedical and chemical analysis. The three major modes of CE are capillary zone electrophoresis (CZE), micellar electrokinetic capillary chromatography (MECC), and capillary isotachophoresis (CITP). The addition to CE of appropriate cyclodextrins as chiral selectors can provide a simple and inexpensive approach for the separation of enantiomers.

In forensic and clinical toxicology, the CZE and MECC techniques have been validated by comparison to other established drug-screening and confirmation techniques. A number of published studies employed CZE and MECC to screen and/or confirm a variety of abused and therapeutic drugs in various biological fluids. Recent developments in CE techniques include the combination of CE with an immunoassay or the coupling of CE and MS for confirmatory testing. At the present time, CE is not as widely used as GC or HPLC for separation of drug components in biological fluids.

5. MASS SPECTROMETRY

5.1. Fundamental Mass Spectrometry

The fundamentals of MS for drug analysis involve (1) charging of the sample components (with or without the breaking-up of the various molecular species) and (2) the detection of the charged molecular and atomic fragments in order to identify the original sample. The process of molecular structure identification depends on the comparison of compound-specific fragmentation fingerprints in a particular mass spectrum with those in databases, and occasionally elemental analysis based on relative isotope abundance. The charged fragments or ions of a single mass can be isolated by manipulation of the electromagnetic fields within a mass analyzer to produce a mass-to-charge ratio (m/z). Although the variety of MS instruments is diverse in the type of apparatus and mechanical processes, the general scheme involves (1) a sample inlet, an ionization source, (2) a vacuum system, (3) a mass analyzer to accelerate and filter ions by mass, (4) a detector, and (5) a system to collect data (computer).

5.1.1. Ion Source

The sample must be introduced in a gas phase to the sample inlet (which is kept at a high temperature to guarantee a gaseous sample) before it is converted to an ion in the ionization chamber. Many approaches to ionize samples have been developed. The most commonly used ionization techniques for drug analysis are electron ionization or electron impact (EI) and chemical ionization (CI). EI is a "hard" ionization technique whereas CI is a "soft" ionization technique. For the interface of LC and MS, soft ionization techniques such as ESI and APCI have been developed.

For ionization by EI, electrons produced by thermoionic emission from a tungsten filament are accelerated in a collimated beam by a high voltage (typically +70 eV) and impact the gaseous analyte molecules, shattering the molecules into fragments and causing each molecule to give up an electron. The resulting energetic cation radical is called the "molecular ion" (or parent ion) M^+. The molecular ion can undergo a predictable and relatively reproducible fragmentation, forming a radical and a cation called the "fragment ion," which is generated from bond cleavage reactions.

In CI, a reagent gas such as methane is typically ionized to radical forms, which impact the analyte molecules in the GC effluent and chemically generate molecular ions and some daughter ions and neutral fragments. The most common type of CI reactions resulting in positive ions are proton transfers of fragmentations with the positive charge being retained by the part with a greater ionizability. Negative ions (NICI) can be generated either by reaction with proton-abstracting reagents or by electron capture of thermalized electrons.

EI and CI methods may be used to complement each other, as the softer CI technique produces less fragmentation and ensures the production of molecular ions, whereas the harder EI technique can give more detailed information about the molecular structure of the sample.

ESI is a newer soft ionization approach for MS and involves the pneumatic nebulization of the analyte solution to produce charged droplets that are sprayed from a capillary tip by means of an applied potential (+4 kV). Solvent evaporation and coulombic repulsion forces eventually lead to the formation of charged analyte ions. A softer but more energetic ionization method than ESI is APCI, in which the analyte solution is directly injected into the CI plasma, where analyte ions are generated from ion-molecule reactions taking place at atmospheric pressure. An electric discharge between the spray capillary and a counter electrode sustains the CI plasma.

5.1.2. Mass Analyzer and Vacuum System

The mass analyzer uses a controlled range of magnetic and/or electric field strengths to filter positively charged molecules by mass-to-charge ratio (m/z) and accelerate the ion of interest in a vacuum to the detector by the influence of an accelerating voltage. Techniques to achieve this separation include quadrupole mass filters (quadrupole mass spectrometer [QMS]), ion traps (quadrupole ion traps [QIT]), Selective Ion Monitoring (SIM), magnetic sector, time-of-flight, and so on.

The quadrupole mass filter is the most commonly used mass analyzer for MS because of its good reproducibility, low cost, and compact nature. Only ions of the desired m/z value can follow a stable trajectory to the detector between four parallel rods, which create electric fields controlled by a fixed direct current (DC) and alternating radio frequency (RF) voltages. The quadrupole mass analyzer is limited in terms of resolution and mass discrimination (peak heights as a function of mass). Conversely, the ion trap boasts high mass resolution but suffers from a limited dynamic range, required low-pressure conditions, space charge effects (ion–ion repulsion), and ion molecule reactions. Three hyperbolic electrodes form a three-dimensional storage space where ions are trapped in a stable oscillating trajectory by the applied RF potentials. Alternation of the voltages causes ions of different m/z to be successively ejected from the exit lens into the detector. SIM is another technique that improves sensitivity in trace analysis, and differs from those previously mentioned in that only ions with the desired m/z values are selected and monitored to enhance the signal-to-noise ratio. Confirmation is normally performed in the SIM mode because only particular compounds have to be identified. For MS-MS, this approach is called *selected reaction monitoring* (SRM).

A vacuum system is used to ensure that the ions in the mass analyzer do not collide with any other molecule during interaction with the magnetic or electric fields. A number of systems can be used for these purposes, a including mechanical vacuum, a high-vacuum pump such as diffusion pump, turbomolecular pumps, and cryopumps.

5.1.3. Detectors and Computer

As desired ions from the mass analyzer strike the detector, a representative signal is produced that is proportional to the number of impinging ions. These signals (fragment mass over detected charge) are amplified by cascading electron emissions and sent to the computer, where the electrical impulses are converted to visual output for further analysis.

The visual output is presented as a mass spectrum of the sample, where each peak is graphed by fragment m/z along the x-axis and abundance, or the quantity of detected fragments for that mass, along the y-axis (therefore corresponding to peak height). A total ion chromatogram (TIC) is obtained by plotting the sum of abundances of all ions in the mass spectrum as a function of elution time. The parent mass, or the detected mass associated with the unfragmented analyte molecule, indicates the molecular mass of the analyte and is usually the largest peak on the spectrum. The remaining peaks provide precise clues to the molecular structure, as their associated fragments can be pieced together to form the original molecule, and identification of the sample can be confirmed by comparison to reference spectra via library search *(200–202)*. The ion with the highest abundance in a mass spectrum is considered the base peak and is normalized to 100%. Other ion fragment abundances are then reported as percentages of the base peak height. For identification purposes, the monitoring of at least three ions and their abundance ratios is required, and it is desirable that one of the ions selected should be the molecular ion.

5.2. The Coupling of Analytical Techniques: GC-MS, LC-MS, CE-MS, and TLC-MS

The coupling of GC, LC, or CE and MS is a powerful technique for the chemical analysis of mixtures of compounds. An emerging development that utilizes TLC and direct on-spot matrix-assisted laser desorption/ionization time-of-flight MS has been applied for fast screening of low-molecular-weight compounds with nearly matrix-free mass spectra using a UV-absorbing ionic liquid matrix *(203)*. In essence, the first system enables separation of the components of a mixture and determines their particular retention times. Molecules entering the MS are ionized and may undergo fragmentation; consequently, the sensitive detector in the MS device provides information for the identification of components by determining their mass spectra. A computer serves as the data collector to record and process the mass spectra obtained *(200–202)*.

Although GC/MS is recognized as the standard procedure for confirming positive immunoassay screening results of drugs of abuse, targeted GC-MS analysis does have limitations. The following section contains an overview of the technique and limitations of both GC and MS separately and of the combined technique of GC-MS. Any analytical technique has its limitations; GC is limited by unequal detector responses to equal amounts of two different samples, the presence of residual impurities, the choice of a carrier gas, the life of an injection port septum, and the crucial temperature range of the injection port. For each analyte of interest, the problem posed by unequal detector responses to equal amounts of different samples is overcome by the calculation of a response factor for each analyte. This response factor is defined as the response of the analyte (peak area or height) divided by the weight (or volume) of the analyte injected. The proper choice of a carrier gas and its purity are vital to the success of the analysis. The gas filter should be changed regularly, and a stable gas flow rate should be maintained to avoid false peaks and a drifting baseline. The lifespan of a septum will be shortened by higher injection-port temperatures. It is essential that the injection port be kept within the correct temperature range to completely vaporize the sample; a lower temperature will result in poor separation and broad or no peak development, whereas a higher temperature may cause the sample to decompose or alter structure and thereby skew the analysis results.

The potential limitations of MS include resolution, interior pressure of the device, high scan rate, the skills of the technician, the locating of the parent mass when present, and the comparison of the analyte identification with that of a standard sample. Resolution refers to the degree of separation of adjacent peaks in a mass spectrum, and is defined as $R = m/\Delta m$, where m is from the observed m/z ratio and Δm is the difference in mass between the two peaks. An MS instrument with low resolution may poorly characterize a sample with large molecular mass, such as body fluids. Just as important as high resolution is maintaining high vacuum conditions within the device in order to minimize collisions between analyte fragments. Such collisions may foster recombination of analyte fragments to make new molecules, thus producing spectral peaks alien to the authentic mass spectrum of the analyte. The tradeoff of the ability of MS instruments to rapidly scan multiple fragment masses is decreased resolution, which may produce unreliable results for quantitative analysis.

The analyses and interpretation of the mass spectra plays an essential role in the accurate determination of the original molecular structure of the sample. The importance of the human element involved in the decision between possible answers outweighs the assistance computers and libraries can provide. Also, the occasional difficulty in recognizing the appropriate parent peak in the mass spectrum may introduce analytical error, since the establishment of the associated parent mass is important for the qualitative decision about the molecular structure of the analyte. In addition, such a parent peak may not even be observed for samples of sufficiently high molecular mass, such as drugs in body fluids. One solution is the use of CI as the ionization source for MS, which helps to ensure the appearance of the parent peak in the mass spectrum. Finally, it is essential that a standard sample of the presumed identity of the analyte be prepared and run under identical conditions both prior to and after the analyte run. Discrepancies between the mass spectra of the sample and the standard indicate a questionable identification.

In practice, GC-MS is regarded by many scientists as the conclusive *modus operandi* for the reliable identification of substances by chemical analysis. For all of the positive attributes of GC-MS, however, even an authoritative technique has limitations. A capillary column interface serves as the connection between the GC column and the MS device, which concentrates the GC sample effluent by removing the gas carrier and then feeds the sample to the MS. The accuracy of the MS technique is dependent on the purity of this effluent; background noise may appear in the mass spectrum as a result of incomplete chromatographic separation of the compounds in the sample. In addition, failure to deflect the carrier gas of the GC device from entering the MS device likewise may cause contamination. To assess the performance of GC-MS analysis, an internal standard (IS) can be added prior to any extraction step so that the IS can undergo the same manipulations, from sample preparation to result analysis, as the sample. For MS decisions, a compound, either structurally related to the analyte of interest, or an analyte labeled with a stable isotope such as deuterium, is generally used as an internal standard.

The performance expectation and limitations of GC-MS as well as solutions to overcome some of the identified limitations have been subjected to a number of reviews *(204–208)*. In addition, The Clinical and Laboratory Standards Institute has developed "Approved Guidelines (C43-A) for GC-MS Confirmation of Drugs." The document provides guidance to routine instrument and method performance verification, calibration, result interpretation, quality control, and quality assurance. The certified laboratories also are subject to periodic surveys with proficiency testing samples provided by specific organizations. The College of American Pathologists (CAP/AACC) has been conducting quarterly surveys and year-end critique for certified laboratories.

The percent coefficient variance from the different laboratories can be assessed from these surveys. In the near future, the proposed new federal Guidelines for WDT will include regulations on the requirements for certified laboratories to validate their confirmatory drug testing (GC-MS, LC-MS, GC-MS-MS, and/or LC-MS-MS) before the laboratory can use it to test specimens *(69)*.

5.3. MS/MS and MSn

The potential of mass spectral analysis is amplified by using a series of MS analyzers in tandem, or MS-MS and MSn. This affords a higher degree of sensitivity, lowers the possibility of interference from contaminants, and aids in structural identification of the molecule for the chemical analysis; but it also adds substantially to the cost of the procedure. The general process most commonly used in MS-MS is similar to linking multiple quadrupoles together and assigning each a separate function. Described as MS-MS in space, three quadrupoles are typically set to analyze the sample in series. The first quadrupole filters the analyte ions in the traditional sense of a mass analyzer by allowing only the ion with the desired *m/z* to pass. Fragmentation of the chosen ion, referred to as the *precursor ion*, occurs in the second quadrupole by impact with collision gas molecules to form product ions. These product ions can then be scanned by the third quadrupole or selectively allowed into the detector. Alternatively, MS-MS may be performed by MS-MS in time, which uses the ion trap as its mass analyzer. After the ejection of all but the desired precursor ion from the trap, the fragmentation of ions with *m/z* values that resonate with the particular applied voltage occurs to generate product ions. This multistage entrapment and fragmentation of ions can hypothetically continue as many times as desired, but is usually unnecessary and cost prohibitive. Nevertheless, the multiple steps of MS-MS virtually eliminate contamination by undesired compounds that may co-elute from the GC column and enable the fragmentation analysis of isolated ions. These are both positive results that will help untangle complex molecular structures and raise the confidence of identification.

6. CONCLUSIONS

The two-stage drug-testing strategy requires the use of analytical methodologies with different chemical principles. Analytical methodologies for drug testing can be grouped into three major categories. Each of these technology categories can be further broken down into multiple selections for instrumentations and methods. Bio-affinity-based binding assays such as immunoassays are commonly used for screening. Separation techniques such as chromatography or electrophoresis, as well as their coupling with powerful detectors such as mass spectrometers, can be effectively used for confirmatory testing of preliminary positive results or systematic analysis of generally unknown toxic compounds. The analytical technologies afford a powerful means toward the detection, identification, and quantification of the presence of abused drugs in biological specimens. Nevertheless, measurement uncertainties and experimental variations always exist. Therefore, the interpretation of analytical results requires the understanding of the performance characteristics and limitations of the techniques used for analysis. In addition, the overall interpretation of drug-testing results has to be considered in the context of both the reasons and the scenarios for testing *(209–212)*. Substance abuse can play various roles in different cultural and occupational settings; hence it is important to understand the nature of drugs-of-abuse testing and how to correlate results from one situation to another.

REFERENCES

1. Armbruster DA, Schwarzhoff RH, Pierce BL, and Hubster EC. Method comparison of EMIT II and ONLINE with RIA for drug screening. J Forensic Sci 1993; 38:1326–1341.
2. Armbruster DA, Schwarzhoff RH, Hubster EC, and Liserio MK. Enzyme immunoassay, kinetic microparticle immunoassay, radioimmunoassay, and fluorescence polarization immunoassay compared for drugs-of-abuse screening. Clin Chem 1993;39:2137–2146.
3. Armbruster DA, Hubster EC, Kaufman MS, and Ramon MK. Cloned enzyme donor immunoassay (CEDIA) for drugs-of-abuse screening. Clin Chem 1995;41:92–98.
4. Beck O, Lin Z, Brodin K, Borg S, and Hjemdahl P. The Online screening technique for urinary benzodiazepines: comparison with EMIT, FPIA, and GC-MS. J Anal Toxicol 1997;21:554–557.
5. Baselt RC. Urine drug screening by immunoassay: interpretation of results, in Advances in Analytical Toxicology, Volume 1 (Baselt, RC, ed), Biomedical Publications, Foster City, CA: 1984; pp. 81–123.
6. Cone EJ, Presley L, Lehrer M, et al. Oral fluid testing for drugs of abuse: positive prevalence rates by Intercept immunoassay screening and GC-MS-MS confirmation and suggested cutoff concentrations. J Anal Toxicol 2002;26:541–546.
7. Ferrara SD, Tedeschi L, Frison G, et al. Drugs-of-abuse testing in urine: statistical approach and experimental comparison of immunochemical and chromatographic techniques. J Anal Toxicol 1994;18:278–291.
8. Gronholm M and Lillsunde P. A comparison between on-site immunoassay drug-testing devices and laboratory results. Forensic Sci Int 2001;121:37–46.
9. Hammett-Stabler CA, Pesce AJ, and Cannon DJ. Urine drug screening in the medical setting. Clin Chim Acta 2002;315:125–135.
10. Jenkins AJ and Goldberger BA. (eds). On-Site Drug Testing,. Humana Press, Totowa, NJ: 2002.
11. Kacinko SL, Barnes AJ, Kim I, et al. Performance characteristics of the Cozart RapiScan Oral Fluid Drug Testing System for opiates in comparison to ELISA and GC/MS following controlled codeine administration. Forensic Sci Int 2004; 141:41–48.

12. Kerrigan S and Phillips WH, Jr. Comparison of ELISAs for opiates, methamphetamine, cocaine metabolite, benzodiazepines, phencyclidine, and cannabinoids in whole blood and urine. Clin Chem 2001;47:540–547.
13. Kroener L, Musshoff F, and Madea B. Evaluation of immunochemical drug screenings of whole blood samples. A retrospective optimization of cutoff levels after confirmation-analysis on GC-MS and HPLC-DAD. J Anal Toxicol 2003;27:205–212.
14. Moore KA, Werner C, Zannelli RM, Levine B, and Smith ML. Screening postmortem blood and tissues for nine classes [correction of cases] of drugs of abuse using automated microplate immunoassay. Forensic Sci Int 1999;106:93–102.
15. Smith ML, Hughes RO, Levine B, Dickerson S, Darwin WD, and Cone EJ. Forensic drug testing for opiates. VI. Urine testing for hydromorphone, hydrocodone, oxymorphone, and oxycodone with commercial opiate immunoassays and gas chromatography–mass spectrometry. J Anal Toxicol 1995;19:18–26.
16. Smith ML, Shimomura ET, Summers J, et al. Detection times and analytical performance of commercial urine opiate immunoassays following heroin administration. J Anal Toxicol 2000;24:522–529.
17. Walsh JM, Flegel R, Crouch DJ, Cangianelli L, and Baudys J. An evaluation of rapid point-of-collection oral fluid drug-testing devices. J Anal Toxicol 2003;27: 429–439.
18. Drummer OH. Chromatographic screening techniques in systematic toxicological analysis. J Chromatogr B Biomed Sci Appl 1999;733:27–45.
19. El Mahjoub A and Staub C. High-performance liquid chromatographic method for the determination of benzodiazepines in plasma or serum using the column-switching technique. J Chromatogr B Biomed Sci Appl 2000;742:381–390.
20. Maier RD and Bogusz M. Identification power of a standardized HPLC-DAD system for systematic toxicological analysis. J Anal Toxicol 1995;19:79–83.
21. Staub C. Chromatographic procedures for determination of cannabinoids in biological samples, with special attention to blood and alternative matrices like hair, saliva, sweat and meconium. J Chromatogr B Biomed Sci Appl 1999;733:119–126.
22. Tracqui A, Kintz P, and Mangin P. Systematic toxicological analysis using HPLC/DAD. J Forensic Sci 1995;40:254–262.
23. Valli A, Polettini A, Papa P, and Montagna M. Comprehensive drug screening by integrated use of gas chromatography/mass spectrometry and Remedi HS. Ther Drug Monit 2001;23:287–294.
24. Dawling S and Widdop B. Use and abuse of the Toxi-Lab TLC system. Ann Clin Biochem 1988;25:708–709.
25. Jain R. Utility of thin layer chromatography for detection of opioids and benzodiazepines in a clinical setting. Addict Behav 2000;25:451–454.
26. Jarvie DR and Simpson D. Drug screening: evaluation of the Toxi-Lab TLC system. Ann Clin Biochem 1986;23 (Pt 1):76–84.
27. Lillsunde P and Korte T. Comprehensive drug screening in urine using solid-phase extraction and combined TLC and GC/MS identification. J Anal Toxicol 1991;15: 71–81.
28. Otsubo K, Seto H, Futagami K, and Oishi R. Rapid and sensitive detection of benzodiazepines and zopiclone in serum using high-performance thin-layer chromatography. J Chromatogr B Biomed Appl 1995;669:408–412.

29. Lemos NP, Bortolotti F, Manetto G, Anderson, RA, Cittadini F, and Tagliaro F. Capillary electrophoresis: a new tool in forensic medicine and science. Sci Justice 2001;41:203–210.
30. Manetto G, Crivellente F, and Tagliaro F. Capillary electrophoresis: a new analytical tool for forensic toxicologists. Ther Drug Monit 2000;22:84–88.
31. Kapnissi CP and Warner IM. Separation of benzodiazepines using capillary electrochromatography. J Chromatogr Sci 2004;42:238–244.
32. Tagliaro F, Turrina S, Pisi P, Smith FP, and Marigo M. Determination of illicit and/or abused drugs and compounds of forensic interest in biosamples by capillary electrophoretic/electrokinetic methods. J Chromatogr B Biomed Sci Appl 1998; 713:27–49.
33. Thormann W. Progress of capillary electrophoresis in therapeutic drug monitoring and clinical and forensic toxicology. Ther Drug Monit 2002;24:222–231.
34. Wernly P and Thormann W. Analysis of illicit drugs in human urine by micellar electrokinetic capillary chromatography with on-column fast scanning polychrome absorption detection. Anal Chem 1991;63:2878–2882.
35. Bogusz MJ, Maier RD, Kruger KD, and Kohls U. Determination of common drugs of abuse in body fluids using one isolation procedure and liquid chromatography— atmospheric-pressure chemical-ionization mass spectromery. J Anal Toxicol 1998; 22:549–558.
36. Bogusz MJ. Hyphenated liquid chromatographic techniques in forensic toxicology. J Chromatogr B Biomed Sci Appl 1999;733:65–91.
37. Bogusz MJ. Liquid chromatography–mass spectrometry as a routine method in forensic sciences: a proof of maturity. J Chromatogr B Biomed Sci Appl 2000;748: 3–19.
38. Breindahl T and Andreasen K. Validation of urine drug-of-abuse testing methods for ketobemidone using thin-layer chromatography and liquid chromatography– electrospray mass spectrometry. J Chromatogr B Biomed Sci Appl 1999;736: 103–113.
39. Dams R, Murphy CM, Lambert WE, and Huestis MA. Urine drug testing for opioids, cocaine, and metabolites by direct injection liquid chromatography/tandem mass spectrometry. Rapid Commun Mass Spectrom 2003;17:1665–1670.
40. Dams R, Murphy CM, Choo RE, Lambert WE, De Leenheer AP, and Huestis MA. LC-atmospheric pressure chemical ionization–MS/MS analysis of multiple illicit drugs, methadone, and their metabolites in oral fluid following protein precipitation. Anal Chem 2003;75:798–804.
41. Goldberger BA and Cone EJ. Confirmatory tests for drugs in the workplace by gas chromatography–mass spectrometry. J Chromatogr A 1994;674:73–86.
42. Hoja H, Marquet P, Verneuil B, Lotfi H, Penicaut B, and Lachatre G. Applications of liquid chromatography–mass spectrometry in analytical toxicology: a review. J Anal Toxicol 1997;21:116–126.
43. Kintz P and Cirimele V. Testing human blood for cannabis by GC-MS. Biomed Chromatogr 1997;11:371–373.
44. Lehrer M. The role of gas chromatography/mass spectrometry. Instrumental techniques in forensic urine drug testing. Clin Lab Med 1998;18:631–649.

45. Marquet P. Progress of liquid chromatography–mass spectrometry in clinical and forensic toxicology. Ther Drug Monit 2002;24:255–276.

46. Maurer HH. Liquid chromatography-mass spectrometry in forensic and clinical toxicology. J Chromatogr B Biomed Sci Appl 1998;713:3–25.

47. Maurer HH. Systematic toxicological analysis procedures for acidic drugs and/or metabolites relevant to clinical and forensic toxicology and/or doping control. J Chromatogr B Biomed Sci Appl 1999;733:3–25.

48. Maurer HH. Role of gas chromatography–mass spectrometry with negative ion chemical ionization in clinical and forensic toxicology, doping control, and bio-monitoring. Ther Drug Monit 2002;24:247–254.

49. Maurer HH, Kraemer, T, Kratzsch, C, Peters, FT, and Weber, AA. Negative ion chemical ionization gas chromatography–mass spectrometry and atmospheric pressure chemical ionization liquid chromatography–mass spectrometry of low-dosed and/or polar drugs in plasma. Ther Drug Monit 2002;24:117–124.

50. Moeller MR, Steinmeyer S, and Kraemer T. Determination of drugs of abuse in blood. J Chromatogr B Biomed Sci Appl 1998;713:91–109.

51. Moeller MR and Kraemer T. Drugs of abuse monitoring in blood for control of driving under the influence of drugs. Ther Drug Monit 2002;24:210–221.

52. Nordgren HK and Beck O. Multicomponent screening for drugs of abuse: direct analysis of urine by LC-MS-MS. Ther Drug Monit 2004;26:90–97.

53. Peat MA. Advances in forensic toxicology. Clin Lab. Med 1998;18:263–278.

54. Peters FT, Kraemer T, and Maurer HH. Drug testing in blood: validated negative-ion chemical ionization gas chromatographic–mass spectrometric assay for determination of amphetamine and methamphetamine enantiomers and its application to toxicology cases. Clin Chem 2002;48:1472–1485.

55. Polettini A, Groppi A, Vignali C, and Montagna M. Fully-automated systematic toxicological analysis of drugs, poisons, and metabolites in whole blood, urine, and plasma by gas chromatography–full scan mass spectrometry. J Chromatogr B Biomed Sci Appl 1998;713:265–279.

56. Polettini A. Systematic toxicological analysis of drugs and poisons in biosamples by hyphenated chromatographic and spectroscopic techniques. J Chromatogr B Biomed Sci Appl 1999;733:47–63.

57. Saint-Marcoux F, Lachatre G, and Marquet P. Evaluation of an improved general unknown screening procedure using liquid chromatography–electrospray–mass spectrometry by comparison with gas chromatography and high-performance liquid-chromatography–diode array detection. J Am Soc Mass Spectrom 2003;14: 14–22.

58. Solans A, Carnicero M, de la Torre R, and Segura J. Comprehensive screening procedure for detection of stimulants, narcotics, adrenergic drugs, and their metabolites in human urine. J Anal Toxicol 1995;19:104–114.

59. Song SM, Marriott P, Kotsos A, Drummer OH, and Wynne P. Comprehensive two-dimensional gas chromatography with time-of-flight mass spectrometry (GC x GC-TOFMS) for drug screening and confirmation. Forensic Sci Int 2004;143:87–101.

60. Venisse N, Marquet P, Duchoslav E, Dupuy JL, and Lachatre G. A general unknown screening procedure for drugs and toxic compounds in serum using

liquid chromatography–electrospray–single quadrupole mass spectrometry. J Anal Toxicol 2003;27:7–14.

61. Weinmann W, Vogt S, Goerke R, Muller C, and Bromberger, A. Simultaneous determination of THC-COOH and THC-COOH-glucuronide in urine samples by LC/MS/MS. Forensic Sci Int 2000;113:381–387.

62. Yonamine M, Tawil N, Moreau RL, and Silva OA. Solid-phase micro-extraction–gas chromatography–mass spectrometry and headspace-gas chromatography of tetrahydrocannabinol, amphetamine, methamphetamine, cocaine and ethanol in saliva samples. J Chromatogr B Analyt Technol Biomed Life Sci 2003;789:73–78.

63. Barcelo-Barrachina E, Moyano E, and Galceran MT. State-of-the-art of the hyphenation of capillary electrochromatography with mass spectrometry. Electrophoresis 2004;25:1927–1948.

64. Lazar IM, Naisbitt G, and Lee ML. Capillary electrophoresis–time-of-flight mass spectrometry of drugs of abuse. Analyst 1998;123:1449–1454.

65. Kosnoski EM, Yolton RL, Citek K, Hayes CE, and Evans RB. The Drug Evaluation Classification Program: using ocular and other signs to detect drug intoxication. J Am Optom Assoc 1998;69:211–227.

66. Heishman SJ, Singleton EG, and Crouch DJ. Laboratory validation study of drug evaluation and classification program: ethanol, cocaine, and marijuana. J Anal Toxicol 1996;20:468–483.

67. Heishman SJ, Singleton EG, and Crouch DJ. Laboratory validation study of drug evaluation and classification program: alprazolam, d-amphetamine, codeine, and marijuana. J Anal Toxicol 1998;22:503–514.

68. Mandatory guidelines for federal workplace drug testing programs. Fed Regist 59, 29908 (http://www.health.org/workplace/GDLNS-94.htm) or (http://workplace.samhsa.gov/fedprograms/MandatoryGuidelines/HHS09011994.pdf), 1994.

69. Proposed Revisions to Mandatory Guidelines for Federal Workplace Drug Testing Programs. Fed Regist 2004;69:19,673–19,732; http://a257.g.akamaitech.net/7/257/2422/14mar20010800/edocket.access.gpo.gov/2004/pdf/04-7984.pdf.

70. Braithwaite RA, Jarvie DR, Minty PS, Simpson D, and Widdop B. Screening for drugs of abuse. I: Opiates, amphetamines and cocaine. Ann Clin Biochem 1995;32 (Pt 2):123–153.

71. Simpson D, Braithwaite RA, Jarvie DR, et al. Screening for drugs of abuse (II): cannabinoids, lysergic acid diethylamide, buprenorphine, methadone, barbiturates, benzodiazepines and other drugs. Ann Clin Biochem 1997;34:460–510.

72. Chang TL, Chen KW, Lee YD, and Fan K. Determination of benzodiazepines in clinical serum samples: comparative evaluation of REMEDi system, aca analyzer, and conventional HPLC performance. J Clin Lab Anal 1999;13:106–111.

73. Drummer OH. Methods for the measurement of benzodiazepines in biological samples. J Chromatogr B Biomed Sci Appl 1998;713:201–225.

74. Schwenzer KS, Pearlman R, Tsilimidos M, et al. New fluorescence polarization immunoassays for analysis of barbiturates and benzodiazepines in serum and urine: performance characteristics. J Anal Toxicol 2000;24:726–732.

75. Burnley BT and George S. The development and application of a gas chromatography–mass spectrometric (GC-MS) assay to determine the presence of 2-oxo-3-hydroxy-LSD in urine. J Anal Toxicol 2003;27:249–252.

76. Cody JT and Valtier S. Immunoassay analysis of lysergic acid diethylamide. J Anal Toxicol 1997;21:459–464.
77. Hoja H, Marquet P, Verneuil B, Lotfi H, Dupuy JL, and Lachatre G. Determination of LSD and N-demethyl-LSD in urine by liquid chromatography coupled to electrospray ionization mass spectrometry. J Chromatogr B Biomed Sci Appl 1997; 692:329–335.
78. Schneider S, Kuffer P, and Wennig R. Determination of lysergide (LSD) and phencyclidine in biosamples. J Chromatogr B Biomed Sci Appl 1998;713:189–200.
78a. Plaut O, Girod C, and Staub C. Analysis of methaqualone in biological matrices by micellar electrokinetic capillary chromatography. Comparison with gas chromatography–mass spectrometry. Forensic Sci Int 1998;92:219–227.
79. Frost M, Kohler H, and Blaschke G. Enantioselective determination of methadone and its main metabolite 2-ethylidene-1,5-dimethyl-3,3-diphenylpyrrolidine (EDDP) in serum, urine and hair by capillary electrophoresis. Electrophoresis 1997;18: 1026–1034.
80. Lakso HA and Norstrom A. Determination of dextropropoxyphene and nordextropropoxyphene in urine by liquid chromatography–electrospray ionization mass spectrometry. J Chromatogr B Analyt Technol Biomed Life Sci 2003;794: 57–65.
81. McNally AJ, Pilcher I, Wu R, et al. Evaluation of the OnLine immunoassay for propoxyphene: comparison to EMIT II and GC-MS. J Anal Toxicol 1996;20: 537–540.
82. Hendrickson RG and Morocco AP. Quetiapine cross-reactivity among three tricyclic antidepressant immunoassays. J Toxicol. Clin Toxicol 2003;41:105–108.
83. Schwartz JG, Hurd IL, and Carnahan JJ. Determination of tricyclic antidepressants for ED analysis. Am J Emerg Med 1994;12:513–516.
84. de Boer D and Bosman I. A new trend in drugs-of-abuse; the 2C-series of phenethylamine designer drugs. Pharm World Sci 2004;26:110–113.
85. Ensslin HK, Kovar KA, and Maurer HH. Toxicological detection of the designer drug 3,4-methylenedioxyethylamphetamine (MDE, "Eve") and its metabolites in urine by gas chromatography–mass spectrometry and fluorescence polarization immunoassay. J Chromatogr B Biomed Appl 1996;683:189–197.
86. Kraemer T and Maurer HH. Determination of amphetamine, methamphetamine and amphetamine-derived designer drugs or medicaments in blood and urine. J Chromatogr B Biomed Sci Appl 1998;713:163–187.
87. Marquet P, Lacassie E, Battu C, Faubert H, and Lachatre G. Simultaneous determination of amphetamine and its analogs in human whole blood by gas chromatography–mass spectrometry. J Chromatogr B Biomed Sci Appl 1997;700: 77–82.
88. Maurer HH, Bickeboeller-Friedrich J, Kraemer T, and Peters FT. Toxicokinetics and analytical toxicology of amphetamine-derived designer drugs ('Ecstasy'). Toxicol Lett 2000;112–113:133–142.
89. Moeller MR and Hartung M. Ecstasy and related substances—serum levels in impaired drivers. J Anal Toxicol 1997;21:591.
90. Nordgren HK and Beck O. Direct screening of urine for MDMA and MDA by liquid chromatography–tandem mass spectrometry. J Anal Toxicol 2003;27:15–19.

91. Pizarro N, Ortuno J, Farre M, et al. Determination of MDMA and its metabolites in blood and urine by gas chromatography–mass spectrometry and analysis of enantiomers by capillary electrophoresis. J Anal Toxicol 2002;26:157–165.

92. Ramseier A, Caslavska J, and Thormann W. Stereoselective screening for and confirmation of urinary enantiomers of amphetamine, methamphetamine, designer drugs, methadone and selected metabolites by capillary electrophoresis. Electrophoresis 1999;20:2726–2738.

93. Crouch DJ, Rollins DE, Canfield DV, Andrenyak DM, and Schulties JE. Quantitation of alprazolam and alpha-hydroxyalprazolam in human plasma using liquid chromatography electrospray ionization MS-MS. J Anal Toxicol 1999;23: 479–485.

94. Bogusz MJ, Maier RD, Kruger KD, and Fruchtnicht W. Determination of flunitrazepam and its metabolites in blood by high-performance liquid chromatography–atmospheric pressure chemical ionization mass spectrometry. J Chromatogr B Biomed Sci Appl 1998;713:361–369.

95. ElSohly MA, Feng S, Salamone SJ, and Brenneisen R. GC-MS determination of flunitrazepam and its major metabolite in whole blood and plasma. J Anal Toxicol 1999;23:486–489.

96. ElSohly MA, Feng S, Salamone SJ, and Wu R. A sensitive GC-MS procedure for the analysis of flunitrazepam and its metabolites in urine. J Anal Toxicol 1997; 21:335–340.

97. Moeller MR and Mueller C. The detection of 6-monoacetylmorphine in urine, serum and hair by GC/MS and RIA. Forensic Sci Int 1995;70:125–133.

98. Presley L, Lehrer M, Seiter W, et al. High prevalence of 6-acetylmorphine in morphine-positive oral fluid specimens. Forensic Sci Int 2003;133:22–25.

99. Spanbauer AC, Casseday S, Davoudzadeh D, Preston KL, and Huestis MA. Detection of opiate use in a methadone maintenance treatment population with the CEDIA 6-acetylmorphine and CEDIA DAU opiate assays. J Anal Toxicol 2001;25:515–519.

100. Cirimele V, Kintz P, Lohner S, and Ludes B. Enzyme immunoassay validation for the detection of buprenorphine in urine. J Anal Toxicol 2003;27:103–105.

101. Hoja H, Marquet P, Verneuil B, Lotfi H, Dupuy JL, and Lachatre G. Determination of buprenorphine and norbuprenorphine in whole blood by liquid chromatography–mass spectrometry. J Anal Toxicol 1997;21:160–165.

102. Polettini A and Huestis MA. Simultaneous determination of buprenorphine, norbuprenorphine, and buprenorphine-glucuronide in plasma by liquid chromatography–tandem mass spectrometry. J Chromatogr B Biomed Sci Appl 2001;754:447–459.

103. Caplan YH and Goldberger BA. Alternative specimens for workplace drug testing. J Anal Toxicol 2001;25:396–399.

104. ElSohly MA and Feng S. Delta 9-THC metabolites in meconium: identification of 11-OH-delta 9-THC, 8 beta,11-diOH-delta 9-THC, and 11-nor-delta 9-THC-9-COOH as major metabolites of delta 9-THC. J Anal Toxicol 1998;22:329–335.

105. ElSohly MA, Stanford DF, Murphy TP, et al. Immunoassay and GC-MS procedures for the analysis of drugs of abuse in meconium. J Anal Toxicol 1999;23: 436–445.

106. Feng S, ElSohly MA, Salamone S, and Salem MY. Simultaneous analysis of delta9-THC and its major metabolites in urine, plasma, and meconium by GC-MS using an immunoaffinity extraction procedure. J Anal Toxicol 2000; 24:395–402.

107. Huestis MA, Oyler JM, Cone EJ, Wstadik AT, Schoendorfer D, and Joseph RE, Jr. Sweat testing for cocaine, codeine and metabolites by gas chromatography–mass spectrometry. J Chromatogr B Biomed Sci Appl 1999;733:247–264.

108. Huestis MA, Cone EJ, Wong CJ, Umbricht A, and Preston KL. Monitoring opiate use in substance abuse treatment patients with sweat and urine drug testing. J Anal Toxicol 2000;24:509–521.

109. Jenkins AJ, Oyler JM, and Cone EJ. Comparison of heroin and cocaine concentrations in saliva with concentrations in blood and plasma. J Anal Toxicol 1995; 19:359–374.

110. Kato K, Hillsgrove M, Weinhold L, Gorelick DA, Darwin WD, and Cone EJ. Cocaine and metabolite excretion in saliva under stimulated and nonstimulated conditions. J Anal Toxicol 1993;17:338–341.

111. Kidwell DA, Holland JC, and Athanaselis S. Testing for drugs of abuse in saliva and sweat. J Chromatogr B Biomed Sci Appl 1998;713:111–135.

112. Kidwell DA and Smith FP. Susceptibility of PharmChek drugs of abuse patch to environmental contamination. Forensic Sci Int 2001;116:89–106.

113. Kidwell DA, Kidwell JD, Shinohara F, et al. Comparison of daily urine, sweat, and skin swabs among cocaine users. Forensic Sci Int 2003;133:63–78.

114. Kintz P and Samyn N. Use of alternative specimens: drugs of abuse in saliva and doping agents in hair. Ther Drug Monit 2002;24:239–246.

115. Moore C, Negrusz A, and Lewis D. Determination of drugs of abuse in meconium. J Chromatogr B Biomed Sci Appl 1998;713:137–146.

116. Niedbala RS, Kardos KW, Fritch DF, et al. Detection of marijuana use by oral fluid and urine analysis following single-dose administration of smoked and oral marijuana. J Anal Toxicol 2001;25:289–303.

117. Ostrea EM, Jr. Testing for exposure to illicit drugs and other agents in the neonate: a review of laboratory methods and the role of meconium analysis. Curr Probl Pediatr 1999;29:37–56.

118. Buchan BJ, Walsh JM, and Leaverton PE. Evaluation of the accuracy of on-site multi-analyte drug testing devices in the determination of the prevalence of illicit drugs in drivers, J Forensic Sci 1998;43:395–399.

119. Department of Transportation, National Highway Traffic Safety Administration (NHTSA). Field test of on-site drug detection devices, DOT HS 809 192 (http://www.nhtsa.dot.gov/people/injury/research/pub/onsitedetection/Drug_index.htm), 2000.

120. Jehanli A, Brannan S, Moore L, and Spiehler VR. Blind trials of an onsite saliva drug test for marijuana and opiates. J Forensic Sci 2001;46:1214–1220.

121. Roadside Testing Assessment (ROSITA). Work package 2, Deliverable D2, Inventory of state-of-the-art road side drug testing equipment. (www.rosita.org), 1999.

122. Walsh JM. On-site testing devices and driving-under-the-influence cases, in On-Site Drug Testing (Jenkins AJ and Goldberger BA, eds), Humana Press, Totowa, NJ: 2002; pp. 67–76.

123. European Workplace Drug Testing Society (EWDTS). European Laboratory Guidelines for Legally Defensible Workplace Drug Testing. (http://www.ewdts.org/guidelines.html), 2002.

124. Brendler J and Liu RH. Initial test cutoff selection based on regression analysis of initial test apparent analyte result vs GC/MS test analyte result—evaluation of two radioimmunoassay kits' test data. Clin Chem 1997;43:688–690.

125. Cone EJ, Sampson-Cone AH, Darwin WD, Huestis MA, and Oyler JM. Urine testing for cocaine abuse: metabolic and excretion patterns following different routes of administration and methods for detection of false-negative results. J Anal Toxicol 2003;27:386–401.

126. Huestis MA, Mitchell JM, and Cone EJ. Lowering the federally mandated cannabinoid immunoassay cutoff increases true-positive results. Clin Chem 1994; 40:729–733.

127. Liu RH, Edwards C, Baugh LD, Weng JL, Fyfe MJ, and Walia AS. Selection of an appropriate initial test cutoff concentration for workplace drug urinalysis—Cannabis example. J Anal Toxicol 1994;18:65–70.

128. Luzzi VI, Saunders AN, Koenig JW, et al. Analytic performance of immuno-assays for drugs of abuse below established cutoff values. Clin Chem 2004;50: 717–722.

129. Smith-Kielland A, Skuterud B, and Morland J. Urinary excretion of 11-nor-9-carboxy-delta9-tetrahydrocannabinol and cannabinoids in frequent and infrequent drug users. J Anal Toxicol 1999;23:323–332.

130. Vandevenne M, Vandenbussche H, and Verstraete A. Detection time of drugs of abuse in urine. Acta Clin Belg 2000;55:323–333.

131. Wingert WE. Lowering cutoffs for initial and confirmation testing for cocaine and marijuana: large-scale study of effects on the rates of drug-positive results. Clin Chem 1997;43:100–103.

132. Ensing K, Bosman IJ, Egberts AC, Franke JP, and de Zeeuw RA. Application of radioreceptor assays for systematic toxicological analysis—2. Theoretical considerations and evaluation. J Pharm Biomed Anal 1994;12:59–63.

133. Janssen MJ, Ensing K, and de Zeeuw RA. Improved benzodiazepine radiorecep-tor assay using the MultiScreen Assay System. J Pharm Biomed Anal 1999;20: 753–761.

134. Janssen MJ, Ensing K, and de Zeeuw RA. Fluorescent-labeled ligands for the benzodiazepine receptor. Part 2: The choice of an optimal fluorescent-labeled ligand for benzodiazepine receptor assays. Pharmazie 2000;55:102–106.

135. Nishikawa T, Ohtani H, Herold DA, and Fitzgerald RL. Comparison of assay methods for benzodiazepines in urine. A receptor assay, two immunoassays, and gas chromatography–mass spectrometry. Am J Clin Pathol 1997;107: 345–352.

136. Joseph R, Dickerson S, Willis R, Frankenfield D, Cone EJ, and Smith DR. Inter-ference by nonsteroidal anti-inflammatory drugs in EMIT and TDx assays for drugs of abuse. J Anal Toxicol 1995;19:13–17.

137. Colbert DL. Drug abuse screening with immunoassays: unexpected cross-reactivities and other pitfalls. Br J Biomed Sci 1994;51:136–146.

138. Ward C, McNally AJ, Rusyniak D, and Salamone SJ. [125]I radioimmunoassay for the dual detection of amphetamine and methamphetamine. J Forensic Sci 1994; 39:1486–1496.

139. Hino Y, Ojanpera I, Rasanen I, and Vuori E. Performance of immunoassays in screening for opiates, cannabinoids and amphetamines in post-mortem blood. Forensic Sci Int 2003;131:148–155.

140. Asselin WM and Leslie JM. Use of the EMITtox serum tricyclic antidepressant assay for the analysis of urine samples. J Anal Toxicol 1990;14:168–171.

141. Bogusz M, Aderjan R, Schmitt G, Nadler E, and Neureither B. The determination of drugs of abuse in whole blood by means of FPIA and EMIT-dau immunoassays—a comparative study. Forensic Sci Int 1990;48:27–37.

142. Gjerde H, Christophersen AS, Skuterud B, Klemetsen K, and Morland J. Screening for drugs in forensic blood samples using EMIT urine assays. Forensic Sci Int 1990;44:179–185.

143. Maier RD, Erkens M, Hoenen H, and Bogusz M. The screening for common drugs of abuse in whole blood by means of EMIT-ETS and FPIA-ADx urine immunoassays. Int J Legal Med 1992;105:115–119.

144. Chronister CW, Walrath JC, and Goldberger BA. Rapid detection of benzoylecgonine in vitreous humor by enzyme immunoassay. J Anal Toxicol 2001;25: 621–624.

145. Iwersen-Bergmann S, and Schmoldt A. Direct semiquantitative screening of drugs of abuse in serum and whole blood by means of CEDIA DAU urine immunoassays. J Anal Toxicol 1999;23:247–256.

146. Loor R, Lingenfelter C, Wason PP, Tang K, and Davoudzadeh D. Multiplex assay of amphetamine, methamphetamine, and ecstasy drug using CEDIA technology. J Anal Toxicol 2002;26:267–273.

147. Way BA, Walton KG, Koenig JW, Eveland BJ, and Scott MG. Comparison between the CEDIA and EMIT II immunoassays for the determination of benzodiazepines. Clin Chim Acta 1998;271:1–9.

148. Fraser AD, and Worth D. Monitoring urinary excretion of cannabinoids by fluorescence-polarization immunoassay: a cannabinoid-to-creatinine ratio study. Ther Drug Monit 2002;24:746–750.

149. Baker DP, Murphy MS, Shepp PF, et al. Evaluation of the Abuscreen ONLINE assay for amphetamines on the Hitachi 737: comparison with EMIT and GC/MS methods. J Forensic Sci 1995;40:108–112.

150. Boettcher M, Haenseler E, Hoke C, Nichols J, Raab D, and Domke I. Precision and comparability of Abuscreen OnLine assays for drugs of abuse screening in urine on Hitachi 917 with other immunochemical tests and with GC/MS. Clin Lab 2000;46:49–52.

151. Moody DE and Medina AM. OnLine kinetic microparticle immunoassay of cannabinoids, morphine, and benzoylecgonine in serum. Clin Chem 1995;41:1664–1665.

152. Smith FP, Lora-Tamayo C, Carvajal R, Caddy B, and Tagliaro F. Assessment of an automated immunoassay based on kinetic interaction of microparticles in solution for determination of opiates and cocaine metabolite in urine. Ann Clin Biochem 1997;34 (Pt 1), 81–84.

153. Klotz U. Performance of a new automated substrate-labeled fluorescence immunoassay system evaluated by comparative therapeutic monitoring of five drugs. Ther Drug Monit 1984;6:355–359.

154. Sheehan M and Caron G. Evaluation of an automated system (Optimate) for substrate-labeled fluorescent immunoassays. Ther Drug Monit 1985;7:108–114.

155. Sharma JD, Aherne GW, and Marks V. Enhanced chemiluminescent enzyme immunoassay for cannabinoids in urine. Analyst 1989;114:1279–1282.

156. Caslavska J, Allemann D, and Thormann W. Analysis of urinary drugs of abuse by a multianalyte capillary electrophoretic immunoassay. J Chromatogr A 1999; 838:197–211.

157. Nath N, Eldefrawi M, Wright J, Darwin D, and Huestis M. A rapid reusable fiber optic biosensor for detecting cocaine metabolites in urine. J Anal Toxicol 1999; 23:460–467.

158. Tsai JSC, Deng D, Diebold E, Smith A, Wentzel C, and Franzke S. The latest development in biosensor immunoassay technology for drug assays. LABOLife, 2002;Nr.4/02:17–20.

159. Yu H, Kusterbeck AW, Hale MJ, Ligler FS, and Whelan JP. Use of the USDT flow immunosensor for quantitation of benzoylecgonine in urine. Biosens Bioelectron 1996;11:725–734.

160. Armbruster DA and Krolak JM. Screening for drugs of abuse with the Roche ONTRAK assays. J Anal Toxicol 1992;16:172–175.

161. Beck O, Kraft M, Moeller MR, Smith BL, Schneider S, and Wennig R. Frontline immunochromatographic device for on-site urine testing of amphetamines: laboratory validation using authentic specimens. Ann Clin Biochem 2000;37(Pt 2), 199–204.

162. Klimov AD, Tsai S-CJ, Towt J, Salamone SJ. Improved immuno-chromatographic format for competitive-type assays. Clin Chem 1995;41:1360.

163. Leino A, Saarimies J, Gronholm M, and Lillsunde P. Comparison of eight commercial on-site screening devices for drugs-of-abuse testing, Scand J Clin Lab Invest 2001;61:325.

164. Peace MR, Poklis JL, Tarnai LD, and Poklis A. An evaluation of the OnTrak Testcup-er on-site urine drug-testing device for drugs commonly encountered from emergency departments. J Anal Toxicol 2002;26:500–503.

165. Towt J, Tsai SC, Hernandez MR, et al. ONTRAK TESTCUP: a novel, on-site, multi-analyte screen for the detection of abused drugs. J Anal Toxicol 1995;19: 504–510.

166. Yang JM and Lewandrowski KB. Urine drugs of abuse testing at the point-of-care: clinical interpretation and programmatic considerations with specific reference to the Syva Rapid Test (SRT). Clin Chim Acta 2001;307:27–32.

167. Weiss A. Concurrent Engineering for Lateral-Flow Diagnostics, IVD Technology 1999;5:48–57.

168. Buechler KF, Moi S, Noar B, et al. Simultaneous detection of seven drugs of abuse by the Triage panel for drugs of abuse, Clin Chem 1992;38:1678–1684.

169. International Union of Pure and Applied Chemistry, http://www.iupac.org/ publications/analytical_compendium/

170. Jain R. Utility of thin layer chromatography for detection of opioids and benzo-diazepines in a clinical setting. Addict Behav 2000;25:451–454.

171. Lillsunde P and Korte T. Comprehensive drug screening in urine using solid-phase extraction and combined TLC and GC/MS identification. J Anal Toxicol 1991;15:71–81.

172. Steinberg DM, Sokoll LJ, Bowles KC, et al. Clinical evaluation of Toxi.Prep: a semiautomated solid-phase extraction system for screening of drugs in urine. Clin Chem 1997;43:2099–2105.

173. Gioino G, Hansen C, Pacchioni A, et al. Use of high-performance liquid chro-matography with diode-array detection after a primary drug screening in patients admitted to the emergency department. Ther Drug Monit 2003;25:99–106.

174. Otsubo K, Seto H, Futagami K, and Oishi R. Rapid and sensitive detection of benzodiazepines and zopiclone in serum using high-performance thin-layer chromatography. J Chromatogr B Biomed Appl 1995;669:408–412.

175. Simonovska B, Prosek M, Vovk I, and Jelen-Zmitek A. High-performance thin-layer chromatographic separation of ranitidine hydrochloride and two related compounds. J Chromatogr B Biomed Sci Appl 1998;715:425–430.

176. Hackett LP, Dusci LJ, Ilett KF, and Chiswell GM. Optimizing the hydrolysis of codeine and morphine glucuronides in urine. Ther Drug Monit 2002;24:652–657.

177. Kemp PM, Abukhalaf IK, Manno JE, et al. Cannabinoids in humans. II. The influence of three methods of hydrolysis on the concentration of THC and two metabolites in urine. J Anal Toxicol 1995;19:292–298.

178. Skopp G and Potsch L. An investigation of the stability of free and glucu-ronidated 11-nor-delta9-tetrahydrocannabinol-9-carboxylic acid in authentic urine samples. J Anal Toxicol 2004;28:35–40

179. Bogusz MJ, Maier RD, Schiwy-Bochat KH, and Kohls U. Applicability of vari-ous brands of mixed-phase extraction columns for opiate extraction from blood and serum. J Chromatogr B Biomed Appl 1996;683:177–188.

180. Brown H, Kirkbride KP, Pigou PE, and Walker GS. New developments in SPME, Part 1: The use of vapor-phase deprotonation and on-fiber derivatization with alkylchloroformates in the analysis of preparations containing amphetamines. J Forensic Sci 2003;48:1231–1238.

181. Chiarotti M. Overview on extraction procedures. IntForensic Sci Int 1993;63: 161–170.

182. Garside D, Goldberger BA, Preston KL, and Cone EJ. Rapid liquid-liquid extrac-tion of cocaine from urine for gas chromatographic–mass spectrometric analysis. J Chromatogr B Biomed Sci Appl 1997; 692:61–65.

183. Gerlits J. GC/MS quantitation of benzoylecgonine following liquid-liquid extrac-tion of urine. J Forensic Sci 1993;38:1210–1214.

184. Soriano T, Jurado C, Menendez M, and Repetto M. Improved solid-phase extrac-tion method for systematic toxicological analysis in biological fluids. J Anal Tox-icol 2001;25:137–143.

185. Yonamine M, Tawil N, Moreau RL, and Silva OA. Solid-phase micro-extraction–gas chromatography–mass spectrometry and headspace-gas chroma-tography of tetrahydrocannabinol, amphetamine, methamphetamine, cocaine and

ethanol in saliva samples. J Chromatogr B Analyt Technol Biomed Life Sci 2003;789:73–78.

186. Lisi AM, Kazlauskas R, and Trout GJ. Gas chromatographic–mass spectrometric quantitation of urinary 11-nor-delta 9-tetrahydrocannabinol-9-carboxylic acid after derivatization by direct extractive alkylation. J Chromatogr 1993;617: 265–270.

187. Lisi AM, Kazlauskas R, and Trout GJ. Gas chromatographic–mass spectrometric quantitation of urinary buprenorphine and norbuprenorphine after derivatization by direct extractive alkylation. J Chromatogr B Biomed Sci Appl 1997;692:67–77.

188. Maurer HH, Tauvel FX, and Kraemer T. Screening procedure for detection of non-steroidal anti-inflammatory drugs and their metabolites in urine as part of a systematic toxicological analysis procedure for acidic drugs and poisons by gas chromatography–mass spectrometry after extractive methylation. J Anal Toxicol 2001;25:237–244

189. Cremese M, Wu AH, Cassella G, O'Connor E, Rymut K, and Hill DW. Improved GC/MS analysis of opiates with use of oxime-TMS derivatives. J Forensic Sci 1998;43:1220–1224.

190. Melgar R and Kelly RC. A novel GC/MS derivatization method for amphetamines. J Anal Toxicol 1993;17:399–402.

191. Segura J, Ventura R, and Jurado C. Derivatization procedures for gas chromatographic–mass spectrometric determination of xenobiotics in biological samples, with special attention to drugs of abuse and doping agents. J Chromatogr B Biomed Sci Appl 1998;713:61–90.

192. Liu RH, Foster G, Cone EJ, and Kumar SD. Selecting an appropriate isotopic internal standard for gas chromatography/mass spectrometry analysis of drugs of abuse—pentobarbital example. J Forensic Sci 1995;40:983–989.

193. ElSohly MA, Little TL, Jr, and Stanford DF. Hexadeutero-11-nor-delta 9-tetrahydrocannabinol-9-carboxylic acid: a superior internal standard for the GC/MS analysis of delta 9-THC acid metabolite in biological specimens. J Anal Toxicol 1992;16:188–191.

194. Foster DJ, Somogyi AA, and Bochner F. Stereoselective quantification of methadone and its major oxidative metabolite, 2-ethylidene-1,5-dimethyl-3,3-diphenylpyrrolidine, in human urine using high-performance liquid chromatography. J Chromatogr B Biomed Sci Appl 2000;744:165–176.

195. Yanagihara Y, Ohtani M, Kariya S, et al. Stereoselective high-performance liquid chromatographic determination of ketamine and its active metabolite, norketamine, in human plasma. J Chromatogr B Biomed Sci Appl 2000;746:227–231.

196. Bogusz M and Erkens M. Influence of biological matrix on chromatographic behavior and detection of selected acidic, neutral, and basic drugs examined by means of a standardized HPLC-DAD system. J Anal Toxicol 1995;19:49–55.

197. Bogusz MJ. Large amounts of drugs may considerably influence the peak areas of their coinjected deuterated analogues measured with APCI-LC-MS. J Anal Toxicol 1997;21:246–247.

198. Dams R, Huestis MA, Lambert WE, and Murphy CM. Matrix effect in bioanalysis of illicit drugs with LC-MS/MS: influence of ionization type, sample preparation, and biofluid. J Am Soc Mass Spectrom 2003; 14:1290–1294.

199. Muller C, Schafer P, Stortzel M, Vogt S, and Weinmann W. Ion suppression effects in liquid chromatography–electrospray-ionisation transport-region collision induced dissociation mass spectrometry with different serum extraction methods for systematic toxicological analysis with mass spectra libraries. J Chromatogr B Analyt Technol Biomed Life Sci 2002;773:47–52.

200. Aebi B and Bernhard W. Advances in the use of mass spectral libraries for forensic toxicology. J Anal Toxicol 2002;26:149–156.

201. Gergov M, Weinmann W, Meriluoto J, Uusitalo J, and Ojanpera I. Comparison of product ion spectra obtained by liquid chromatography/triple-quadrupole mass spectrometry for library search. Rapid Commun Mass Spectrom 2004;18: 1039–1046.

202. Kratzsch C, Peters FT, Kraemer T, Weber AA, and Maurer HH. Screening, library-assisted identification and validated quantification of fifteen neuroleptics and three of their metabolites in plasma by liquid chromatography/mass spectrometry with atmospheric pressure chemical ionization. J Mass Spectrom 2003; 38:283–295.

203. Santos LS, Haddad R, Hoehr NF, Pilli RA, and Eberlin MN. Fast screening of low molecular weight compounds by thin-layer chromatography and "on-spot" MALDI-TOF mass spectrometry. Anal Chem 2004;76:2144–2147.

204. Armbruster DA, Tillman MD, and Hubbs LM. Limit of detection (LQD)/limit of quantitation (LOQ): comparison of the empirical and the statistical methods exemplified with GC-MS assays of abused drugs. Clin Chem 1994;40:1233–1238.

205. Baselt RC. Commentary on Wu AHB, Hill DW, Crouch D, Hodnett CN, McCurdy HH. Minimal standards for the performance and interpretation of toxicology tests in legal proceedings. J Forensic Sci 2000;45:507.

206. Underwood PJ, Kananen GE, and Armitage EK. A practical approach to determination of laboratory GC-MS limits of detection. J Anal Toxicol 1997;21:12–16.

207. Wu AH. Mechanism of interferences for gas chromatography/mass spectrometry analysis of urine for drugs of abuse. Ann Clin Lab Sci 1995;25:319–329.

208. Wu AH, Hill DW, Crouch D, Hodnett CN, and McCurdy HH. Minimal standards for the performance and interpretation of toxicology tests in legal proceedings. J Forensic Sci 1999;44:516–522.

209. ElSohly MA. Practical challenges to positive drug tests for marijuana. Clin Chem 2003;49:1037–1038.

210. ElSohly MA, and Jones AB. Drug testing in the workplace: could a positive test for one of the mandated drugs be for reasons other than illicit use of the drug? J Anal Toxicol 1995;19:450–458.

211. Kapur BM. Drug-testing methods and clinical interpretations of test results. Bull Narc 1993;45:115–154.

212. Kidwell DA. Discussion: caveats in testing for drugs of abuse. NIDA Res Monogr 1992;117:98–120.

Chapter 4

The Use of Nitrocellulose Membranes in Lateral-Flow Assays

Michael A. Mansfield

SUMMARY

Microporous nitrocellulose membranes are used in lateral-flow assays as the substrate upon which immunocomplexes are formed and visualized to indicate the presence or absence of an analyte in a liquid sample. The pore sizes of membranes used in this application are comparatively large, ranging from 3 to 20 μm. Several attributes have resulted in nitrocellulose being the preferred substrate for lateral-flow assays. First, nitrocellulose adsorbs protein at a high level. Second, chemistries that make the membrane wettable with aqueous solution do not significantly diminish protein adsorption. Third, nitrocellulose membranes can be cast that have pores sufficiently large to allow lateral flow of fluid in a reasonable time. To facilitate the utilization of nitrocellulose in lateral-flow assays, the membrane can be cast directly onto a polyester backing. The backing does not interfere with the function of the nitrocellulose while significantly improving its handling properties. Optimal performance of nitrocellulose membranes requires an understanding of the interactions of test reagents with the nitrocellulose and the effects of reagent location on assay sensitivity.

1. HISTORICAL BACKGROUND

Nitrocellulose has been used industrially for over a century *(1)* and for the production of microporous membranes for well over 75 yr *(2)*. The use of

From: *Forensic Science and Medicine: Drugs of Abuse: Body Fluid Testing*
Edited by R. C. Wong and H. Y. Tse © Humana Press Inc., Totowa, NJ

nitrocellulose membranes as a substrate for the formation of biochemical complexes has been commonplace in biochemical applications since the 1970s with the publication of techniques for Southern blotting *(3)*, Northern blotting *(4)*, and Western blotting *(5)*. In the 1980s, the principles of immunodetection were applied in such a way that an immunochemical reaction on the surface of a nitrocellulose membrane could be used as a rapid technique for the detection of an analyte in a liquid sample *(6–8)*. This led to development of a host of convenient and inexpensive on-site or point-of-collection testing (POCT) devices, including testing of drugs of abuse. The immunochemical principles used in a lateral-flow format are similar to those used in other immunoassays. Many tests on the market today require only a single step: application of a liquid sample to the assay device. Their simplicity, however, is sometimes offset by the limited sample volume accommodated within the strip.

Lateral-flow membranes comprise a subset of the nitrocellulose membranes that are currently available. This chapter is intended to provide an assay developer with an understanding of the properties of these membranes and their use in lateral-flow assays. It should be kept in mind that the membrane is but a single material in a lateral-flow test. The integration of the membrane with the other materials and chemistries and the application of appropriate manufacturing techniques are essential to making a functional test *(9,10)*.

The basic design of a lateral-flow test strip (Fig. 1) consists of four porous materials *(10)*. The sample pad usually contains buffering agents, salts, and surfactants that make the sample compatible with the assay. The conjugate pad contains a detector particle, such as a colloidal gold or latex. The membrane is striped with capture reagents that lead to the production of a visual signal through the formation of an immunocomplex. The absorbent pad, located at the distal end of the strip, serves as a sink for the sample as it migrates through the strip. Whereas the membrane is a microporous structure made from nitrocellulose, the pad materials are typically nonwoven materials made from glass fiber or cellulose. Contact points between these materials are included so that there is a continuous flow path from the sample pad to the end of the absorbent pad. During manufacturing (*see* Chapter 6), the materials are aligned on an adhesive card to hold them in place. The card is cut into individual strips and then placed into a plastic housing. The housing serves to isolate the sample pad as the point for sample application and also contains a viewing window to permit visualization of the test and control lines. The entire assembly is stored under desiccation.

When a sample is applied to the sample port, it enters the sample pad, dissolving any soluble compounds. The sample then migrates into the conjugate pad, simultaneously solubilizing and mixing with the detector particles. The mixture then migrates through the membrane and into the absorbent pad. Once

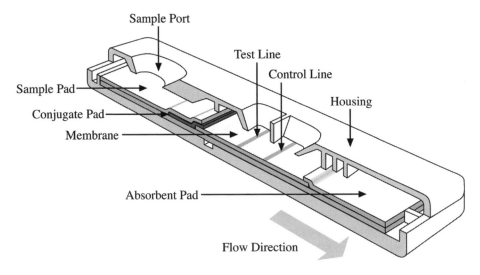

Fig. 1. Diagrammatic view of a lateral flow test (courtesy of Millipore Corporation).

the absorbent pad is saturated, the test will not accommodate any additional sample volume.

2. MANUFACTURING NITROCELLULOSE MEMBRANES

2.1. Nitrocellulose Polymer

Nitrocellulose is manufactured by treating refined cellulose with nitric acid *(1)*. This causes the substitution of hydroxyls on the glucose rings with nitro groups. In practice, the maximum nitration ratio is 2.3 substitutions per ring. Above this ratio, the polymer spontaneously decomposes. Whereas cellulose and cellulose acetate do not adsorb protein, nitrocellulose is highly adsorptive, making it a suitable polymer for membranes requiring immobilization of proteins *(2,10)*. Describing the characterization of nitrocellulose polymer is beyond the scope of this chapter. It should be pointed out that membrane manufacturers obtain nitrocellulose from companies that specialize in its manufacture.

2.2. Nitrocellulose Lacquers

The first step in producing membranes is the preparation of a lacquer *(2)*, which consists of nitrocellulose polymer dissolved in a mixture of solvents and nonsolvents. Nitrocellulose would be insoluble in the nonsolvents if they were included at a sufficiently high concentration. Nevertheless, they are necessary for the formation of a microporous structure and are included at a concentration low enough to ensure the solubility of the nitrocellulose. The mixture must also be chemically stable for the duration of a casting run, which can last several days.

2.3. Membrane Casting

In simple terms, casting a membrane is the controlled precipitation of nitrocellulose from the lacquer. Technologically, however, the equipment required to achieve uniform precipitation is complex (2), in part because the process must be continuous to achieve a high level of production efficiency. The first step in the casting process is the spreading of a thin, uniform layer of lacquer on a moving belt. The belt carries the lacquer into a series of chambers where air flow, temperature, and humidity are adjusted to control the evaporation rate of the solvents from the lacquer. As the solvents evaporate, the nitrocellulose strands migrate within the liquid phase, eventually reaching a concentration where they precipitate. The size of the pores within the structure is dictated by the evaporation rate, with more open structures achieved by reducing the evaporation rate. Overall, the casting process is slow, running at a rate of <2 linear ft/min. Because a single casting run may be hundreds of linear meters long, the casting equipment must be capable of maintaining constant conditions for several days.

Nitrocellulose is inherently hydrophobic (2,10), and membranes made solely from it would be incompatible with the aqueous systems used to apply reagents and run samples. For this reason, the casting process must include a technique for introducing a wetting agent into the membrane. This can be done through inclusion of the wetting agent in the lacquer or by application of the wetting agent to the membrane in a separate step. Regardless of the technique used, the final product must be uniformly wettable so that it allows even adsorption of reagent solutions and uniform lateral flow of samples.

2.4. Membrane Backing

Nitrocellulose membranes are inherently brittle and break easily under tension. Tensile strengths for lateral-flow membranes are usually <2 lb/in, making them very difficult to handle, especially in automated processes. To compensate for the weakness, the membrane can be cast directly onto a polyester film (10). This virtually eliminates all of the handling issues associated with breakage of the membrane, making it easier to manufacture and then process into test strips. The nitrocellulose adheres to the polyester without any additional components being added to the lacquer or the surface of the film. Another advantage of casting on a film is that the composite structure is much less flammable than the nitrocellulose alone.

Membranes are typically cast on polyester films that are either 2 mil or 4 mil thick. This is how the market has developed over the past 15 yr, as opposed to limiting membrane manufacturing. Also, most of the films that are used are either transparent or semi-transparent. The choice of a 2-mil or 4-mil backing is dictated primarily by the design of the test strip and the housing in which it will be placed. The internal compression points of the housing have to be matched to the thickness of the strip at all contact points so that the flow path is maintained without crushing any of the porous components. In theory, the thickness and opacity of the film can be modified as needed for a particular design. Custom-made membranes, however, may be significantly more expensive than standard products.

A disadvantage of backed membranes is that reagents can be applied to only one side of the membrane *(10)*. The air side of the membrane (the surface from which the solvents are evaporated during casting) may have structural inconsistencies that affect the consistency with which capture reagents are laid down and the uniformity of sample flow when the test is run. These inconsistencies arise during the casting process as a result of variation in the precipitation of nitrocellulose at the membrane's surface when compared with the bulk of nitrocellulose through the depth of the membrane. Many of these inconsistencies are visible macroscopically and can be culled by visually checking the surface quality and uniformity (discussed later). On an unbacked membrane, the belt side, which was in contact with the moving belt during casting, is free of these defects. Obviously, during the development process, a decision has to be made as to whether the handling difficulties of an unbacked membrane outweigh the advantage of surface uniformity. Most test manufacturers use backed membranes.

3. CHARACTERIZING NITROCELLULOSE MEMBRANES

The challenge in characterizing nitrocellulose membranes for lateral-flow tests is devising methods that are reflective of the way that they are used. Lateral-flow membranes have pore sizes ranging from 3 to 20 µm *(10,11)*. Below this range, the lateral flow rate is too slow to be practical in this format. Above this range, it is currently technologically impossible to make the membranes. Many of the traditional methods used to characterize membranes reflect their use for liquid filtration. Pore-size rating and flow time are two such methods. Although they work well, their relevance to lateral flow is limited because the pore structure is being assessed through the plane of the membrane. These parameters may have no relationship to how the membrane performs as it is used in a lateral flow format, where liquid movement is parallel to the plane of the membrane. They also cannot be measured on backed membranes. The most important characteristics of lateral-flow membranes are capillary flow time, thickness, and surface quality.

3.1. Capillary Flow Time

Arguably, the most important aspect of membrane performance in a lateral flow test is capillary flow time—the time required for a liquid sample to migrate through the pores in the lateral direction *(10)*. Capillary flow time is synonymous with wicking time *(2)*. The flow time affects the appearance of the lines when they are applied during strip manufacture and the sensitivity of the final test when the strip is run. Capillary flow time is expressed in terms of time per distance, with the length of the strip kept constant. (Millipore reports capillary flow time as s/4-cm distance *[10]*.) One end of the strip is placed in a liquid reservoir, and the time that it takes for the liquid to wet out the strip by capillary flow is measured. The flow front of the liquid should be uniform across the strip. Unevenness of the flow front indicates uneven wetting of the pores, which could arise from variation in wettability or pore structure. Many lateral-flow tests incorporate membrane strips that are 2 to 2.5 cm in length. Although lateral flow times can be measured on strips this short, the precision of the measurements is typically lower because of difficulties in handling small coupons. Longer strips are easier to handle, and the endpoint is easier to visualize.

Capillary flow times span a wide range. The fastest membranes have flow times of approx 60 s/4 cm; the slowest membranes have flow times of 240–300 s/4 cm *(10)*. The choice of flow time for a given assay depends on the requirements for sensitivity and specificity, the availability of the critical immunoreagents, and the required time to reach endpoint. Faster-flowing membranes reach endpoint more quickly but require more reagents and may lack the required sensitivity. Slower membranes can be used when reagents are in limited supply or costly, with the tradeoff that it will take longer to run the test.

3.2. Thickness

Membrane thickness is important for several reasons *(10)*. First, thickness, in combination with the porosity (the % air in a porous structure), allows prediction of how much liquid is necessary to fill the pore structure. Second, thickness variations can affect strip manufacture if the processing steps cannot accommodate the variation. Third, the thickness of the membrane has to be matched to the thickness of the other strip components and the housing to avoid overcompression in the assembled device. Thickness is straightforward to measure using gages that do not crush the membrane. If the membrane is unbacked, only the membrane is measured. If the membrane is cast onto a polyester film, however, the reported thickness is that of the composite structure. Variations can result from the membrane, the film, or both. Manufacturers have specifications on the thickness of the polyester film as a raw material; its thickness is normally more consistent than that of the membrane.

3.3. Surface Quality

Surface quality is a subjective assessment made by manufacturers on the basis of historical experience *(2,10)*. Because the uniformity of the membrane's structure is related to the consistency of solvent evaporation, variations in the process are frequently manifested as artifacts on the air side of the membrane. These artifacts have been described using nonscientific terms such as "stucco" and "orange peel," which, nevertheless, accurately describe the appearance of the membrane.

Ideally, the air side of the membrane is smooth. This ensures the highest probability of uniform deposition of the capture reagents on the membrane. When surface roughness occurs, the structures that contribute to the roughness can cause the reagent line to be irregular. They may alter the uniformity of liquid absorption as the line is applied or cause nonuniform adsorption of the capture reagent. Both problems are manifested in the final test strips as nonuniform signal lines when samples are run.

Another artifact that can affect test-strip performance is powder, which is comprised of small particles of nitrocellulose scattered across the surface of the membrane. These particles arise when a fraction of the nitrocellulose precipitates independently of the mass of nitrocellulose comprising the porous structure. Most nitrocellulose membranes have powder, although at a low level it does not significantly impact test-strip production. When there is a high level of powder, it can be dislodged from the membrane, causing a build-up of powder on production equipment. If capture reagents have been applied, they will be dislodged with the powder. Powder arising from a precipitation artifact should not be confused with powder comprising pieces of membrane that break away from the membrane edges. Cutting processes that are not optimized for nitrocellulose can cause significant edge damage, including breakaway of flecks of membrane.

4. PROTEIN-BINDING PROPERTIES

In relation to lateral flow tests, protein binding is often incorrectly equated with signal intensity at the test line. More appropriately, protein binding should be equated with the adsorption of protein-based capture reagents to the membrane *(2,10,11)*. Because the capture reagent is the first molecule in the immunocomplex, it must be adsorbed to the membrane irreversibly if the entire immunocomplex is to contribute to the signal. The capture reagent must also retain biological activity with the reactive sites available to the analyte.

4.1. Binding Capacity

Nitrocellulose has a high capacity for adsorbing protein (2,5,10–12). Initial attraction of a protein molecule to the polymer involves interaction between the dipoles of the nitro groups on the polymer and the carbonyl groups in peptide bonds. Adsorption is further enhanced by the interaction between the nitrocellulose and hydrophobic domains within the protein (11). The immunoglobulin (Ig)G binding capacity of lateral-flow membranes exceeds 100 $\mu g/cm^2$. Considering that a typical reagent line is 1 mm wide, there is approx 10 μg of binding capacity available per cm of line length. Because IgG is normally applied at a rate of 1–2 $\mu g/cm$, the binding capacity of the membrane is 5- to 10-fold greater than needed. The adsorption capacity for bovine serum albumin (BSA), which is commonly used as a carrier for drug conjugates, ranges from 60 to 80 $\mu g/cm^2$. These values are based on static adsorption assays where the surface is saturated with the protein (12).

4.2. Adsorption and Retention

Regardless of how much protein is applied to the membrane, it must be retained at the point of application to contribute to the signal. Although the capture reagent is localized at the point of application simply as a consequence of evaporation of the water, whether it remains in place when the sample is run depends on how tightly it is adsorbed to the nitrocellulose (10,11). The effectiveness of adsorption is in turn a function of the other solutes used in the reagent buffer and their interaction with the nitrocellulose and capture reagent. Chemistries used to preserve biological activity can be detrimental to adsorption. Surfactants, such as Tween-20, commonly used to prevent aggregation, interfere with adsorption by preventing the protein from coming into contact with the nitrocellulose at the molecular level (10,11). Also, water can interfere with adsorption when not completely evaporated after reagent application. Albumin conjugates may require more aggressive desiccation than antibodies.

4.3. Orientation

To participate in a binding reaction, the active sites of a capture reagent must be exposed to the sample stream. Relative to the initial adsorption event, this is impossible to control. Molecular orientation is essentially random. Nevertheless, a sufficiently large proportion of the applied molecules are oriented properly for biological recognition to take place.

4.4. Reactivity

Compared with aqueous-based immunoassays, lateral-flow tests require that the capture reagents remain biologically active after being desiccated on the nitrocellulose for months to years. Many capture reagents meet this criterion, but not without consideration of the chemistry of the buffers used to apply them *(10)*. In general, the reagent buffers should be kept as simple as possible: (1) buffer molarity <10 mM, (2) sodium chloride and other salts eliminated, (3) surfactants and detergents eliminated, and (4) other additives eliminated. Evaporation of the water used in the carrier buffer concentrates other solutes around and onto the capture reagent. The concentration of the buffer and other salts increases as a larger proportion of the water is evaporated, potentially denaturing proteins. The buffer and salts eventually crystallize and may mask the capture reagent. Larger crystals can also clog the pores of the membrane, retarding sample flow. In either case, the net effect is reduction of the ability of the capture reagent to participate in the immunoreaction. Thus, the reagent buffer should contain only those constituents necessary and sufficient to retain biological activity.

Although the application buffer should be kept as simple as possible, the lability of a particular reagent may require a more complex buffer for retaining biological activity or solubility during its preparation. In this case, factors that may compromise adsorption to the membrane must be considered, with the recognition that some reagents may not be usable in a lateral-flow format.

Relative to drug-of-abuse assays, reactivity can be problematic. Drug-of-abuse assays are modeled after competitive and inhibition assays, and often there is only a single antibody available. If the antibody is unreactive when adsorbed to the membrane, it will have to be conjugated to the detector particle. The drug conjugate then has to be used as the capture reagent on the membrane. Because a drug's structure is not subject to denaturation like a protein molecule, the carrier would only need to have sufficient mass to adsorb effectively and prevent steric hindrance by the nitrocellulose polymer. The reagent buffer will have to be tailored to the specific chemical properties of the drug conjugate.

5. THE CAPTURE REAGENT LINES

Capture reagents must be applied to the membrane as a distinct line so that the signal can be clearly read *(10,11)*. The concentration of the capture reagent in the application buffer and the dispensing rate determine the mass of capture reagent that is applied per unit of length. If the mass applied remains constant, then the width of the line will determine the intensity of a signal. Intuitively, spreading the same mass of capture reagent across a wider line makes the signal appear weaker. Whereas assessment of strong signals is not adversely affected by wider lines, a weak signal may be impossible to see because the color is too diffuse. In general, the lines should be as thin as possible.

5.1. Reagent Application Methods

The interaction between the dispensing mechanism and the membrane affects line width *(10)*. Dispensing mechanisms can be categorized as contact and noncontact. In contact systems, a flexible tip is placed in contact with the membrane. The reagent solution is dispensed through the tip as the membrane is pulled underneath or as the tip is dragged across the membrane; the engineering of the dispenser dictates whether the tip or the membrane moves. In either case, contact of the tip with the membrane introduces the opportunity to damage the surface of the membrane. If the downward pressure of the tip is too great, the tip will emboss a groove in the membrane. Although the groove may not affect distribution of the capture reagent, it introduces a discontinuity in the sample stream that can physically entrap detector particles when a sample is run. For systems using latex detector particles, grooves as shallow as a few microns can be problematic.

The other application mechanisms are categorized as noncontact and involve the dispensing of a liquid stream or aerosol onto the membrane. The initial width of the line is dictated by the diameter of the liquid stream or aerosol when it contacts the membrane. For liquid-dispensing systems, a gap height that is too large will cause breaks in the fluid stream that appear as gaps in the line on the membrane. If the gap is too small, there is a risk that the tip will scrape into the nitrocellulose. For aerosol dispensers, the tip normally is too high to come into contact with the membrane. The major consideration for the gap height is how high the tip should be, because the aerosol spreads out as it moves farther from the tip.

Regardless of the type of dispenser used, variation in material thickness must be taken into account. Engineering of the dispensing equipment allows the gap between the dispenser tip and platform to be fixed (Fig. 2). The thickness of the materials between the tip and platform, however, can vary. Mounting a backed membrane on an adhesive card results in a composite of up to four layers: membrane, polyester film, adhesive, and plastic card. Variation in one or more of these layers will affect the consistency of the final gap height between the membrane and tip. Additional variation will arise if the materials are not laminated together smoothly or if the plastic card does not lie flat on the platform. If at all possible, thickness specifications (means and ranges) should be obtained for all of the materials, especially when changing vendors.

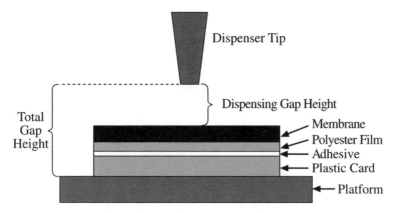

Fig. 2. Configuration of a noncontact dispensing mechanism.

5.2. Effect of Capillary Flow Time

The capillary flow time of the membrane affects the appearance of the lines by its impact on the rate with which the liquid spreads when the capture reagent solution is dispensed onto the membrane *(10)*. When the liquid stream contacts the membrane, it moves both into the depth of the membrane and laterally. As the flow time of the membrane decreases (i.e., flow rate increases), the lateral spread of the liquid increases. Depending on the rate with which the capture reagent adsorbs to the nitrocellulose, this can cause the applied reagent to also spread into a wider line. To overcome this problem, the reagent can be dispensed at a higher concentration in a lower volume to apply the same mass. If adsorption occurs at the point of the dispensing, the buffer may actually spread farther than the capture reagent.

5.3. Effect of Chemical Interactions

The width of the reagent lines is affected by the wettability of the membrane, which is a function of the chemistries in the membrane *(2,10,11)*. If the membrane is completely wettable, the reagent solution should be easily absorbed into the pore structure. If, however, the membrane is not completely wettable, the reagent solution can bead up on the surface of the membrane and be absorbed slowly or not at all. This causes irregularities in the appearance of the line.

Slow wettability can be caused by several factors *(10,11)*. The most significant is insufficient wetting agent in the membrane. In addition to the adverse effect on reagent dispensing, this is likely to affect the lateral-flow properties of the membrane when the test is run. Another cause of slow wettability is high surface tension of the reagent buffer. Buffers with high surface tension tend to be absorbed more slowly, especially if the amount of the wetting agent in the membrane is at the low end of its specified range. A third cause is static charge on the membrane. The charge repels the liquid stream in contact dispensers and can cause deflection of the droplets from an aerosol dispenser. In all cases, the line will not be uniform.

Beyond uniform absorption of the reagent line, chemical interactions affect the adsorption of the capture reagent to the membrane (discussed under Subheading 4). Ideally, the protein will adsorb to the nitrocellulose within the width of the dispensed liquid stream and have a uniform distribution from edge to edge *(10,11)*. Chemical conditions that reduce long-term adsorption usually prevent immediate adsorption at dispensing. When this occurs, the capture reagent will be carried laterally as the buffer is absorbed into the membrane, ultimately resulting in a more diffuse signal. Depending on the interactions among the capture reagent, the buffer chemistry, and the membrane chemistry, the capture reagent may be distributed irregularly *(11)*. Concentration of the capture reagent at the edges gives the line a bipartite appearance. Concentration at the edges coupled with a concentrated central zone produces a tripartite appearance. The edges of the line can also be highly irregular when adsorption is not optimized.

One of the confounding problems with poor line quality is that it is not normally detectable during the dispensing process. The capture reagents normally have no inherent color, and the width and quality of the liquid line are not predictive of capture-reagent distribution. During product development, irregularities in capture-reagent distribution can be detected by staining the membrane for protein *(10)*. In production, however, they usually are not seen until the completed test strips are subjected to quality-control testing. Because of the costs associated with manufacturing completed test strips, capture reagent striping can be useful as an incoming quality-control method.

6. SIGNAL DEVELOPMENT

6.1. Uniformity of Liquid Flow

When a test is developed, the signals at the test and control lines should have a uniform intensity across the width of the strip *(2,10,11)*. This requires that the liquid flow evenly through the membrane and that the detector particles be evenly distributed across the strip. Achievement of these goals is a function of liquid flow through the sample and conjugate pads and the consistency with which the sample is transferred onto the membrane. This is in turn related to the consistency of the materials used for the pads and the uniformity with which they are assembled into finished test strips. Uneven detector particle distribution causes uneven color development at the test and control lines. It is important to recognize that the membrane cannot correct flow and distribution problems arising in the pads.

6.2. Sensitivity

Sensitivity is a function of the position of the line on the membrane *(10)*. Because sample flow is unidirectional, the formation of the immunocomplex is a nonequilibrium reaction. Interaction of the detector particle with the capture reagent is related to the length of time that the two are sufficiently close at the molecular level. Once a detector particle has passed beyond the capture reagent, it no longer has the potential to contribute to a signal. Therefore, increasing the flow rate of the membrane increases the speed with which the detector particle passes the capture reagent, reducing the probability of an interaction and, consequently, the sensitivity.

Sensitivity is also affected by the change in flow rate as the sample moves along the membrane *(10)*. The flow rate decays exponentially as the liquid front moves through the membrane (Fig. 3). When the sample front reaches the capture reagent line, the overall rate at which the detector particles pass is dictated by the flow profile distal to the test line, not by the faster flow profile between the conjugate pad and the test line. Placement of the line closer to the conjugate pad results in lower sensitivity because, in total, the detector particles move past the capture reagent more rapidly. This aspect of sensitivity presents a major challenge when a single test strip is being used to screen for several drugs of abuse. For each capture reagent line, the corresponding detector particles have a different flow rate profile, requiring that the concentration of each pair be optimized for its position on the membrane.

Also, variation in the release of the detector particle from the conjugate pad between test strips introduces variation into the sensitivity *(10)*. A test strip exhibiting rapid release of the detector particle will produce lower sensitivity because most of the particles pass the test line at a relatively fast rate. If release of the detector particles is delayed, they pass the test line at a slower rate, resulting in a greater probability of interaction with the capture reagent. Although this phenomenon can increase sensitivity, it can also cause false positives resulting from nonspecific interactions. For these reasons, it is important to design the strip so that detector particle release is consistent.

7. MEMBRANE BLOCKING

Blocking of the membrane is sometimes used to minimize nonspecific binding of the analyte and detector particle or to improve the flow properties of the membrane *(10,11)*. Blocking agents used in other immunoassays can be

A   Reduced Sensitivity

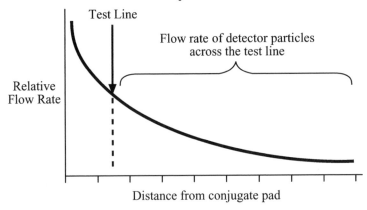

B   Increased Sensitivity

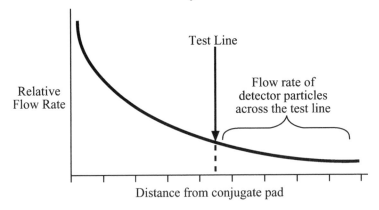

Fig. 3. Relationship between capture line placement and sensitivity.

used successfully in lateral-flow tests, although for large-scale manufacturing an ample and consistent supply must be available. Also, application of the blocking agent represents an additional processing step in manufacturing. It is important that the blocking agent not be applied in excess, because any molecules not adsorbed to the nitrocellulose can dry down as crystals in the pores, reducing or blocking sample flow.

An excess of blocking agent can be avoided by titrating to the minimum amount required or by washing the membrane after blocking to remove any excess. Often, it is simpler to impregnate a blocking agent into the sample pad to be mobilized when the sample is applied to the test.

8. FINAL COMMENTS

Nitrocellulose membranes were the first membrane to be used commercially in lateral-flow tests and continue to be the overwhelming choice for new tests being brought to market. They can be manufactured with the appropriate combination of surface quality, lateral-flow consistency, and protein-binding capacity to be suitable for large-scale production. Through an understanding of the properties of nitrocellulose membranes, the product development process can be successfully optimized.

REFERENCES

1. Miles FD. Cellulose Nitrate. Interscience, New York, NY: 1955.
2. Beer HH, Jallerat E, Pflanz K, and Klewitz TM. Qualification of cellulose nitrate membranes for lateral-flow assays. IVD Technology 2002;8:35–42.
3. Southern EM. Detection of specific sequences among DNA fragments separated by gel electrophoresis. J Mol Biol 1975;98:503–517.
4. Goldberg DA. Isolation and partial characterization of the *Drosophila* alcohol dehydrogenase gene. Proc Natl Acad Sci USA 1980;77:5794–5799.
5. Towbin H, Staehelin T, and Gordon J. Electrophoretic transfer of proteins from polyacrylamide gels to nitrocellulose sheets—procedure and some applications. Proc Natl Acad Sci USA 1979;76:4350–5354.
6. Zuk R and Litman DJ. Immunochromatographic assay with support having bound "MIP" and second enzyme. US Patent 4,435,504 1984.
7. Campbell RL, Wagner D.B, and O'Connell JP. Solid phase assay with visual read-out. US Patent 4,703,017, 1987.
8. Rosenstein RW, and Bloomster TG. Solid phase assay employing capillary flow. US Patent 4,855,240. 1989.
9. Weiss A. Concurrent engineering for lateral-flow diagnostics. IVD Technology 1999;5:48–57.
10. Millipore Corporation. Rapid Lateral Flow Test Strips: Considerations for Product Development. Lit. No. TB500EN00. Bedford, MA: 2002.
11. Jones KD. Troubleshooting protein binding in nitrocellulose membranes. IVD Technology 1999;5:32–41.
12. Pitt AM. The nonspecific protein binding of polymeric microporous membranes. J Parenteral Sci Tech 1987;41:110–113.

Chapter 5

Antibody–Label Conjugates in Lateral-Flow Assays

Paul Christopher, Nikki Robinson, and Michael K. Shaw

SUMMARY

In addition to the dry parts of a lateral-flow assay, there are also the biological components that allow the visualization of the results. Because of the relatively small size of a drug-of-abuse molecule, a competitive immunoassay with an antibody molecule conjugated to a colloidal gold particle is used. Antibodies can be polyclonal or monoclonal. In all cases, the antibodies have to be purified before use. Gold colloids are formed by the reduction of gold tetrachloric acid through a "nucleation" process. The size and shape of the colloids depend on the type and amount of reducer used. An accurate and reproducible lateral-flow assay requires the use of high-quality gold conjugates. The most common size of colloidal gold particle used is 40 nm. Conjugation of colloidal gold particles and antibodies depends on the availability and accessibility of three amino acid residues—lysine, tryptophan, and cysteine. Once a high-quality antibody–gold conjugate is formed, it can be applied to the conjugate pad either by soaking or by spraying. The drying process that follows is essential. It is affected by temperature, humidity, air flow, and pad thickness. Typically, forced-air systems are employed in conjunction with elevated temperature in the drying process. Finally, the proper functioning of a lateral-flow assay also depends on other nonbiological components, such as surfactants, blocking reagents, and buffers.

From: *Forensic Science and Medicine: Drugs of Abuse: Body Fluid Testing*
Edited by R. C. Wong and H. Y. Tse © Humana Press Inc., Totowa, NJ

1. INTRODUCTION

Since the early 1980s, home-use pregnancy tests have played an important catalytic role in the applications of lateral-flow immunoassays in point-of-collection (POC) drugs-of-abuse (DOAs) testing. Today, the worldwide market demand for DOA testing devices is enormous, and the diverse application of these testing systems continues to increase. Such devices have the advantage of easy application as compared with instrumented devices, and the results are available immediately. A lateral-flow test strip typically consists of four parts: the sample pad, the conjugate pad, the nitrocellulose membrane, and the absorbent wick. The assembly and characteristics of these dry parts are discussed in other chapters (*see* Chapters 4 and 6). The proper functioning of the device, however, depends on the maintenance of the right conditions of the chemical buffers, the surfactants, and other molecules. Finally, there are also the biological components—the proteins and specific antibodies that allow visualization of the results. This chapter will describe the principles of this detection system and precautions to take in its preparation.

2. THE DETECTION SYSTEM IN LATERAL-FLOW ASSAYS

Most rapid tests consist of two antibodies—one labeled with a visual tag such as colloidal gold or colored latex, and one used as capture material immobilized on the nitrocellulose membrane. However, with DOA assays, the size of the drug molecule to be detected is relatively small, with perhaps only one immunogenic epitope. In this case, the luxury of a two-antibody detection system does not exist. Therefore, the most common type of rapid test is an inhibition assay. In this type of test, the colloidal gold-labeled antibody is used as the detector reagent, and a drug–carrier protein conjugate is used as the capture material. Whereas the antibody is incorporated into the conjugate pad and is free-flowing, the drug–carrier protein conjugate is immobilized on the nitrocellulose membrane in the form of a narrow line (*see* Chapter 4). In the absence of drug in a testing specimen, labeled antibodies freely migrate into the nitrocellulose membrane and form antibody–antigen complexes with the immobilized drug–protein conjugates, thereby forming a colored line visualized through the results window. In the presence of drug in the testing specimens, labeled antibodies in the conjugate pad readily recognize and bind to the in-flowing free drug molecules, rendering them saturated in their antigen binding site, and they are are thus unable to bind to the immobilized drug–carrier conjugate when the antibody–drug complexes reach the nitrocellulose membrane. This results in the absence of a colored line in the results window. Note that the appearance of a colored line in the results window correlates with a negative test and the absence of a colored line in the window indicates a positive drug test.

Competition assays where the drug–carrier molecule is conjugated to the label and the antibody is used as the capture agent are also feasible, but are not widely employed. This may be a result of the unlikely success of linking the drug–carrier complex to the label in such a way that the drug is always available to bind to the capture antibody. Any blockade of antibody–antigen binding will undoubtedly result in a lowering of the test sensitivity and possible false-negative results.

Drug detection assays often have different specifications for detection limits depending upon whether they are urine or saliva/sweat based. In addition, the drug metabolite to be detected may be different in each system. It is not necessarily the case that an assay developed for the detection of cannabis in urine, for example, will work satisfactorily with saliva or sweat. Therefore, one must carefully consider the specifications of the assay before progressing to the stage of selecting the biological materials. These types of tests rely on minimal batch variation to achieve the specified level of cut-off consistently. Small variation is inevitable because of the nature of the biological materials used; however, the manufacturer may minimize this variation by choosing quality raw materials.

2.1. The Antibody Component

By virtue of their high levels of specificity and binding affinities, antibodies are the ideal choice of agent for drug detection. Antibodies are produced by the immune system as weapons to eliminate invading pathogens (1). Antibodies to a specific DOA can be produced by immunizing animals with the selected DOA conjugated to a carrier protein. A carrier protein is necessary because small chemicals (DOAs) by themselves are usually not immunogenic enough (as a hapten) to elicit an antibody response (2–6). Common protein carriers for this purpose include bovine serum albumin (BSA) and keyhole limpet hemocyanin (KLH). However, this technique is not as simple as it sounds and is not for the amateur protein chemist. The type of linker used, the length of the linker used, the molar ratio of the drug to the carrier protein, and the type of carrier protein to be used are only some of the factors that must be carefully considered to achieve effective conjugation.

Once immunized, the host animal will then produce antibodies to areas of the whole complex antigen. It is likely that there will be antibodies to the drug, to areas formed by the drug and the carrier, and to the carrier. All of these antibodies in the antibody preparation will bind to the colloidal gold label and cause unwanted cross-reactions. This type of unwanted cross-reactivity is often observed in an inhibition assay as a failure to block a signal even when levels of free drug are taken above the normal working range. This does not always occur, but should be considered possible if cut-off is difficult to achieve. To circumvent this problem, the antibodies of unwanted specificity must be "absorbed out" by mixing the sera with the carrier protein and recovering the unbound antibodies. Alternatively, it is sensible to use one drug–carrier (e.g., KLH) to raise the antibody and to use a different drug–carrier (e.g., BSA) for the capture complex.

2.1.1. Polyclonal vs Monoclonal Antibodies

Antibodies can be produced polyclonally or monoclonally. Polyclonal antibodies are derived from blood sera of animals immunized with an antigen and, as the name implies, consist of a mixture of antibodies produced by different B-cell clones, each with a different specificity and binding affinity. Monoclonal antibodies, on the other hand, are derived by immortalization of a specific antibody-producing cell (a B-cell hybridoma) *(7,8)* such that its progeny produce antibodies of a single specificity. Production of monoclonal antibodies is not a trivial exercise. Laboratories not equipped to produce their own monoclonal antibodies are advised to subcontract the job to commercial sources. Polyclonal antibodies have the advantage of being simple to produce. Small animals such as mice and rats can be used to produce polyclonal antibodies for initial specificity testing. Larger animals such as rabbits, horses, and cows can yield large amounts of antisera. The fact that polyclonal antisera contain multiple antibody specificities may prove useful for some end users who have to detect drugs with related structures, e.g., methylenedioxyamphetamine (MDA) and methylenedioxymethamphetamine (MDMA). A monoclonal antibody, on the other hand, is specific for a single epiotpe. The screening and isolation of a monoclonal antibody-secreting cell line is labor intensive. In addition, monoclonal antibodies can be made only in rodents (mice, rats, and hamsters) because fusion partners (myeloma cells) *(7)* from large animals are presently not available. Once a monoclonal-secreting line is identified, antibodies are produced by growing the cell line and antibodies purified from culture supernatants. Large quantities of monoclonal antibodies can also be produced by injecting hybridoma cell lines into the peritoneal cavity of pristine-primed mice and collecting ascite fluids for further purification.

2.1.2. Purification of Antibodies

All antibodies, whether monoclonal or polyclonal, should be purified before use. Besides antibodies, sera and ascitic fluids *(7)* all contain extraneous blood proteins, which may interfere with antibody binding. Monoclonal antibodies grown in culture usually will have similar proteins derived from culture supplements such as fetal calf serum. Purification has the added benefit of concentrating the antibody preparation, which aids in the stability of the antibody protein.

Simple methods of antibody purification include DEAE or Sephadex column separation, or precipitation with a solution of saturated ammonium sulfate. In addition to immunoglobulins, the purified preparation will contain a mass of proteins. All of these proteins will compete for binding sites on the surface of the labeled gold colloid. Those with the greatest level of the three residues controlling protein binding to colloid—cysteine, tryptophan, and lysine—will conjugate most readily to the naked negatively charged colloid (discussed later), and these may not be the proteins required to drive the assay. This will result in a low degree of sensitivity of the detector reagent in the assay. More specific purification of antibodies can be achieved with protein A or protein G derivatives *(9–10)*. These bacterial cell-wall proteins have high binding affinity for the Fc region of immunoglobulins, making them the ligands of choice for antibody isolation. Protein A or protein G can be coupled to sepharose beads and antibody-containing preparations (sera, ascite fluids, culture supernatants) can be passed through a chromatographic column. Bound antibodies are then eluted with acidic buffers. Protein A and G can bind immunoglobulins from many animal species, including large animals commonly used for polyclonal antibody preparation (e.g., sheep, goat). It should be noted that protein A and protein G do not bind all immunoglobulin isotypes and subtypes equally. For example, protein A does not bind immunoglobulin G (IgG) or IgA subclasses efficiently. For these isotypes, protein G and protein L are appropriate choices, respectively. Furthermore, because the binding specificities of protein A and protein G are the Fc region of immunoglobulins, all immunoglobulins, irrespective of their antigen specificities, will be bound to the column and eluted with the DOA-specific antibodies. Monoclonal antibody culture supernatants, while containing the majority of specific antibodies, also contain fetal calf serum as a culture supplement. Naturally occurring calf immunoglobulins will co-purify with the DOA-specific antibodies and, as pointed out above, will bind to the gold colloid and lower the level of sensitivity of the DOA assay.

The highest degree of purity comes from affinity purification. In this case, the DOA of choice is coupled to a specific matrix. Antibody-containing preparations are passed over the drug-matrix column, which binds only those antibodies specific for the DOA. All other immunoglobulins and nonspecific proteins are washed through the column. The specific antibodies are then eluted by altering the salt or pH of the column buffer. Affinity purification may be costly in terms of time, money, and serum, but produces a quality conjugate, which should be considered as a key raw material for any assay.

2.2. The Labeling Component

In order to visualize the binding of specific antibodies to drug molecules in DOA testing, the antibody component is often conjugated (labeled) to a color medium. For this purpose, a number of particulate conjugates have been used, with varying degrees of success. Latex was among the earliest used. Latex particles offer high visibility (in a variety of colors), low cost, and ease of preparation and conjugation. Its natural tendency to aggregate after binding to the ligands makes latex the ideal choice in agglutination assays, but not in rapid tests, in which stability of the antibody conjugates for an extended period of time is essential. Other media for color detection such as enzyme-linked immunosorbent assays (ELISAs) are commonly incorporated into clinical test kits. These assays offer high sensitivity and visibility, but the requirement for multiple color-development steps makes this approach not suitable for rapid tests. Inert particulates such as gold, silver, and carbon have been used in many applications, and offer considerable advantages in rapid tests. All three are stable, low-cost conjugates that are easy to prepare in large scale. Colloidal gold probably offers the highest visibility, sensitivity, and reproducibility, and has thus become the most commonly used conjugate for rapid tests *(11)*.

2.2.1. Colloidal Gold Conjugates

Gold colloids are formed by the reduction of gold tetrachloric acid ($HAuCl_4$) through a nucleation process, in which central icosahedral gold nuclei of eleven atoms are first formed. Further reduction reaction causes the remaining gold atoms to bind to the nuclei to eventually form the colloid state *(12)*. Common reducing agents include sodium thiocyanate, sodium citrate, and sodium borohydride. The size and shape of the colloids depend on the type and amount of reducer used *(13)*. A larger amount of reducer will allow formation of a larger number of nuclei and hence a smaller size of the particles.

To make a high-quality and reproducible label, it is essential that a good-quality gold colloid and high-purity antibody be used *(12)*. Although it is considered easy to make a gold conjugate, it is not easy to manufacture a good gold conjugate with consistent reproducibility. To start with, the gold colloid should always be uniform in shape with an even distribution of single particles (as shown in Fig. 1). Poor-quality gold will contain particles with irregular morphologies. These particles will be prone to aggregation even before the addition of the detector reagent. In addition, irregular sizes and shapes will affect the amount of antibody that can be loaded onto each particle, and this will directly affect the performance of each batch of finished conjugate.

Once the ligand has been conjugated, the quality of the gold conjugate must be assessed before incorporation into the rapid-test assay. Usually, electron microscopy is employed as a quality-control measure. Figures 1 and 2 compare the appearance of a good-quality gold sample with that of a poor-quality gold sample. Note the size and shape of the particles. The presence of clusters in a gold conjugate is indicative of a poorly optimized product. With time, the frequency of these clusters and the number of particles per cluster

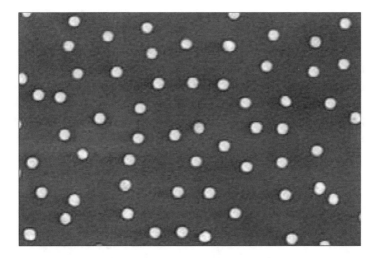

Fig. 1. Good quality gold particles. Note the regular size and shape of the particles.

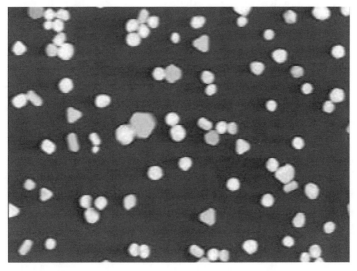

Fig. 2. Poor quality gold particles. Note the irregular shape and size distribution of the particles. Also notice the aggregation of particles.

can increase. In inhibition assays, this results in false negatives *(14)* and poor stability of the final product. Any excess antibody present will compete with labeled antibody for binding sites with the capture reagents, and this will lead to reduced sensitivity and potentially false-positives.

Gold particles can be produced that range in size from 5 to 100 nm in diameter. In a rapid test, the colloidal gold particle must be large enough to be seen. The most common size used is 40 nm. This size gives maximum visibility with the least steric hindrance in the case of IgG conjugation. Other sizes from 5 nm to 100 nm have been conjugated with success. However, 5-nm particles do not have the bright red color of the large-size particles and hence give only a very weak to no signal at the detection line, no matter how many particles are used. Only particles larger than 20 nm give a meaningful signal. On the other hand, 100-nm particles are too large compared with the antibody molecule. An IgG antibody has a molecular weight of 160 kDa and a length of approx 8 nm, of which only 4 nm extends out from the surface of the colloidal gold particle. This size differential creates steric hindrance and makes it difficult for the short surface antibody to interact with other molecules.

It is accepted that three amino acid residues play an important role in the conjugation of proteins to gold particles *(15)*. These are: lysine, which ishighly positively charged, and is attracted to the negatively charged gold particle; tryptophan, which binds through hydrophobic interactions; and cysteine, which forms the strongest attachments via dative bonds through the formation of sulfur bridges with the gold surface, such that the antibody and gold particles share electrons.

The success of the conjugation in terms of performance in the assay depends on the location of these amino acid residues in the protein to be conjugated. If they should be located in a region of the antibody near the antigen combining site (the Fab region) *(1)*, then the gold label can interfere with the binding capacity of the antibody. This is termed *steric hindrance*, and is almost impossible to overcome without compromising the integrity of the molecule supplied for conjugation. For optimal sensitivity of the assay, the three amino acids—lysine, tryptophan and cysteine—should be located in the Fc region (the constant portion) of the antibodies, and for antigens should be topologically isolated from the working reactive epitopes.

3. Application of Gold Conjugates to the Test Strip

After conjugation, the gold-labeled antibody will be dried down onto a pad. The method in which the gold is applied to the pad, the buffer it is supported in, and the method of drying will affect performance. The detector or conjugate reagent in a lateral-flow assay systems can be presented in a variety of ways—for example, as a ready to use liquid or as a lyophilized reagent that is reconstituted before use—but is predominantly incorporated as part of the dry assay strip. In use, the sample or a chase buffer in the system is typically used to reconstitute a dried conjugate reagent as part of the lateral-flow assay system. There are many ways that the drying of the conjugate reagent may be achieved; this is largely dependent on the scale of the manufacturing process, and ranges from simple hand application of the reagent with passive drying to semi- or fully automated application and forced drying.

3.1. Application of Conjugate Reagent to Pads

Conjugate reagent may be successfully applied to the pad in a number of ways, depending on the process scale and the degree of dosing control required. The required scale of the process will be directly linked to projected sales of the final product. The degree of dosing control required is related the robustness of the assay system, and tends to be more critical for semi-quantitative assay systems than for qualitative assays, in which conjugate reagent is typically used in excess.

Conjugate reagent can be soaked in sheet or band form in a manual soaking process. This typically involves simply soaking a sheet or a band of conjugate pad material in a defined volume of conjugate reagent under defined conditions. This results in a fully wetted conjugate sheet or band that must then be dried. This method is simple and cost-effective at small scale but may not be as reproducible as the alternatives below.

Conjugate may be soaked using a more automated process that the above, in which conjugate pad is in roll form and a reel-to-reel soaking method is used. This typically involves feeding the pad material from the roll to a collector via a soaking tank where the conjugate pad is immersed in the conjugate reagent. Conjugate reagent is absorbed into the pad material, which is then subject to an in-line drying process. This method does require some sophisticated equipment but is deemed to have the advantage of being more reproducible than a manual system.

Conjugate reagent may be applied using a spraying or dispensing technique. This is performed using a special-purpose dispensing system—for example, with equipment employing a positive-displacement syringe with air-spraying nozzle. Typically, the conjugate reagent is applied to the pad as the pad is moved under the dispense head. This application technique can be used as a semi-manual or semi-automated process. This method is considered to be capable of controlling the conjugate dose more effectively than soaking, but the performance of the process is dependent to a large extent on the physical properties of the conjugate pad material in terms of absorption capacity, wicking rate, and consistency both within and between lots of material.

3.2. Drying of Conjugate Pads

The drying process employed for the conjugate pads must be considered alongside the dosing method, as the two processes are inexorably linked. The aim of the drying process is not only to remove the moisture from the pads, but also to do this in a controlled way to ensure a stable, reproducible end product. A key requirement for the dried conjugate is that it can be readily and completely reconstituted following the drying process. The conjugate application medium and choice of pad material are important considerations for both the drying and release of conjugate. The drying process is simple in principle—i.e., the removal of water or moisture from the pad. In practice, this is affected by the normal factors that affect any drying process—temperature, humidity, air flow, and pad thickness. The consistency of the drying process under the selected conditions must be determined and process capability and validation performed to ensure that the drying process is capable of producing consistent product.

The drying process is easiest to perform at a defined temperature around ambient room temperature—e.g., 18–25°C—under a range of ambient humidities—e.g., 30–60% relative humidity (RH). The limitation of this technique is that the ambient conditions will vary, leading to potential variation in dried components.

Control of the temperature and humidity during the drying process is advantageous and will lead to a more stable process to yield a more consistent product. Raised temperature will lead to a more rapid and efficient drying process. Elevated temperature can be achieved using drying cabinets or drying rooms, or by the use of more localized drying tunnels or stacks where the component or product is passed through a series of heaters. Typically, forced air systems are employed in conjunction with elevated temperature in the drying process. The drying tunnels described above will normally be equipped with a fan arrangement to force heated air over the component as it passes through the dryer.

Control of the relative humidity during the drying process is also advantageous. Lowered humidity will lead to a more rapid and efficient drying process. Often, the combination of elevated temperature, use of forced air, and control of relative humidity will be used in the drying process.

There are other methods that can be successfully employed for drying. For example, freeze drying has the advantage of being rapid and in theory more consistent. Freeze drying, however, can be costly and difficult to scale up, and requires a detection reagent that is not damaged by the freezing process.

The storage of the components and/or final product can also contribute to the strip drying process. Typically, intermediate components and final product are stored in pouches with very low vapor transmission rates (e.g., aluminum foil with a desiccant material such as silica gel or molecular sieve). This storage method is designed to protect the dry strip from moisture that could affect performance, and is also conducive to the further drying of the strip.

The reproducibility of the drying process is likely to directly impact the reproducibility of the final assay device; therefore, the drying process conditions, including time, temperature, humidity, and air flow, are key parameters with which to achieve the required control over the process, thus ensuring that a stable and reproducible component is produced.

3.3. Non-Biological Assay Components

In addition to the biological components of the assay system, there are also a range of reagents that will directly impact on the performance of the assay system. These include surfactants, blocking reagents, and buffers, which are typically used to condition the system to achieve the desired functional performance.

3.3.1. Surfactants

Surfactants are routinely used in DOA assays and contribute to assay performance in a number of ways. Surfactants typically used include both anionic and cationic groups. The effects of surfactants on immunoassay systems include sample conditioning to aid antigen epitope presentation and effects on antigen–antibody binding characteristics, which are key aspects that affect the performance of the system in terms of detection limit and in terms of controlling the rate of false-positive and/or -negative results *(14)*.

Surfactants also play a key role in some of the physical aspects of the lateral-flow system. The flow of liquid through the system, the reconstitution of dried reagents, and the mixing of the assay reagents can all be affected by surfactant content. This in turn will affect the time to test result, the clarity of the test result, and other performance aspects. Additionally, depending on the choice of support membrane in the system (normally nitrocellulose), surfactant can be required to aid in membrane blocking. Typically, nonspecific binding of proteins or other components in the system to the membrane can be reduced or controlled by the use of surfactants, thereby avoiding or reducing potential false-positive or false-negative results.

4. FUTURE DIRECTIONS

Future advances in rapid test technology may increase the sensitivity limits of gold conjugates. At present, the limit of sensitivity in a visual assay, even with high-quality antibodies, is in the region of 1 ng/mL. However, the use of readers and, in the future, perhaps alternative labels such as magnetic particles and fluorescent quantum dots, may increase this further and lead to the development of quantitative or semi-quantitative assays.

5. CONCLUSIONS

Conjugation of proteins to colloidal gold is a process that should not be undertaken lightly. In DOA rapid tests, the sensitivity and reliability of the assay are generally determined by the quality of reagents used in its development. Colloidal gold labels and antibodies form the major detection components. Other physical factors, such as drying and use of surfactants, should also be carefully controlled. Future technologies should aim at improving the consistency and reproducibility of these assays.

REFERENCES

1. Corley RB. Antibodies, in Immunology, Infection and Immunity (Pier GB, Lyczak JB, and Wetzler LM, eds), ASM, Washington, DC: 2004; pp. 113–143.
2. Anacker RL, Finkelstein RA, Haskins WT, et al. Origin and properties of naturally occurring hapten from *Escherichia coli*. J Bacteriol 1964;88:1705–1720.
3. Korosteleva TA and Skachkov AP. Study of carcinogenic aromatic amines as haptens. Fed Proc Transl Suppl 1965;24(5):873–876.
4. Berrens L. A possible function of hapten-amino acid conjugates in the process of sensitization for simple chemical allergens. Dermatologica 1965;131(3):287–290.
5. Makela O. Assay of anti-hapten antibody with the aid of hapten-coupled bacteriophage. Immunolgy 1966;10(1): 81–86.
6. Dutton RW and Bullman HN. The significance of the protein carrier in the stimulation of DNA synthesis by hapten-protein conjugates in the secondary response. Immunology 1964;26:54–64.
7. de StGroth SF and Scheidegger D. Production of monoclonal antibodies: strategy and tactics. J Immunol Methods 1980;35:1–21.
8. Scharff MD, Roberts S, and Thammana P. Hybridomas as a source of antibodies. Hosp Pract 1981;16(1):61–66.
9. Elisson M, Andersson R, Osllson A, Wigzell H, and Uhlen M. Differential IgG-binding characteristics of staphylococcal protein A, streptococcal protein G and a chimeric protein AG. J Immunol 1989;142:575–581.
10. Akerstrom B, Brodin T, Reis K, and Bjorck L. Protein G: a powerful tool for binding and detection of monoclonal and polyclonal antibodies. J Immunol 1985;135(4):2589–2592.
11. Chandler J, Gurmin T, and Robinson N. The place of gold in rapid tests. IVD Technologies 2000; March:37–49.
12. Chaudhuri B and Raychaudhuri S. Manufacturing high-quality gold sol. IVD Technologies 2001;March:46.
13. Frens G. Controlled nucleation for the regulation of particle size in monodisperse gold solutions. Nature 1973;20:241.
14. Chandler J, Robinson N, and Whiting K. Handling false signals in gold-based rapid tests. IVD Technologies 2001;March: 34–45.
15. Robinson N. Immunogold conjugation for IVD applications. IVD Technologies 2002;March:33.

Chapter 6

Lateral-Flow Assays
Assembly and Automation

David Carlberg

SUMMARY

This chapter discusses materials selection, product design and tolerancing, and automated manufacturing processes to help in the efficient and cost-effective design and manufacture of lateral-flow assays. Raw materials including filter materials, membranes, and adhesives are discussed. A detailed discussion on properly dimensioning and tolerancing a typical lateral-flow laminate is provided. Several illustrations are provided to help in the understanding of proper dimensioning practices and to illustrate potentially problematic housing designs. The chapter concludes with six automation imperatives—six ideas that will help to ensure the successful and cost-effective implementation of automated manufacturing processes for the high-volume manufacturing environment.

1. INTRODUCTION

The development of lateral-flow assays has provided a convenient and inexpensive means for identification of target substances in biological specimens. The market for lateral-flow assays is enormous and growing. These test strips and devices have found numerous applications in testing of drugs of abuse, infectious diseases, and pregnancy, just to name a few. New tests and applications are being developed virtually on a daily basis. A test strip typically consists of a plastic backing holding together a sample pad for deposition of sample fluids, a conjugate pad pretreated with sample detection particles (*see* Chapter 5), a microporous membrane (*see* Chapter 4) containing sample

From: *Forensic Science and Medicine: Drugs of Abuse: Body Fluid Testing*
Edited by R. C. Wong and H. Y. Tse © Humana Press Inc., Totowa, NJ

capturing reagents, and an absorbent pad at the distal end serving to collect excess fluids. The enormous demand for such testing devices necessitates a good understanding of the tenets of manufacturing and automation. This chapter provides a comprehensive discussion on many of these issues.

It is understandably important, during the development stage of a product's evolution, to evaluate and carefully consider all aspects of its manufacture. These include scalability, the efficient transition from lab scale to clinical and limited-manufacturing scale to fully automated commercial-scale manufacturing. Each material, each procedure, each process must be compared and contrasted to ensure that the end product is functional, reliable, and rugged. In the extremely competitive marketplace of lateral-flow assays, it is a virtual certainty that automated manufacturing processes will be a necessity and not a luxury. With automation comes improved efficiencies, lower scrap rates, higher yields, and lower manufacturing costs. Automation also provides opportunities for automated inspections, thus greatly improving overall quality of the finished product.

In planning for automation, one may want to consider consulting with one or more quality automation equipment suppliers early in the development phase. Most reputable automation companies are willing to discuss design and development issues relating to product or process at little or no cost. It is best when considering automation vendors to find ones with knowledge and experience specific to the application. Test-strip manufacturing is not as simple as it appears on the surface; failure to select a company with specific experience may be costly or even disastrous in the long run.

2. DESIGNING FOR AUTOMATION

Good product design includes a number of factors, such as materials selection, component tolerances, manufacturing process tolerances, and designs that allow efficient manufacture through automated processes. Failure to recognize the importance and interrelationship of these elements could spell the failure of new product development activities.

2.1. Materials Selection

It is not our intent to discuss materials selection as it relates to product function, but rather to discuss manufacturing issues related to these materials. As described previously, lateral-flow assays are generally a combination of filter materials and membranes supported by a plastic backing, all of which are held together by a layer of pressure-sensitive adhesive. These materials are generally selected for their functionality within the test matrix, i.e., filter characteristics, flow rates, and so on. However, when there is a choice between two or more materials, each of which suits these primary product design criteria, then the secondary material selection criteria should be on manufacturing efficiency and the elimination of potential manufacturing problems.

A good example of this is in the selection of the membrane material. Although a large variety of membrane materials are available, nitrocellulose remains the most widely used membrane for lateral-flow assays (*see* Chapter 4). Nitrocellulose membranes provide a variety of flow-rate options depending on test requirements. The membrane is provided in two different configurations, supported and unsupported (backed and unbacked). Unsupported nitrocellulose is very fragile. It breaks quite easily and is very difficult to guide in reel-to-reel applications, making it extremely difficult to process on automated manufacturing equipment. Additionally, unsupported nitrocellulose typically comes from the manufacturer with an interleaf paper that separates the layers of the roll and must be removed and discarded. This adds complexity and cost to the manufacturing process. Supported nitrocellulose membrane, on the other hand, is cast directly onto a polyester backing web. This gives the membrane structural support and integrity and provides for much more efficient processing, making it the ideal choice for use in lateral-flow assays.

The filters used for sample pads, conjugate pads, and absorbent pads come in a variety of materials. Sample and absorbent pads are usually paper-based products. Conjugate pads may also be paper based, but glass fiber or polypropylene materials are also common. As mentioned previously, it is important to determine first what material performs best within the test-strip matrix. But when optimizing design, the limitations of each material should be carefully evaluated and compared for maximum efficiency on automated equipment. Paper products generally have low tensile properties, especially when wet. This can result in handling problems, especially in web-coating or laminating processes. Glass fiber materials can be difficult to slit or cut and cause significant wear on cutting blades and shears. In addition, nonwoven glass fiber materials generally have poor tensile properties and can be difficult to process on web systems.

The backing material used in the majority of test strips is generally polyvinyl chloride (PVC), polystyrene, or polyester with a pressure-sensitive adhesive layer on one side. The pressure-sensitive adhesive typically includes a release liner that is removed prior to laminating the filter and membrane materials onto it. There are two major considerations when selecting the backing material for the strip—material thickness and adhesive. The backing material should be thick enough to provide structure and support to the strip but should not be so thick as to create cutting problems. Generally speaking, the backing material should be slightly thicker if the strip will not be assembled into a plastic housing, allowing the free strip to have a feeling of quality and integrity. A typical backing material for a free strip might be 0.015 to 0.020 in (0.4 to 0.5 mm) thick. A strip that will be assembled into a plastic housing would have a backing material in the range of 0.008 to 0.015 in (0.2 to 0.4 mm). This thickness should be considered carefully and discussed with a reputable provider of cutting equipment to ensure that the combined thickness and toughness of the strip does not create problems when attempting to cut the material into individual test strips. It should be noted that thicker backing materials tend to result in higher cutting forces, causing undesirable marks along the edges of the strips or improper fluid flow when the test strip is used. Another potential hazard is that the forces required to cut it can actually damage the cutting equipment. This is especially true if rotary shearing processes are used to cut the strips.

Perhaps the most overlooked and most troublesome material in all of test-strip manufacturing is the adhesive itself. Adhesive can frequently build up on the surfaces of the equipment. Strips can stick to each other. Balls of adhesive can collect and interfere with efficient processing or even end up adhered to the strips in the final product. For this reason, it is very important to consider adhesives very carefully. It is generally best to use as little as possible, opting for minimal thickness and for adhesives that are the least aggressive but that are sufficient to hold the components together. There are a number of reputable manufacturers of pressure-sensitive adhesives who have extensive knowledge and experience with lateral-flow assays. It is advisable to evaluate alternatives at length and to test them in actual use. Reliable adhesives should hold the strip components together and not tend to ooze out and create sticky strip edges when they are cut.

One final concern regarding material selection is that of material availability. It is best to not become sole-sourced to one supplier. It is disastrous if a test-strip product is in full-scale manufacture and the supplier of one of the components suddenly discontinues the material.

2.2. Test-Strip Design and Tolerancing

Once a test-strip matrix has been established, it is then necessary to optimize it and develop the requisite protocols for its efficient and cost-effective manufacture. This discussion will focus only on the mechanical design of the test strip and not on the chemistry or the mechanics of the test itself.

It is necessary to first understand the manufacturing process as it relates to materials and tolerances. Each component of the test, including membrane, backing substrate, and each of the pad materials, has a defined dimension and an associated dimensional tolerance. For example, assume a membrane with a nominal width of 25 mm. The membrane has a manufacturing tolerance associated with it. Depending on the process utilized to produce the membrane, this tolerance could be as low as ±0.10 mm to as much as ±1.00 mm. In the former case this means that the material can be between 24.90 mm and 25.10 mm wide and still be within its specified tolerance range. In the latter case, the material can have an allowable width between 24.00 mm and 26.00 mm. There is a big difference between these two sets of dimensions.

The lamination process for test strips involves the layering of the materials in such a way as to produce defined interfaces between components. It may be necessary that the conjugate pad overlap the nitrocellulose membrane, for example, by a defined amount of 1 mm. Depending on the tolerances of the materials and the means by which they are laid down in the lamination process, this overlap could, in fact, end up as a gap.

Tolerances play an important role in the function of the end product, and it is critical that their role be well understood. If material tolerances are specified too tightly, then material costs will be high. If process tolerances are specified too tightly, then yields will be low and manufacturing equipment costs will be high. If material and process tolerances are specified too loosely, then the product may not function as desired. It is important, therefore, to strike a balance in the specifications of both the material and process tolerances. It is also important, in the process, to discuss tolerances with materials suppliers and determine what tolerances can be held and the costs associated with those tolerances. There are trade-offs associated with these decisions. Tighter material tolerances generally allow somewhat looser manufacturing tolerances. Looser manufacturing tolerances allow higher yields, lower equipment costs, and lower product costs. It is probably safe to say that most tolerances for web materials will fall in the range of ±0.1 mm if they are produced from hard tooling, to ±0.25 mm to as much as ±1.00 mm if from adjustable tooling. It is usually best to hold material tolerances as tight as is practical and cost effective, as this will allow higher yields from the lamination process.

As mentioned previously, the lamination process will provide defined overlaps of the materials generating a flow path for the test fluid. In defining the dimensional and tolerance requirements for this process, it is critical to understand that all of the dimensioning and tolerancing must be established from a single reference or datum edge. This reference datum is typically one edge of the backing substrate. Regardless of whether the product is being laminated in a continuous web process or in discrete sheets, one edge of the substrate material should always be considered the datum reference point. Lamination dimensions should not be defined between the different layers of

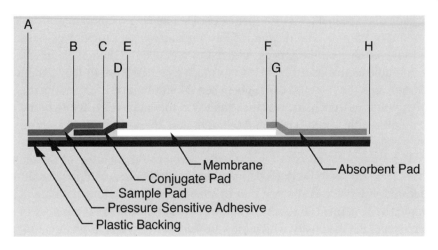

Fig. 1. Side view of test-strip construction.

the laminate; they should be defined from the reference edge of the substrate. As illustrated in Fig. 1, the left end (position A) would be considered the datum edge, or datum 0.

2.2.1. Understanding Dimensioning and Tolerancing

Every material has dimensional tolerances. Every process has dimensional tolerances. It is important to understand these tolerances and their interrelationship. A thorough understanding of dimensioning and tolerancing will help avoid some very common pitfalls in the design of lateral-flow assays.

Referring to Fig. 1, the following assumptions are made regarding the materials:

Material	Dimension	Tolerance	Dimensional range
Sample pad	12 mm	± 0.25 mm	11.75 mm to 12.25 mm
Conjugate pad	8 mm	± 0.25 mm	7.75 mm to 8.25 mm
Membrane	25 mm	± 0.25 mm	24.75 mm to 25.25 mm
Absorbent pad	12 mm	± 0.25 mm	11.75 mm to 12.25 mm
Plastic backing	49 mm	± 0.25 mm	48.75 mm to 49.25 mm

It is further assumed that the equipment accuracy for the placement of each of the materials is ±0.25 mm. This is the process tolerance. In this example, A is considered the 0 reference point, or "0 datum." This is the edge of the plastic backing material. Because this is the primary element in the assembly of the laminate, it must always be the starting point for dimensioning the locations of the other materials.

In most typical lateral-flow assays, the sample pad is intended to be coincident with the edge of the plastic backing material. This means that its left edge would be coincident with datum 0. Because this has a process tolerance of ±0.25 mm, the left edge of the sample pad is truly at a position from –0.25 mm to +0.25 mm. Its right edge (C) is at a nominal dimension of 12 mm ± 0.25 mm. However, considering that the left edge is at 0 ± 0.25 mm, C therefore is actually at 12 mm ± 0.50 mm (the sum of the two ±0.25 mm tolerances).

In the next step, the specified overlap of the sample pad over the conjugate pad (B – C) is defined to be 6 mm ± 0.25 mm. This is not possible because position C is only accurate to within ±0.50 mm, and because the accuracy of the equipment to place the edge of the material is only ±0.25 mm, the overlap can only be within ±0.75 mm if the conjugate pad is placed with respect to its left edge (B). The overlap tolerance would be ±1.0 mm if the equipment were referencing the right edge (E) of the conjugate pad because its material tolerance (±0.25 mm) must also be taken into consideration.

Next, if a 1-mm overlap of the conjugate pad onto the membrane is desired, depending on the edge from which the previous two materials are referenced as they are laminated, the location of E is known only to within ±0.75 or ±1.0 mm. If the edge (D) of the membrane is used for registration (tolerance of ±0.25 mm), then its location is within ±1.0 or 1.25 mm of nominal. This means that there could be as much as 2.25 mm overlap (1 mm defined dimension plus 1.25 mm total positional tolerance), or there could actually be a 0.25 mm gap between materials (1 mm defined overlap dimension minus 1.25 mm tolerance).

Obviously, the sample pad, the conjugate pad, and the membrane are not laminated in the order described above, as the membrane must be placed first so that the other materials can be made to overlap. But this illustrates the close attention to the tolerances required when dimensioning the product.

The proper way to dimension the lamination is to first determine the most important relationship. Keep in mind that one edge of the plastic substrate material must always be the primary reference point (datum 0). If the most important relationship is a 1.0-mm overlap of the conjugate pad over the membrane, then relative to datum 0, the equipment must register the edges of the material that define this dimension—D for the membrane and E for the conjugate pad. One can then determine the dimensional relationships of the other materials accordingly, making sure to reference each of the other dimensions from the datum edge of the backing material. If the next most important relationship is the overlap of the absorbent over the membrane, then define the location of the absorbent (F) relative to datum 0 (A). The location of G can be determined only by adding the dimensions D plus its process tolerance (±0.25 mm) and the nominal width of the membrane (25 mm) plus its mater-

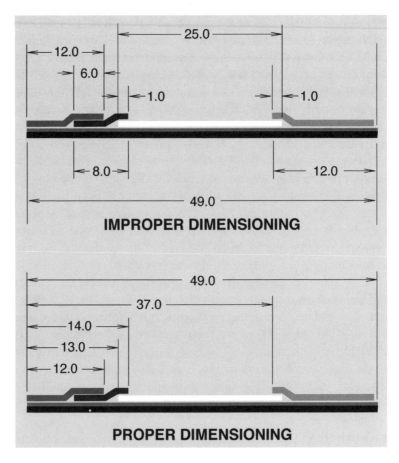

Fig. 2. Proper and improper dimensioning of the laminate.

ial tolerance (±0.25 mm). Refer to Fig. 2 for examples of proper and improper dimensioning of the laminate.

2.3. Housing Design

Often the design of the plastic housing is much too trivialized. It is frequently assumed that as long as the strip itself functions according to plan, the housing is just a package for the strip and it doesn't really matter much what it looks like or how it is designed. On the other extreme, Marketing may decide that the housing is the most important element of the product and what matters most is a fancy and unique shape. How the housing relates to the strip or the means by which it will be manufactured are often ignored.

The sizes and shapes of devices currently on the market vary widely. Rectangular, circular, square, oval, triangular, and freeform shapes are all commonplace. There are molded plastic housings, strips laminated between layers of plastic much like a credit card, fancy curved surfaces, and bright colors. It is important to realize that, in addition to simply enclosing the strip, the housing must support the strip properly to allow for proper fluid flow. The strip has to be accurately positioned endwise so that the test and control lines are clearly visible in the read window. The strip must also fit snugly within registration features so that it does not slide around during the assembly process and to ensure that its edges remain hidden under the sides of the read window. Proper housing design should also ensure that the layers of the lamination are pressed together just enough but not so tight as to create a restriction of fluid flow. Additionally, the housing must be designed so that it can be easily and efficiently assembled in an automated process.

In this discussion we will focus on the injection-molded plastic housing, the most common in the industry. In addition, we will focus on housing designs that allow for the simplest, lowest-cost automation processes. These housings are not particularly elegant or fancy; they are simple, symmetric rectangular elements.

To allow for the lowest possible assembly cost, the lower housing should be designed with straight parallel sides and a flat bottom. Figure 3 illustrates three different housing designs.

Housing B in this illustration is the simplest to automate because its sides are straight and parallel. Housings A and C are more difficult to align in automated assembly systems because their sides do not provide a simple, straight reference edge for accurately registering the part.

It is acceptable to have pockets or recesses in the under surface of the housing, as long as they do not prevent the housing from sitting flat. The design should include raised edges to help keep the housing stiff and prevent warpage or twisting. The lower housing should include a strip nest. The purpose of this nest is to properly align the strip in the housing in both the lengthwise and sidewise axes. This nest can be comprised of short sections of raised walls, small pins, or it can be a recess in the floor of the housing. A good rule of thumb is to have the height of the walls of the nest at least two-thirds of the maximum thickness of the strip. The strip should be a press fit in the nest with an interference of approx 0.003 to 0.008 in (0.075 to 0.20 mm). Lengthwise, the strip should have a clearance of approx 0.010 in (0.25 mm). The floor of the nest may require stepped elevations to properly present the surface of the membrane to the underside of the read window in the mating upper housing. The edges of the strip nest should be designed to be parallel to the outer edge of the housing. This allows for simple registration when placing the strip in the hous-

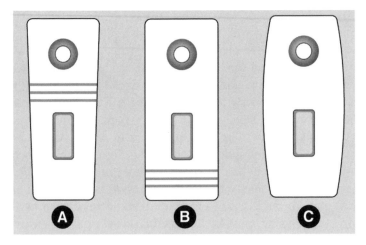

Fig. 3. Three types of housing design.

ing by automated processes. The lower housing should include at least six pins for securing the upper housing. These pins should be at least 0.040 in (1 mm) in diameter and should include a chamfer of approx 0.010 in × 45° (0.25 mm × 45°). The pins should be positioned asymmetrically to prevent the upper housing from being assembled backwards on the lower housing.

One element that is frequently overlooked in the design of the lower housings is a means by which to detect the orientation of the part when employing automated assembly processes. The upper housings are generally easy to orient, as they typically have openings through the part (sample well and read window) that can be easily identified with optical sensors; but the lower housings are usually relatively flat and symmetric parts. For this reason, the lower housings are generally much more difficult to orient automatically and at high speed. It is very important, therefore, to provide a defining feature. This feature must be prominent and it must be located in an asymmetric position on the housing. The feature should be located on the top surface of the part and it should include a height difference from the floor of the housing of at least 0.080 in (2 mm) so that it can be easily detected by an optical sensor even if the part has some warpage.

As discussed previously for the lower housing, the upper housing should also be rectangular. As for the lower housing, the upper housing should also include raised edges to help maintain flatness and provide some stiffness. The housing should be designed such that when placed on a flat surface with its open side down (the side that mates to the lower housing), it is stable and does not rock. As with the pins on the lower housing, the mating sockets on the upper housing should include a lead-in chamfer of approx 0.010 in × 45°

(0.25 mm × 45°). These chamfers on the pins and sockets will provide easier alignment of the housings during the assembly process. These pins and sockets are the main structures that hold the assembly together. The fit of the pins into the sockets must be worked out very carefully with the housing designer and the molder. If the fit is too tight, the pins will break during the assembly process. If they are too loose, the assembly will not be held together securely enough.

When dimensioning the plastic housings, one edge and one end of the housing should be chosen as the datum edge. This edge should be the same for both the lower and the upper housing (i.e., when the parts are assembled together, the datum edges should be at the same locations on both components).

One very important dimension on the plastic parts—one that it seems is quite often overlooked—is a flatness specification. When plastic parts are molded, they can twist and warp if the mold process is not controlled properly. Warped parts are difficult to process at high speeds in automatic equipment and can cause frequent and annoying machine jams. A reasonable flatness specification for molded housing components should be in the range of 0.03 inch (0.75 mm). This means that when the plastic part is laid on a flat surface, the part should not bow or rock by more than this amount.

3. AUTOMATED PROCESSES

Because the manufacture of lateral-flow assays is done in such significant volumes, many of the processes can and should be done automatically. With automaton comes higher quality, higher yields, lower scrap rates, and lower overall product costs. And, since the automated processes reduce the number of assembly personnel required, these processes generally require less manufacturing space.

There are a number of processes in the manufacture of lateral-flow assays for which automated processing equipment is available. These include dispensing of chemical reagents, lamination of the components that create the strips, the cutting of these laminated materials into strips, and the assembly and packaging of the devices.

3.1. Low- to Moderate-Volume Manufacturing

Most of the lab-scale instruments currently available in the industry are fully capable of producing test strips in a low- to moderate-volume manufacturing environment. When selecting instruments for this application, there are two primary factors to watch for: equipment quality and scalability.

As with most things in life, the quality and durability of the tools used to produce a product will more than pay for themselves over time. Quality equipment usually costs a little bit more initially, but the real cost of ownership is more dependent on how reliable and stable it is in extended use. Problematic equipment can cost more in repairs and lost production than the original cost of purchase. As product demand increases, so too will the demand on the machinery used to produce it. For this reason, it is very important to maintain a view toward scale-up in the early stages of product development.

3.1.1. Dispensing

Lab-scale to moderate-volume liquid reagent-dispensing instruments generally consist of a small bench-top module that secures the membrane in place and moves it beneath several precision dispense tips. An individual sheet of membrane is placed on a flat surface (platen) and secured by vacuum. Precision liquid-metering pumps are utilized to deliver a very precise and uniform volume per unit time of reagent to the individual dispense tips. Then, as the vacuum platen is moved uniformly beneath these dispense tips, fine lines are dispensed onto the surface of the membrane. Once a sheet of membrane has been successfully dispensed, it must be removed from the instrument and dried. This can generally be done by allowing it to sit for an extended period of time in ambient atmosphere. Alternatively, drying can be accelerated by placing each sheet in a heated drying chamber.

3.1.2. Lamination

Small-scale lamination systems provide a means to accurately place the various filters and membranes to create a laminated card containing a multitude of individual test strips. Commercially available card laminators are usually designed to secure pre-cut sections of the components on a vacuum platen. Each individual component must be manually positioned using precision guide features on the instrument. Once accurately positioned, each component is secured in place by vacuum and then assembled onto the exposed adhesive of the plastic backing material while maintaining its precision alignment. Such small-scale lamination systems are not particularly high throughput instruments, but they do serve to create accurate laminations so long as the operator is careful to accurately place each component relative to the guide surfaces provided.

3.1.3. Test-Strip Cutting

There are two different approaches to test-strip cutting—guillotine shear cutting and rotary slitting. Each process has distinct advantages and disadvantages relative to the other. Guillotine shear cutting has a distinct advantage over rotary in that it is highly flexible—strip widths can be changed at will. In a matter of seconds, a different strip width can be entered via a programming keypad. It is this flexibility that makes guillotine shear cutters such an important part of every development lab. One problem with guillotine cutters is that adhesive can build up very quickly on the cutting surfaces, causing significant problems and requiring frequent cleaning. Depending on the type and amount of adhesive present in the product, this problem can be quite severe and can be disastrous in a production environment. Another issue with guillotine cutters is that of blade sharpening. Because each strip produced comes from one blade action, there is a one-to-one correlation of blade cycles to test strips produced—millions of blade actions are required to produce millions of strips. The blade wears down over time, especially if the laminate being cut contains glass fibers or other tough or abrasive materials. As the blade wears, adhesive buildup problems become more acute, requiring more frequent cleaning. Ultimately, the blade must be removed and sharpened.

Rotary shear cutters mitigate the two primary issues with guillotine shears. However, this too comes at a cost. Rotary shears are inflexible—to change a strip width requires a change of tooling. Rotary cutters are dedicated to a specific strip width. As such, they are extremely accurate and repeatable, but they are designed to cut only one strip width. Rotary shears are designed to cut many strips at one time—as many as 50 strips. This means less adhesive buildup, because for one action of the shear, 50 strips are produced as opposed to only 1 from a guillotine. Additionally, the strips are not cut at the same place on the rotary shear blades each time. This means the adhesive buildup is even less. So, whereas in extreme cases (depending on adhesive) a guillotine blade may require cleaning after as few as 2500 to 5000 strips (10 to 20 min), a rotary shear module might require cleaning after 500,000 strips (8 h) or even more. On the other hand, the guillotine blade can be cleaned in a minute or two, whereas, the rotary cut module may require as much as 30 min or more to clean. The same goes for sharpening—the guillotine shear blade may require sharpening as frequently as every other month or so, whereas the rotary cut module may go a year or more between sharpenings. All this obviously depends upon usage and types of materials being cut.

Another significant advantage of rotary shear cutting is the tremendous output capability of the process. Assuming 50 strips per card and 20 cards per minute being processed, output is easily 1000 strips per minute. Compare this to guillotine cutting—the fastest guillotine cutter on the market cuts 360 strips per minute. Allowing for manual placement of cards and the trimming of the leading and trailing ends of each card, the net output is no better than about 250 strips per minute from a guillotine shear.

3.2. High-Volume Manufacturing

Once product demand has reached the point where high-volume manufacturing is required, it is time to consider highly engineered, sophisticated process equipment. In most cases, this will be custom-designed equipment developed specifically for the application. This of course comes at a significant cost, both in capital and time. As discussed earlier in this chapter, consideration should have been made in the early stages of product development to allow for the efficient scale-up to high-volume manufacturing. Now it is time to reap the rewards of that forward thinking.

3.2.1. Dispensing

Once done in discreet sheets, high-throughput dispensing should now be considered. This means a continuous reel-to-reel process. Due to the much lower labor content, the end result is a higher-quality product. In addition, any production process such as this should include real-time 100% in-process inspection to cull out any discontinuities or other anomalies in the dispensed lines. Such a process includes a computerized inspection system to continually analyze the product relative to a set of programmed line-quality parameters and a means by which the membrane is marked to identify these reject zones. Reel-to-reel dispensing systems generally include a means of mounting a roll of raw membrane, a region for dispensing the various reagents, a vision inspection and reject marking module, an inline dryer module, and a means for rewinding the dispensed web.

3.2.2. Laminating

Diagnostic laminations are usually too thick and stiff to be rewound into a roll after lamination. Such a process tends to crack or tear the components within the lamination. For this reason, we do not generally see reel-to-reel processes for lamination of lateral-flow tests. Instead, the process is from reel to card. Reel-to-card laminators provide a means of supporting individual rolls of each of the components of the laminate and guiding them each to a point where they are laminated onto the exposed adhesive of the plastic support web. A rewind spindle is used to take up the spent release liner from the support web. Best manufacturing practice suggests that a vision inspection system be employed to inspect the laminate as the process continues, ensuring that all of the components are properly positioned within their specified tolerance ranges. Any sections that fail the vision inspection should be marked with a permanent mark indicating that that section has been identified as reject.

Finally, the output of the lamination process is a shear module that cuts the laminated web into individual cards of a predetermined length.

3.3. Automated Device Assembly

The automated assembly of the product is probably the most cost effective of all the automated processes in producing a test-strip device. This process includes the coming together of all the raw materials, including dispensed and laminated cards, and upper and lower plastic housings. Undoubtedly the most labor-intensive component of the entire manual or low-volume test-strip manufacturing process is that of cutting the strips and assembling them into a plastic housing. If done by hand, this requires many assemblers and a large amount of manufacturing space in order to produce large quantities of strips. Yields are low because of all of the handling required. Product quality is dependent on visual inspection by the assemblers. Fatigue and inattention can lead to poor quality output.

The automated assembly line generally includes a means by which to supply the process with a continuous supply of pre-dispensed, pre-laminated cards. Upper and lower plastic housings are fed from bulk supply hoppers to vibratory or centrifugal feeder bowls where they are properly oriented and delivered to the assembly process. Since it is assumed that the equipment will be custom designed specific to the product and application, any detailed discussion of the equipment would be inconsequential. It is probably only important to suggest that any such automated assembly system should provide a means for rejecting sections of the raw materials that were identified as reject on upstream equipment, and that the process should include automated vision inspection points as deemed appropriate for the final product. The details of the implementation, the mechanisms for achieving each specific function, and the control architecture for the system are best left up to the designer and builder of the equipment.

4. Six Automation Imperatives

The following are six imperatives that, if fully understood and followed, will help ensure a positive outcome when undertaking any project for custom-built automated manufacturing equipment:

1. *Define the project.* This means writing a complete equipment and process specification outlining exactly what the equipment will be required to do, what the expected machine throughput should be, and so on. Also included within the project specification should be a complete definition of the materials to be processed, including drawings that clearly define all dimensional requirements and tolerances.

2. *Have realistic expectations.* Recognize that automated manufacturing systems are expensive and you get what you pay for. It is not necessarily best to go with the cheapest price. A cheap price often means poor or nonexistent after-delivery support. Recognize also that because this is custom-designed equipment, it will likely not be perfect upon installation—there may be problematic areas that need addressing over time. A well-qualified, reputable equipment supplier should be willing to work through these issues until they are fully resolved.

3. *Recognize the need for in-house support staff.* Sophisticated manufacturing systems will require dedicated in-house technical support. This includes well-trained equipment operators as well as service and maintenance technicians.

4. *Recognize the need for spare parts.* Parts wear out, sometimes even during shipment or initial startup of the equipment. It is important to obtain a list of recommended spare parts from the equipment supplier and if at all possible purchase the spare parts and have them available upon arrival of the equipment. This will save valuable time and help avoid potential problems during the equipment startup. It will also be very important long after the equipment is operational and in production.

5. *Choose equipment supplier carefully.* This means checking references. It means asking others knowledgeable in the industry about the supplier's reputation for providing robust equipment and after-installation support and service. It means checking into the financial stability of the company—it would be disastrous to have them go out of business in the middle of the project, or even afterwards when their service and support is critical. It also means having a good feeling about the people with whom you will be working.

6. *Stay involved throughout the project.* Do not expect to simply write a contract and then sit back and wait for the equipment to show up. Successful projects require attention. They require constant communication between customer and equipment supplier. Insist upon at least monthly progress reports. Maintain telephone or email communication, asking pertinent questions relating to schedule, technical issues, problems encountered, and corrective actions taken during the equipment development, assembly, and debug activities.

5. CONCLUSIONS

The introduction of the lateral-flow test strip revolutionized the way body fluids are tested. It opened vast new areas for testing, making it faster, easier, and cheaper to obtain results. Now we are seeing tremendous commoditization of test-strip products. Competition is driving prices ever lower. For these reasons, survival in the market will be dependent on (1) well-planned, well-designed products that incorporate simple, efficient design principles and (2) automated manufacturing processes that include appropriate in-process inspection to provide the highest-quality, lowest-cost product possible.

Chapter 7

Oral-Fluid Drug Testing Using the Intercept® Device

R. Sam Niedbala and Keith W. Kardos

SUMMARY

Numerous devices are becoming available for collection and testing of oral fluids. The Intercept® device (Orasure Technologies), along with its associated immunoassays, is one of the first to be approved for commercial sale in the United States. This chapter presents clinical and nonclinical information on the principles of operation and performance of the Intercept device. This chapter specifically reviews the physiology of the oral cavity as it relates to the use of the Intercept device to collect specimens for analysis. Once a sample is prepared for analysis, performance data for numerous assays are reviewed. This includes analytical performance of various aspects of Intercept immuoassays used, including cross-reactivity, precision, limits of detection, and effects of interferents. Finally, clinical field data are included demonstrating the use of the Intercept device from large population prevalence studies.

1. ORAL FLUID AS A MATRIX FOR DRUGS-OF-ABUSE TESTING

The results of substance abuse deeply affect individuals, families, and society at large. One solution has been to test individuals for the presence of drugs of abuse (DOA). Such tests may be administered to job applicants and parolees, as well as immediately after accidents and along the roadside by police.

Many countries have legislation in place or pending for drug testing. This legislation defines when, where, and how drug testing should be performed

From: *Forensic Science and Medicine: Drugs of Abuse: Body Fluid Testing*
Edited by R. C. Wong and H. Y. Tse © Humana Press Inc., Totowa, NJ

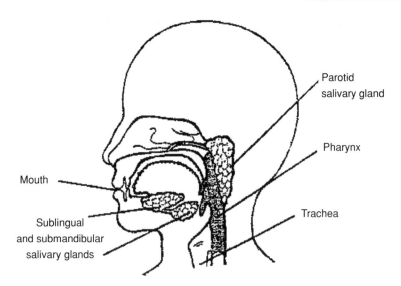

Fig. 1. Major glands of the mouth. Breakdown of materials contributed by various saliva glands: 65% submandibular, 23% parotid, 4% sublingual, and 8% minor glands.

(1–3). The first country to enact such legislation was the United States. This model allowed the use of urine as the primary testing matrix. Urine testing, however, has limitations, including the need for special facilities for collection and a witness to prevent the samples from being adulterated. Furthermore, urine testing does not reflect recent drug use, which therefore limits its value toward judging impairment.

With the advance of technology, newer, more sensitive analytical techniques have allowed the use of alternative body fluids such as saliva—or oral fluid—in DOA testing. "Oral fluid" has become the more common term for a sample collected from the mouth for diagnostic purposes *(1)*. It is the combination of fluids excreted by the glands of the mouth along with other debris.

The mouth is composed of many glands, the primary ones being the parotid and submandibular glands *(4–7)*. Figure 1 shows a diagram of the major glands of the mouth. The parotid ducts are located in the upper bucal cavity and produce fluids that are primarily low in viscosity. The submandibular glands are located in the lower bucal cavity and produce a mucous mixture. These fluids and their components have several purposes, including wetting of food matter to facilitate swallowing; infection control; maintenance of healthy teeth; and wetting of the oral mucosa. Given all of these functions, the mouth is a complex entry into the body with a diverse set of mechanisms. Therefore, as one considers DOA testing using oral fluids, one should consider these dynamics

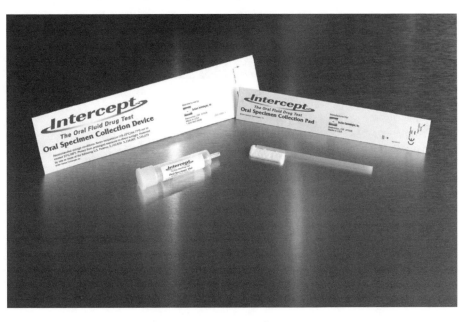

Fig. 2. The Intercept® device.

and anticipate them when collecting samples to be used for substance-abuse analysis.

2. METHOD OF COLLECTING AND TESTING USING THE INTERCEPT® DEVICE

This chapter is primarily focused on describing the use of a new method to collect and test oral fluids for drugs of abuse. The Intercept® device (Orasure Technologies) (Fig. 2) has been tested and used for a variety of abused drugs. The collection device consists of an absorbent cotton fiber pad impregnated with a salt and affixed to a nylon stick, and a preservation solution (0.8 mL) in a plastic container. The collection device pad is placed between the lower gum and cheek for 2–5 min. While resident in the oral cavity, the pad will absorb a passive sample of oral mucosal transudate (OMT). The OMT is composed of collected fluids resident in the oral cavity as well as a small amount of blood components drawn into the pad transmucosally. The result is an enriched sample that allows analysis of small molecules such as drugs or large proteins such as antibodies. With this device, an average of 0.4 mL of oral fluid is collected. The collection device pad is then placed in the preservative solution. The resulting total volume is approx 1.2 mL (0.4 mL specimen and 0.8 mL

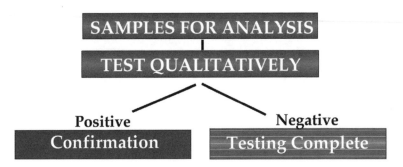

Fig. 3. Qualitative assay testing algorithm.

preservative solution). Consequently, the oral fluid specimen is diluted by a factor of 3. All testing is performed on the dilute specimen, and concentrations are reported based on the final diluted specimen.

3. SCREENING TESTS FOR INTERCEPT

Collected oral fluid specimens have routinely been analyzed using algorithms that are similar to those of urine testing. Figure 3 shows a diagram for the qualitative determination of drugs using the Intercept collector. After field collection, a sample is shipped to a primary testing laboratory using chain-of-custody procedures. An initial screen is completed using microtiter-based immunoassay for each target drug. An initial presumptive positive is then followed by confirmation testing using a combination of gas chromatography (GC) and mass spectrometry (MS) (GC-MS or GC-MS-MS). This same approach is currently used for urine testing by laboratories following US federal guidelines for performing DOA analysis. This algorithm is technically and legally defensible because initial screening tests that rely solely on immunoassay are subject to the varying levels of cross-reactivity of the antibodies used in such tests. The combination of an immunoassay that can broadly identify the potential presence of an abused substance followed by a highly specific and sensitive mass spectrometric confirmation technique provides assurance of correct identification of positive samples. Thus, the testing of oral fluids can mirror the existing algorithm for testing urine, providing a similar logic to ensure accuracy.

The following procedures are typical of a microplate-based enzyme immunoassay (EIA) using tetrahydrocannabinol (THC) as an example (Fig. 4). Briefly, 25 µL of specimen, calibrator, or control is added to each well of an anti-THC-coated plate (immobilized sheep anti-cannabinoids polyclonal antibody) followed by addition of 25 µL of buffer and incubation for 60 min at

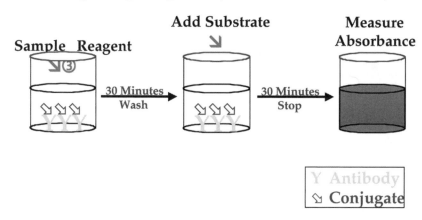

Fig. 4. Enzyme immunoassay.

room temperature (RT). After incubation, 50 µL of THC enzyme conjugate (horseradish peroxidase labeled with THC derivative) is added and the plate is incubated for an additional 30 min at RT. The plate is then washed six times with 0.3 mL of distilled water, followed by addition of 0.1 mL substrate reagent (tetramethylbenzidine) and incubation for 30 min at RT. After incubation, 0.1 mL of stopping reagent (2 N sulfuric acid) is added. Absorbance is measured at 450 nm and 630 nm within 15 min of stopping the reaction. The specific signal is measured at 450 nm while the 630 nm measurement is used to blank the sample. The final color signal developed is inversely proportional to the amount of drug present in a sample. Mean values of specimens are compared to the mean value of the calibrator (1 ng/mL, $N = 4$). Specimens with absorbance less than or equal to the calibrator were considered positive and specimens with responses greater than the calibrator were considered negative *(8–10)*.

EIA technologies are inexpensive and provide sufficient analytical sensitivity for routine analysis of oral fluid specimens. Future technological enhancements are expected to introduce new homogeneous immunoassay techniques that require no wash or separation steps, which will further simplify the screening process. Once such techniques are available, oral-fluid screening may be automated on large-scale analyzers.

4. CHARACTERISTICS OF SCREENING TESTS

Each of the microplate immunoassays has specific performance characteristics that are critical to the effectiveness of the overall Intercept system of collection and testing. Some of the most critical analytical parameters deserve more detailed discussions.

Table 1
Limit of Detection (LOD), Range of Calibrators,
and Cutoff for Each Intercept® Assay

Assay*	LOD (ng/mL)	Assay calibrator range (ng/mL)	Cutoff (ng/mL)
Amphetamine	25.5	0–200	100
Barbiturate	8.2	0–40	20
Methamphetamine	8.0	0–80	40
Cannabinoid (THC)	0.37	0–2.0	1.0
Benzodiazepine	0.2	0–2.0	1.0
Cocaine Metabolite	1.5	0–10	5.0
PCP	0.49	0–10	5.0
Methadone	0.50	0–10	5.0
Opiates	1.4	0–20	10

*Note: All values shown as calculated for Intercept and not whole oral fluids. Multiply the values by 3 to obtain whole oral fluid values.
TCH, tetrahydrocannabinol.

4.1. Analytical Sensitivity/Limit of Detection

The limit of detection (LOD) is defined from the signal-to-noise ratio at the zero-drug concentration as the mean zero absorbance (A_0) minus three times the noise level (LOD = A_0 – 3SD). The LOD was determined by obtaining the average absorbance value for 80 readings of blank oral-fluid diluent and calculating the standard deviation (SD) and three times the standard deviation (3SD) of the absorbance. The absorbance value minus 3SD was then extrapolated from the curve and represents the sensitivity of the assay. The LOD range of calibrations and cutoff for each Intercept assay are listed in Table 1. The assay cutoffs are separately determined through clinical testing. It is important to note the separation of the cutoffs used from the LOD. It would not be appropriate for a routine screening technique to use the LOD also as its cutoff, because other performance characteristics such as precision would most likely not be acceptable at the LOD.

4.2. Precision

The precision of the OraSure Technologies Inc. (OTI) Intercept Micro-Plate EIAs was assessed by testing oral-fluid diluent containing various concentrations of the target drug. The intra-assay precision was determined by analyzing each level 16 times per run for four runs. The inter-assay precision was determined by analyzing two samples at each level twice per day for 5–20 d, depending on the assay. The oral-fluid diluent used for these tests is carried in a phosphate buffer, which adjusts collected oral-fluid specimens to neutral pH. All tests were performed at room temperature. It should be noted that absolute absorbance values for microplates will be affected by room temperature; this should be considered when performing inter-assay or inter-day precision analysis. The results of this testing are shown in Table 2.

4.3. Cross-Reactivity

The cross-reactivity was determined for each assay for analogous and ubiquitous compounds. Analogous compounds that were cross-reactive in each of the Intercept assays are shown in Fig. 5. Cross-reactivity was determined by spiking various concentrations of each tested compound into the Intercept diluent fluid. A sample that showed a response was compared with each assay standard curve in order to calculate the percent cross-reactivity. For example, a test compound that showed equal immunoassay response to the cutoff concentration in a particular assay would be judged as showing 100% cross-reactivity. Some compounds shown have calculated cross reactivities that are very low. These values are included to show that extraordinarily large concentrations of such drugs would be required to elicit a response in the immunoassay. Thus, those performing a secondary confirmation by GC-MS-MS would not target confirming such compounds in presumptively positive clinical specimens.

4.4. Interferents

The effect of interfering substances or adulterants was examined in the Intercept Micro-Plate EIAs. Testing interferents by spiking them into buffer or some other artificial matrix is not relevant. Therefore, samples from volunteers were used after they consumed a potential interferent. In this experiment, five subjects consumed 1 oz of each adulterant, and oral-fluid samples were collected from each volunteer using the Intercept oral-fluid collection device after a 5-min and 10-min period following consumption. Samples were processed and pooled for each interferent and collection time. Aliquots from each sample pool were spiked with various concentrations of target drug and tested in the assay. The signals obtained for samples containing only the adulterants were used to assess any effects that may lead to false-positive results. The signals of samples containing drug in the presence of each adulterant were used to assess the overall effects of the adulterant. The substance was considered not to interfere if, after the 10-min waiting period, the samples containing 0 or the cutoff level of drug produced absorbance readings greater than the cutoff and if the samples containing 1.5 and 2.0 times the cutoff produced absorbance readings less than the cutoff. Data generated for an Intercept secobarbital assay are

Table 2
Precision of Intercept® Micro-Plate Enzyme Immunoassays

	Concentrations ng/mL	Intra-assay %CV ($n = 64$)	Inter-assay %CV ($n = 4/d$, 20 d)
Amphetamine	0	3.9	6.7
	50	3.5	6.7
	100	4.0	7.5
	150	4.5	7.7
	200	6.4	7.9
Secobarbital	0	4.1	8.5
	10	4.4	8.9
	20	3.8	8.9
	30	7.1	8.9
	40	4.9	9.4
Methamphetamine	0	7.8	7.5
	20	7.0	7.7
	40	6.2	7.9
	60	7.8	7.5
	80	6.4	8.4
Δ^9-THC	0	4.7	8.7
	0.5	4.5	9.3
	1.0	5.2	11.0
	1.5	5.5	11.6
	2.0	4.6	10.8
Nordiazepam	0	5.1	7.6
	0.5	6.1	10.4
	1.0	6.5	11.0
	1.5	4.9	11.4
Benzoylecgonine	0	3.7	8.0
	2.5	3.4	9.0
	5.0	4.3	9.6
	7.5	7.6	10.5
PCP	0	7.2	10.7*
	0.5	6.1	11.8*
	1	7.1	14.0*
	1.5	8.8	18.5*
Methadone	0	6.3	9.9
	2.5	6.6	12.3
	5.0	6.7	12.9
	7.5	6.8	13.6
Morphine	0	3.6**	7.5***
	5	6.4**	8.9***
	10	6.6**	9.5***
	20	6.9**	8.7***

* %CV ($n = 4/d$, 14 d).
** %CV ($n = 20$).
*** %CV ($n = 20/d$, 5 d).
THC, tetrahydrocannabinol; PCP, phencyclidine.

A

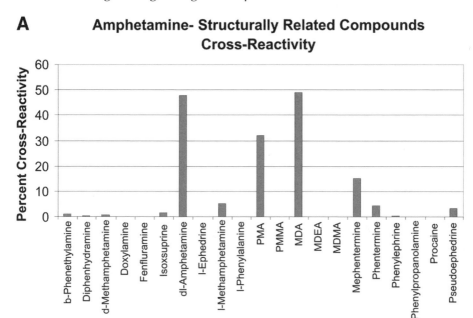

B

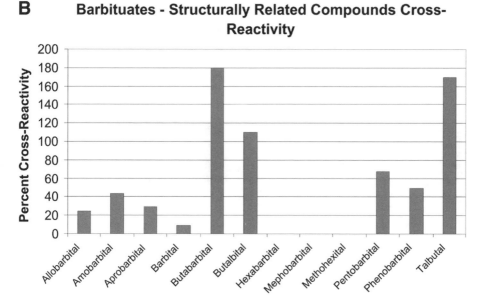

Fig. 5. Drugs-of-abuse cross-reactivity results for structurally related compounds tested using Intercept® immunoassays.

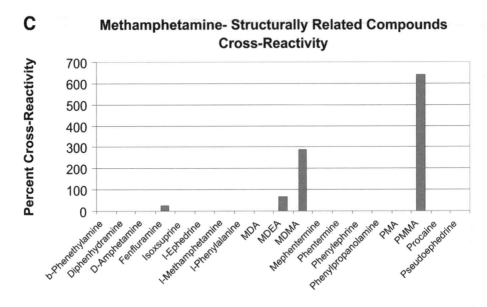

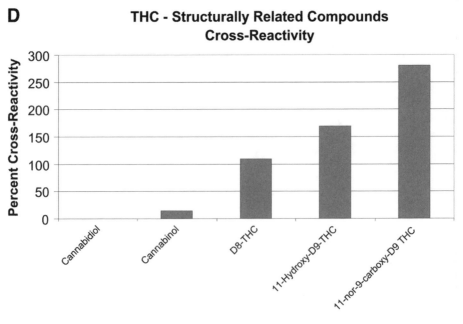

Fig. 5. *(continued)*

E

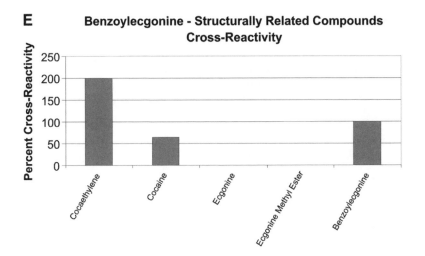

Benzoylecgonine - Structurally Related Compounds Cross-Reactivity

F

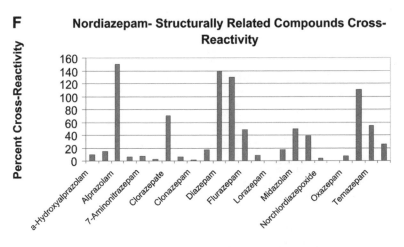

Nordiazepam- Structurally Related Compounds Cross-Reactivity

G

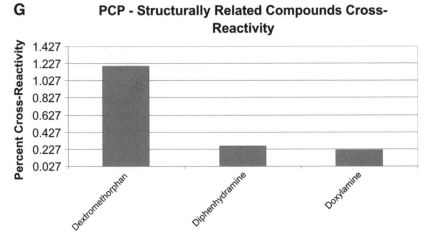

PCP - Structurally Related Compounds Cross-Reactivity

Table 3
Effects of Adulterants on Intercept® Enzyme Immunoassays

Substance	EIA Result at 10 min. (adulterant only)	EIA Result at 10 min. (adulterant + secobarbital)
Sugar	No effect	No effect
Toothpaste	No effect	No effect
Cranberry Juice	No effect	No effect
TUMS®	No effect	No effect
Orange Juice	No effect	False negative
Cola	No effect	No effect
Cough Syrup	No effect	False negative
Antiseptic	No effect	No effect
Water	No effect	No effect

shown in Table 3. The exact mechanism for some adulterants affecting the EIA assays is not known; but most likely this is an effect of pH. It should be noted that particular attention should be given to waiting 5–10 min prior to collection, which will remedy these effects.

5. INTERCEPT ORAL-FLUID SAMPLE GC-MS CONFIRMATION METHOD

In the algorithm used for Intercept, a presumptive positive specimen requires a GC-MS-MS analysis to assure true positivity. However, the levels to be determined require improved procedures compared with those commonly used for urine testing. Although numerous instruments are available that are capable of performing Intercept confirmations, the general steps and target ions would be the same. Therefore, this section presents a sample procedure used for the most difficult analyte, THC (8), followed by critical factors used to identify other typical DOA targets. Ultimately, each laboratory will validate its equipment and adopted procedures.

Quantitative analysis of THC in oral-fluid specimens can be performed by GC MS MS on a Finnegan TSQ 7000 Triple Stage Quadrupole (ThermoQuest, San Jose, CA) equipped with a 5% phenyl methyl silicone capillary column (15-m × 0.25-mm i.d.). The capillary inlet system can be operated in the split-less mode. Instrumental conditions were as follows: injection port, 275°C; GC temperature program, 100°C for 0.5 min, ramp 45°C/min to 235°C, hold 1.5 min, ramp 45°C/min to 310°C, and hold 1.5 min; transfer line, 250°C; source, 200°C; manifold, 90°C. A total of 200 μL of each oral-fluid specimen was used in the extraction procedure. Initially, internal standard (D3-THC) at a concentration of 0.5 ng/mL was added to each specimen, calibrator, and control sample. Each sample was treated with 2 mL of 0.2 *M* NaOH and 3 mL of hexane:ethyl acetate (9:1 v/v). The tubes were rocked for 30 min and then centrifuged. The upper organic layer was removed, acidified with 3 mL of 0.1 *M* HCl, and rocked an additional 15 min. Following centrifugation, the upper organic layer was removed and evaporated to dryness at 40°C. The residue was derivatized with 30 µL of bis(trimethylsilyl)-trifluoroacetamide (BSTFA) (1% trimethylchlorosilane [TMCS]) and 30 µL of ethyl acetate at 70°C for 30 min. A calibration standard of THC was prepared for each batch at 0.5 ng/mL concentration in artificial saliva (certified blank matrix). The following parent ions were selected for each compound to form product ions: THC, *m/z* 386 and D3-THC, *m/z* 389. The following product ions were selected for quantitation: THC, *m/z* 371 and D3-THC, *m/z* 374. For a specimen to be considered positive for THC, both the parent and product ions had to be present and within 2% of the retention time of the calibrator. In addition, the area of each ion had to be greater than the corresponding area of the ion in the calibration standard. The assay exhibited a between-run precision for THC in oral-fluid specimens of 4.3% at 0.25 ng/mL and 9.5% at 1 ng/mL. The assay limit of quantitation (LOQ)/LOD for THC was 0.2 ng/mL for a 0.2-mL extracted specimen.

Other compounds can be similarly analyzed. For reference, Table 4 lists the target analytes and their target ions that may be detected in oral fluids, and Table 5 shows typical LOQ/LOD values of various drugs of abuse obtained by GC-MS-MS using Intercept diluent. The target analytes, in some cases, are similar to those in urinalysis, but in other cases, such as with THC and cocaine (benzoylecgonine [BE]), they identify the compounds specific to oral fluids. Laboratories working with Intercept samples should validate their own instruments and methods.

Confirmation of presumptively positive specimens is perhaps the single most important procedure for any testing laboratory. The confirmation result will be the focus of any contested tests in a court of law. The defensibility of the procedure will require detailed attention to all aspects of the analysis. Therefore, the above information serves to provide some insight to potential approaches and expected results for confirmation of Intercept samples.

6. ANALYSIS OF INTERCEPT TESTING RESULTS

The Intercept device has been reviewed by the US Food and Drug Administration (FDA) for all of the assays discussed in this chapter. The Intercept system for oral-fluid analysis has been further tested in a large number of studies. The largest study to date includes an overall analysis of 77,000 specimens

Table 4
Ions Monitored for Internal Standard and Analytes

Analyte	Description	Quant Ions
THC d-3	Internal Std	238
THC	Std	238
BE d-3	Internal Std	303
BE	Std	300
PCP d-5	Internal Std	84 + 122
PCP	Std	84 + 117
Codeine d-3	Internal Std	285
Codeine	Std	282
Dihydrocodeine	Std	285
Morphine d-3	Internal Std	269 + 270
Morphine	Std	266 + 267
6-MAM	Std	266 + 267
Methamphetamine d-11	Internal Std	260
Methamphetamine	Std	254
MDMA	Std	254
MDEA	Std	268
Pseudoephedrine	Std	254
Amphetamine d-11	Internal Std	244
Amphetamine	Std	240
MDA	Std	162

THC, tetrahydrocannabinol; BE, benzoylecgonine; PCP, phencyclidine; 6-MAM; 6-monoacetylmorphine; MDMA, 3, 4-methylenedioxymethamphetamine; MDEA, 3,4 methylenedioxyethylamphetamine; MDA, methylenedioxyamphetamine.

submitted to a reference laboratory over a 12-mo period *(11)*. The results for the common five-panel DOA were compared to urine results within the same laboratory and also to the Quest laboratory data base for urine testing. Tables 6–8 show that, overall, oral-fluid results obtained by the Intercept system are comparable to those found with urine testing. This is somewhat surprising considering the shorter window of detection of drugs in oral fluid. Possible reasons for these results include broad use of urine adulterants masking many positives or the fact that many individuals abusing drugs have ingested substances close to the time of their sample collection. In either case, it suggests that oral fluid is a good alternative to urine testing for routine pre-employment testing.

7. CONCLUSIONS

DOA testing has become routine in many aspects of life. An established algorithm, which appears to be universally accepted, utilizes antibody-based tests

Table 5
Typical Limit of Quantitation (LOQ)/Limit of Detection (LOD)
of Various Drugs of Abuse Obtained by GC-MS-MS
Using Intercept® Diluent

Target Analyte	LOQ (ng/mL)	LOD (ng/mL)
Amphetamine	10.0	1.0
Codeine	5.0	2.5
MDMA, MDEA, MDA	1.0	0.5
BE	2.5	1.25
Morphine	5.0	2.5
Methamphetamine	1.0	0.5
PCP	0.5	0.25
THC	0.5	0.25
6-MAM	1.0	0.5

GC-MS-MS, gas chromatography-tandem mass spectrometry; MDMA, 3, 4-methylenedioxymethamphetamine; MDEA, 3,4 methylenedioxyethylamphetamine; MDA, methylenedioxyamphetamine; BE, benzoylecgonine; PCP, phencyclidine; THC, tetrahydrocannabinol; 6-MAM ; 6-monoacetylmorphine.

Table 6
Cutoff Concentrations in Oral-Fluid Specimens Tested
by Intercept® (Whole Saliva) and in GC-MS-MS Confirmation Assays

Assays	Cutoff concentrations oral fluid (ng/mL)
Initial Test (Intercept®)	
THC (Parent Drug and Metabolite)	3
Cocaine Metabolites	15
Opiate Metabolites	30
Phencyclidine	3
Amphetamines	120
Confirmatory Test	
THC (Parent Drug)	1.5
Benzoylecgonine	6
Morphine	30
Codeine	30
6-Acetylmorphine	3
Phencyclidine	1.5
Amphetamine	120
Methamphetamine	120

Table 7
**Overall Confirmed Positive Rates for Oral-Fluid Specimens Tested
in Lab*One* Over a 10-mo Period (Jan. 2001–Oct. 2001)***

Oral fluid specimens (n = 77,218)	Number of specimens	% Positive
Confirmed Positive Tests	3,908	5.06
THC (Parent)	2,486	3.22
Cocaine	865	1.12
Opiates	175	0.23
Phencyclidine	21	0.03
Amphetamine/Methamphetamine	361	0.47

*6-Acetylmorphine was only tested for morphine positives and is not included in the overall total number of positives.

Table 8
**Comparison of Positive Drug Prevalence Rate Found in Oral-Fluid Testing
With Federally Mandated and General Workforce Urine Drug Testing
Programs According to Quest Diagnostics' Drug Testing Index**

Drug Category	Positivity prevalence rate: oral fluid drug testing Jan.–Oct. 2001 (n = 77,218)	Drug testing index: federally mandated urine drug testing* Jan.–Dec. 2001 (n = 1,000,000)	Drug testing index: general workforce urine drug testing* Jan.–Dec. 2001 (n = 5,200,000)
THC	3.22	1.72	3.17
Cocaine	1.12	0.60	0.69
Opiates	0.23	0.26	0.29
Phencyclidine	0.03	0.05	0.02
Amphetamines	0.47	0.29	0.29
TOTAL	5.06	2.92	4.46

*Urine test date according to Quest Diagnostics' Drug Testing Index for workplace drug tests performed January to December, 2001 by Quest Diag. (data source can be found at http://www.questdiagnostics.com/business/b_bus_lab_emp_drugtesting_index.html)

for screening of presumptive positive samples. These presumptive positive samples are then confirmed using a combination of GC and MS. In the early days of drug testing, urinalysis went through a series of changes and modifications until reliable and legally defensible procedures were established. In many ways, oral-fluid testing has followed a similar path, with some exceptions. In oral-fluid testing, significant advances in screening and confirmation technologies have allowed the use of comparatively minute amounts of sample with similarly reliable results. In addition, positive oral-fluid testing can be indicative of a more recent time frame of drug use. It is expected that future technological development will make it possible to correlate oral-fluid testing with drug impairment and not just drug presence, as is currently possible with blood samples *(12–16)*.

REFERENCES

1. Substance Abuse and Mental Health Administration. Mandatory Guidelines for Federal Workplace Programs. Fed Regist 1988;53:11,970–11,989.
2. Verstraete A. Roadside Testing Assessment (www.ROSITA.org), 2000.
3. Road Safety (Drug Driving) Act 2003. Parliament of Victoria, Australia, 2003.
4. Malamud D and Tabak L. Saliva as a diagnostic fluid. Ann NY Acad Sci 1993; 694:276–279.
5. Samyn N, Verstraete A, van Haeren C, and Kintz P Analysis of drugs of abuse in saliva. For Sci Rev 1999;11(1):1–19.
6. Mucklow JC., Bending MR, Kahn GC, and Dollery CT. Drug concentration in saliva. Clin Pharmacol Ther 1978;24:563–570.
7. DiGregorio GJ, Piraino A, Nagle B, and Knaiz E. Basic biological sciences— secretion of drugs by the parotid glands of rats and human beings. J Dental Res 1977;56(5):502–50.
8. Niedbala RS, Kardos KW, Fritch, D. F., et al. Detection of marijuana use by oral fluid and urine analysis following single-dose administration of smoked and oral marijuana. J Anal Toxicol 2001;25:289–303.
9. Niedbala RS, Kardos KW, Fries T, and Davis A. Immunoassay for detection of cocaine/metabolites in oral fluids. J Anal Toxicol 2001;25:62–68.
10. Niedbala RS, Kardos K, Waga J, et al. Laboratory analysis of remotely collected oral fluid specimens for opiates by immunoassay. J. Anal. Toxicol. 2001;25:310–315.
11. Cone E, Presley L, Lehrer M, et al. Oral fluid testing for drugs of abuse: positive prevalence rates by Intercept™ immunoassay screening and GC-MS-MS confirmation and suggested cutoff concentrations. J Anal Toxicol 2003;27:169–172/
12. Cone EJ, Kumor K, Thompson LK, and Sherer M. Correlation of saliva cocaine levels with plasma levels and with pharmacologic effects after intravenous cocaine administration in human subjects. J Anal Toxicol 1988;12, 200–206.
13. Menkes DB, Howard RC, Spears GFS, and Cairns ER. Salivary THC following cannabis smoking correlates with subjective intoxication and heart rate. Psychopharmacology 1991;103:277–279.
14. Chait LD and Zacny JP. Reinforcing and subjective effects of oral Δ^9-THC and smoked marijuana in humans. Psychopharmacology 1992;107:255–262.
15. O'Neal CL, Crouch DJ, Rollins DE, Fatah A, and Cheever ML. Correlation of saliva codeine concentrations with plasma concentrations after oral codeine administration. J Anal Toxicol 1999;23:452–459.
16. Pitts FN, Allen RE, Aniline O, and Yago LS. Occupational intoxication and long-term persistence of phencyclidine (PCP) in law enforcement personnel. Clin Toxicol 1981;18(9):1015–1020.

Chapter 8

Dräger DrugTest®
Test for Illegal Drugs in Oral-Fluid Samples

Stefan Steinmeyer, Rainer Polzius,
and Andreas Manns

SUMMARY

The Dräger DrugTest® System (Dräger Safety) is a competitive, lateral-flow immunoassay for the detection of drugs of abuse in oral fluid. It is a point-of-care system comprised of an oral-fluid sample collector, test cassette, and analyzer, which delivers results read by the instrument for the simultaneous detection of the full National Institute on Drug Abuse (NIDA)-5 panel of drugs in a single oral-fluid sample. Oral-fluid testing has significant advantages over techniques involving blood or urine, such as its noninvasive nature, reduced costs and turnaround time, and reduced risk of sample adulteration; it also allows for accurate drug testing for a full NIDA-5 panel virtually anywhere and a more dignified treatment of test subjectsy. Dräger DrugTest is a product platform based on Up-Converting Phosphor Technology (UPT™; Orasure Technologies) and is used by law-enforcement agencies primarily to test operators and passengers of motor vehicles (i.e., roadside drug testing). This report provides an overview of the design of the system, the technology used, and the field studies in which the system has been tested.

1. INTRODUCTION

The practice of drug testing is undergoing a technological revolution, which is affecting not only the method, but also the location of testing. For on-site testing, such as along a roadside or in an unsecured location, urine drug

From: *Forensic Science and Medicine: Drugs of Abuse: Body Fluid Testing*
Edited by R. C. Wong and H. Y. Tse © Humana Press Inc., Totowa, NJ

screening performance has been limited by the difficulty of specimen collection when no adequate facilities (e.g., police truck with a bathroom) are available and of correlation of test results with drug impairment and blood drug concentration. Some drugs, particularly cannabis, can remain in urine for several weeks, but the impairing effects last a maximum of only 24 h. Therefore, the presence of drugs in urine can only indicate that the individual has been exposed to drugs, but not that he or she is inevitably under the influence. Also, because of privacy issues and potential alteration of a specimen by donors, the development and assessment of alternative test methods continues to be of interest *(1–5)*.

Recent advances in analytical technology have enabled the detection of drugs and drug metabolites in alternative biological specimens, such as in oral fluids, for the purpose of roadside checks, workplace testing, or the testing of individuals under criminal justice supervision *(6)*. Analyzing samples of oral fluid or sweat are relatively new ways for the detection of drug abuse. Oral-fluid analysis is a particularly promising method for the following reasons: An oral fluid sample can be taken directly on site, safeguarding the privacy of the subject. Oral-fluid sampling is not intrusive and guarantees physical safety. Furthermore, there is very little possibility of sample tampering because the operator can monitor the sampling process.

Oral-fluid testing can reveal the presence of pharmacologically active drugs in an individual at the time of testing. Significant correlation has been found between oral-fluid concentrations of drugs of abuse and behavioral and physiological effects *(7)*. Numerous recent studies have proven that oral fluid meets the requirements for drug-of-abuse screening at the workplace, roadside, or other locations *(8–10)*.

In this chapter, the Dräger DrugTest® (Dräger Safety) is described. This system is a point-of-collection (POC) rapid immunoassay intended for the collection of oral fluids and qualitative detection of drugs through the use of the DrugTest Analyzer.

2. DESIGN OF THE SYSTEM

The Dräger DrugTest was developed on the basis of findings relating to drug abuse in road traffic and taking into account the recommendations of the European Roadside Testing Assessment (ROSITA) study *(see* Chapter 17), in which requirements for roadside-testing equipment were identified *(11)*. The device is capable of simultaneously detecting the following classes of drugs: cannabis, amphetamines, methamphetamines, cocaine, opiates, and phencyclidine (National Institute on Drug Abuse [NIDA]-5 panel). In Figs. 1 and 2, the main components of the system are shown:

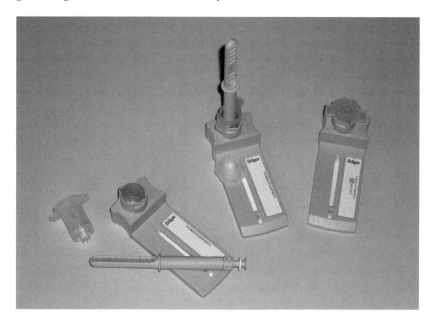

Fig. 1. Dräger DrugTest® Kit for oral fluid samples (collection device, test cassette and inserted sample preparation cartridge).

1. DrugTest Kit for oral fluids: the collection device for taking the oral fluid sample and the test cassette for detecting the drugs;
2. DrugTest Analyzer: portable instrument for reading the test cassette and for data management;
3. Accessories: impact printer and keyboard (accessories not illustrated in Figs. 1 and 2: negative and positive controls, transportation case).

The entire process of analysis, from collecting a sample to the display of the measurement results on the analyzer, takes around 15 min. Under observation, the subject collects an oral-fluid sample by gently moving the collection device from side to side in the mouth for about a minute until the sponge is saturated, as shown in Fig. 3. As a result, an average of 330 ± 130 µL oral fluid is collected, sufficient to allow clinically effective screening and confirmation. The fluid is expressed from the sponge by firm pressing of the collection device into the sample-preparation cartridge (SPC) in the test cassette. The handle can then be removed by counter-clockwise twisting, and a 4-min reaction time is started. The SPC should then be pressed down firmly to start an 8-min development time, when the sample flows up the strip inside the test cassette. The different steps of the process are shown in Fig. 1. After the 8-min development, the cassette can be inserted into the analyzer and a test can be read out

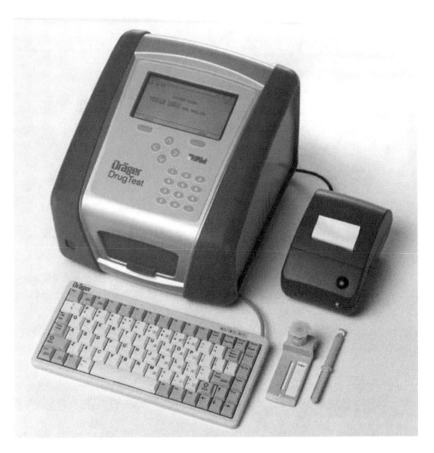

Fig. 2. Dräger DrugTest® Analyzer with keyboard and printer.

according to the screen prompts. Once the analysis of the cassette begins, a progress bar will appear on the Dräger DrugTest Analyzer display. After 3 min of reading, the analyzer reports the results with either a "+" or "−" on the display screen for each drug (Fig. 4). No interpretation is required. There is a greater than 95% confidence level that a positive result will be attained with drug at 250% of its following detection limits (cut-off concentrations; *see* Table 1).

During the procedure, the subject and the operator data can be entered optionally with the keypad, a connected keyboard, and/or a barcode scanner. The results are automatically stored under their respective sample number (there is enough memory for up to 2000 sets of data) and can be displayed, printed out, or sent via an infrared (IR) interface to a personal computer. After the specimen has been tested, the collector sponge, which remains in the SPC,

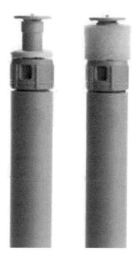

Fig. 3. Collection device before (left) and after (right) completion of the sampling process.

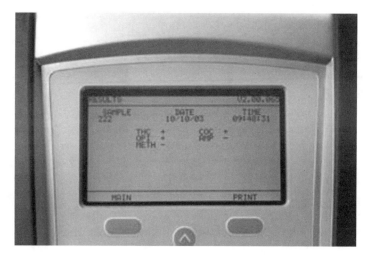

Fig. 4. Measurement results on the analyzer's display.

still contains around 200 µL of the original oral fluid sample, so that this sample can be transported to a laboratory for confirmation. At the laboratory, the collector is pulled out of the SPC in order to remove the sample from the cassette, and the drug is then extracted from the sponge and analyzed by instrumented devices such as gas chromatography (GC)-mass spectrometry (MS).

Table 1
Screening Cut-Offs

Amphetamine	10 ng/mL
Methamphetamines	10 ng/mL
Cocaine metabolic products	5 ng/mL
Opiates	5 ng/mL
Cannabinoids	20 ng/mL
Phencyclidine	10 ng/mL

3. PRINCIPLE OF THE TEST

The detection method is based on a competitive, lateral-flow immunoassay (*see* Chapters 3 and 4), which utilizes highly specific antibodies for the different drug classes and detects simultaneously the different drugs from a single oral-fluid sample. Drug or drug metabolites in the oral fluid compete with the immobilized drug derivatives for limited drug–antibody binding sites. The degree of binding, i.e., the number of complexes formed by the antibodies and the target substance, depends on the concentration of the target substance. A more detailed description of immunological detection can be found elsewhere *(12)*.

To allow analysis of the immunological binding reaction, a patented signal technology, known as Up-Converting Phosphor Technology (UPT™, Orasure Technologies), is used. The antibodies are covalently conjugated with spherical, crystalline submicrometer-sized particles(phosphors), which are able to absorb IR light and subsequently emit photons in the visible range. Upon excitation with low-energy long-wave laser radiation (980 nm, IR range) during the reading process within the DrugTest Analyzer, the phosphors convert the light up to a high-energy visible emission spectrum. The emitted light is registered, amplified, and quantified by a detector, allowing a very sensitive detection of approx 10 green-emitting particles (550 nm) and 100 blue-emitting particles (475 nm). This up-converting process is unique in nature in that the optical properties of the phosphors are unaffected by their environment. Therefore, there is no contribution to test background phosphorescence from the sample matrix and assay interferents *(13,14)*.

The intensity of the emitted light is an indication of the drug concentration in the sample; there is an inverse relationship between the drug or drug metabolite concentration present in the sample and the signal strength at the test zone.

Fig. 5. *(opposite page)* Schematic diagram of a morphine test strip and the reading process if the sample does not contain any drug (above), and if morphine is present in the sample (below).

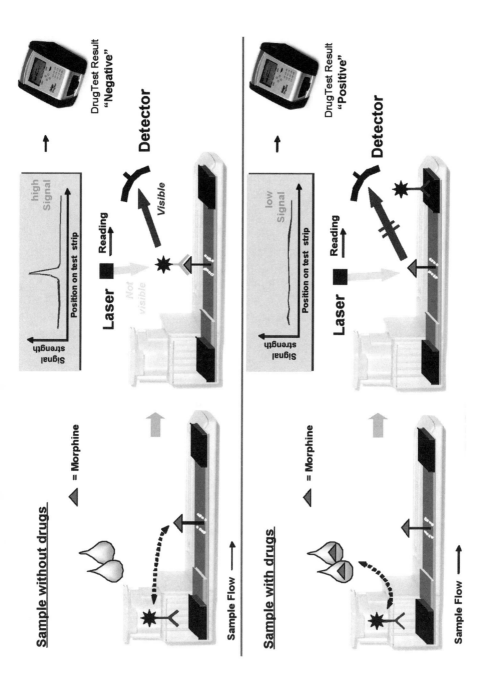

139

Figure 5 shows a schematic diagram of a test strip used for the detection of morphine. After sampling, the collected sample is expressed into the SPC and delivered into the cassette, which contains a lateral-flow strip of nitrocellulose impregnated with test and reference lines. In the lateral-flow strip, phosphor–antibody complexes mix with sample/buffer and move by capillary action along the test strip. If the sample does not contain any morphine, the antibodies cross the membrane and bind with the membrane-fixed morphine molecules in the test zone (Fig. 5, top). When morphine is present in the oral-fluid sample, the drug will complex with the phosphor–antibody conjugate during flow. Upon reaching of the test lines, there is no reaction of the phosphor-antibody conjugate with the membrane-fixed morphine molecules in the test zone, because the active sites on the antibody are already occupied by the drug in the sample. Consequently, the subsequent analysis of the test lines using the Dräger Drug-Test Analyzer will not produce a signal (Fig. 5, bottom). The assay reference band will not be influenced by the presence or absence of drug in the oral fluid and, therefore, will be present in all reactions.

On a multi-analytical test strip, different substances can be detected simultaneously. Figure 6 (left side) shows a schematic diagram of a test strip with three distinct and physically separate test zones to detect, e.g., cannabis, cocaine, and amphetamines. As a result of the immunological detection reaction, the antibodies coupled to the UPT particles will bind exclusively in the test zone corresponding to their drug (cocaine, cannabis, amphetamine). Through the changing of their composition, phosphor particles of varying emission spectra can be produced, allowing multiplexed testing. The use of different phosphors allows differentiation of different binding reactions without necessitating the physical separation of the test zones on the test strip. In the example shown in Fig. 6 (right side), amphetamine-specific antibodies are solely coupled to phosphors that emit green light, whereas cannabis-specific antibodies are fixed to phosphors that emit blue light. By means of clear spectral separation of the two emission spectra using optical filters in the Dräger DrugTest Analyzer, it is then possible to detect separately green and blue light at the same spot and, therefore, the different drugs—in this case amphetamine and cannabis—associated with them. Unlike other labeling technologies (e.g., gold particles), the use of UPT can increase not only the sensitivity, but also the selectivity of the analysis.

Fig. 6. *(opposite page)* Schematic diagram of a test strip with three distinct and physically separate test zones to detect, e.g., cannabis, cocaine, and amphetamines (multi-analytical test strip, left side), and a schematic diagram of a test strip with one test zone, allowing multiplexed testing to detect, e.g., cannabis and amphetamines (right side).

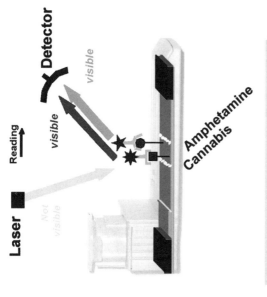
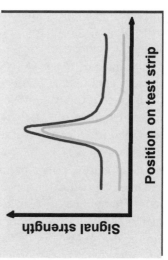
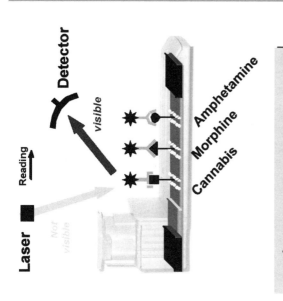
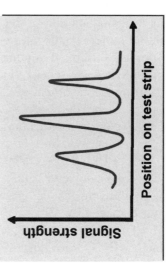

141

4. CLINICAL STUDIES

Right from the start of product development, field trials have been important for testing the system's function and the potential user's acceptance. The oral fluid remaining in the test cassette was subsequently laboratory tested by means of gas chromatography (GC)-tandem mass spectrometry (MS-MS). Through a comparison of the screening results with the results of the confirmation analysis, the system's key performance data (sensitivity, specificity, accuracy) could be determined.

Between August and November 2001, a pilot study by the police force in the German state of Saarland evaluated a prototype of the Dräger DrugTest system and investigated the variability of oral-fluid analysis results in relation to blood/serum *(7)*. For the purposes of this study, oral-fluid and blood samples were taken during police patrol from 177 car drivers and analyzed by GC-MS. The DrugTest collection device was used to obtain oral-fluid samples and was rated by the police officers as simple and user friendly. In all cases, sufficient oral fluid for GC-MS laboratory analysis was provided. Comparing the data from the oral fluid with the serum for amphetamine, methylenedioxymethamphetamine (MDMA), morphine, benzoylecgonine, and tetrahydrocannabinol (THC), the sensitivities were 100%, 97%, 87%, 87%, and 92%, respectively. The overall specificity and accuracy was in the range of 91–98% and the oral-fluid samples and the serum were both negative or positive for any substance 97% of the time. This is proof of oral fluid's suitability for determining recent drug consumption and of the usefulness of the DrugTest sampling device for forensic purposes, allowing both screening and confirmation. Even for THC, known to be excreted minimally into saliva *(15)*, the correlation of serum and oral-fluid data was remarkably good, indicating good recovery in the elution of THC from the adsorbent of the collection device.

In October 2002, a clinical study in Slovenia addressed drug consumption among patients in addiction-treatment programs, with a potentially high rate of polytoxicomanic drug users. Within the study, 92 valid screening results of the Dräger DrugTest System obtained from addicted patients from outpatient clinics were compared with the GC-MS-MS analyses of the oral-fluid samples. The Dräger DrugTest demonstrated very good results for sensitivity, specificity, and accuracy: THC (95.2%, 90.1%, 91.3%), cocaine (87.5%, 96.4%, 95.7%), and opiates (92.9%, 84.4%, 87.0%). Amphetamine (AMP) and methamphetamines (METH) were not included in the test panel at that time, but were the objects of further investigation *(16)*.

From July 12 to 13, 2003, several Dräger DrugTest systems were in use at four different police control sites during one of the world's largest annual techno parties, the "Love Parade" in Berlin. Police from several German states around Berlin checked incoming and outgoing visitors, focusing on drug trafficking and on drivers under the influence of alcohol and drugs. Many young drivers were found to be noticeably under the influence of drugs or alcohol, and a remarkably higher rate of blood samples were taken for driving under the influence of drugs (DUID) (79) than for driving under the influence of alcohol (DUIA) (6). Seventy-two oral-fluid samples were taken with the DrugTest collection device and analyzed on site with the DrugTest. According to the different control locations, the testing environment varied from a fixed station in an open tent to inside of a police car and/or van. All on-site oral-fluid samples were analytically confirmed in a laboratory by GC-MS and GC-MS-MS, and accuracy values of 91.5% (THC), 97.2% (cocaine), 100.0% (opiates), 95.8% (METH), and 74.6% (AMP) were found.

5. CONCLUSIONS

The new on-site drug detection concept presented in this report makes possible another important step towards improved safety standards. Experts and customers in legal medicine and law enforcement, toxicologists, and so on have been involved from the very beginning of the development process for the Dräger DrugTest System. Up until now, more than 1000 real oral-fluid samples, in more than 5000 single assays, have been tested in field studies. These data were and will be part of the continued development of the Dräger DrugTest, and serve as realistic guidelines by which to guarantee the high standard of the system and improve it when necessary. As a result, the system represents a suitable solution for the practical diagnosis of recent drug consumption, for use in the areas of rehabilitation and substitution, workplace investigations, and law enforcement.

REFERENCES

1. Cody JT, Valtier S, and Kuhlman J. Analysis of morphine and codeine in samples adulterated with Stealth. J Anal Toxicol 2001;25(7):572–575.
2. Tsai LS, ElSohly MA, Tsai SF, Murphy TP, Twarowska B, and Salamone SJ. Investigation of nitrite adulteration on the immunoassay and GC-MS analysis of cannabinoids in urine specimens. J Anal Toxicol 2000;24(8):708–714.
3. King EJ. Evaluation of Intect™ test strips for detecting adulteration of urine specimens used for drugs-of-abuse testing. J. Anal. Toxicol. 2000;24(6):456.
4. Wu AH, Bristol B, Sexton K, Cassella-McLane G, Holtman V, and Hill DW. Adulteration of urine by "Urine Luck." Clin. Chem. 45(7), 1051–1057, 1999.
5. King EJ. Performance of AdultaCheck 4 test strips for the detection of adulteration at the point of collection of urine specimens used for drugs-of-abuse testing. J Anal Toxicol 1999;23(1):72.
6. Yacoubian GS Jr, Wish ED, and Perez DM. A comparison of saliva testing to urinalysis in an arrestee population. J. Psychoactive Drugs 33(3), 289–294, 2001.

7. Toennes SW, Steinmeyer S, Maurer H-J, Kauert G, and Moeller MR. Screening for drugs of abuse in oral fluid—correlation of analysis results with serum in forensic cases. J Anal Toxicol, 2005; 29(1): 22–27.
8. Caplan YH and Goldberger BA. Alternative specimens for workplace drug testing. J Anal Toxicol 2001;25(5):396–399.
9. Kintz P and Samyn N. Use of alternative specimens: drugs of abuse in saliva and doping agents in hair. Ther Drug Monit 2002;24(2):239–46.
10. Schramm W, Smith RH, Craig PA, and Kidwell DA. Drugs of abuse in saliva: a review. J Anal Toxicol 1992;16(1):1–9.
11. European Union. ROSITA—EU Project Contract DG VII RO 98-SC.3032 www.rosita.org.
12. Wild D (ed). The Immunoassay Handbook, First Edition. Stockton, New York: 1994.
13. Niedbala RS, Feindt H, Kardos K, et al. Detection of analytes by immunoassay using up-converting phosphor technology. Anal Biochem 2001;293(1):22–30.
14. Hampl J, Hall M, Mufti NA, et al. Upconverting phosphor reporters in immuno-chromatographic assays. Anal Biochem 2001;288(2):176–87.
15. Idowu OR and Caddy B. A review of the use of saliva in the forensic detection of drugs and other chemicals. J Forensic Sci Soc 1982;22(2):123–35.
16. Zorec-Karlovsek M, Niedbala S, Fritch D, Steinmeyer S, and Manns A. The suitability of oral fluid testing in outpatient clinics for treatment of drug addiction. Abstracts of the 3rd European Academy of Forensic Science Meeting. September 22–27, 2003. Istanbul, Turkey. Forensic Sci Int 2003;136 (Suppl 1):309.

Chapter 9

On-Site Oral-Fluid Drug Testing by Oratect®

Raphael C. Wong

SUMMARY

Oral fluids have been generating increased interest as a matrix for abused drug testing. The present chapter describes an oral-fluid on-site detection device, Oratect®, which screens for six drugs simultaneously. Oratect integrates collection, testing, and confirmation sampling into a single device. The collection process is simple, and test results can be obtained within 5 to 6 min. The data collected so far suggest that it is a viable screening test. Recently, the testing has been extended to alcohol, so that a simultaneous determination of drugs and alcohol is possible.

1. INTRODUCTION

Oral fluids offer an attractive alternative matrix for drug testing as a result of several factors including: (a) reduced chances for adulteration; (b) accessibility; (c) non-invasiveness; and (d) better correlation with serum drug levels compared to urine. These factors contribute to the increasing acceptability of oral-fluid drug testing as a valid indicator of drug usage *(1–3)*. As a result, guidelines for performing such testing *(4)* have been established by the US Substance Abuse and Mental Health Services Administration (SAMHSA). There are several notable oral-fluid testing devices on the market. For example, Intercept® (OraSure Technologies, Inc.) is laboratory-based (*see* Chapter 7), whereas Dräger DrugTest® (Dräger Safety AG & Co.) is an on-site instrument-based device (*see* Chapter 8). Noninstrumental on-site drug screens have been available since the

From: *Forensic Science and Medicine: Drugs of Abuse: Body Fluid Testing*
Edited by R. C. Wong and H. Y. Tse © Humana Press Inc., Totowa, NJ

late 1990s. These include Drugwipe® (Securetec Detektions-Systeme AG) (*see* Chapter 10), Oralab™ (Varian Corporation), Oralstat™ (American Bio Medica Corporation), Oral-Screen™ (Avitar, Inc.), and Oratect® (Branan Medical Corporation). Oralab, Oralstat, and Oral-Screen are two-component devices in which oral fluids, collected by a sampling device, are transferred to a separate test device for analysis. Oratect, on the other hand, is a one-step device in which both collection and testing processes are incorporated into a single device.

Certain challenges must be addressed by oral-fluid on-site devices. These include:

1. The collection process must be easy and quick;
2. The testing must overcome the inconsistency of the oral-fluid matrix;
3. The sensitivity of the test must meet the lower drug concentrations present in the oral cavity;
4. The test strip must be able to perform in spite of the slow migration of oral fluid and instability of tetrahydrocannabinol (THC).

This chapter examines the design of the Oratect device *(5)* by addressing some of these issues, and subsequently describing its performance.

2. DESIGN OF THE ORATECT DEVICE

The Oratect device (Fig. 1) is a single, integrated test device capable of collecting and testing an oral-fluid sample and saving a portion of it for confirmation purposes. Oratect is to be operated completely by a donor under the direct observation of a monitoring person who is not required to participate in the collection or testing procedures. As an on-site device, Oratect is noninstrumental, with the collection and testing processes completed within 5 to 8 min.

2.1. Description of the Oratect Device

The Oratect device provides qualitative drug-screen test results and is configured to detect six drugs simultaneously. Because the concentrations of drugs in the oral fluids are generally lower than those in urine, the tests are more sensitive, with lower cut-off concentrations. The detectable drugs and their cut-off (C.O.) levels are shown in Table 1.

The device consists of three components—a cap, a collection pad, and a test device. The cap is a hollow receptacle enclosing the collection pad, which is attached to the test device. Each device has two windows, each accommodating a single test strip capable of testing three drugs.

The cap serves several functions. It protects the collection pad during shipping. In addition, it is used as a pinching device to detach the collection pad from the test device for confirmation purposes. After detachment, it may also serve as a storage compartment for the collection pad.

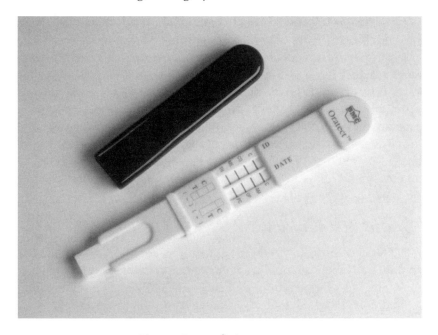

Fig. 1. Oratect® drug screen.

Table 1
Cut-Off Levels of Oratect®

Drug	Cut-off level in ng/mL
Cocaine (COC)	20
Methamphetamine (MET)	50
Amphetamine (AMP)	50
Opiates (OPI)	20
Phencyclidine (PCP)[a]	4
Δ^9-tetrahydrocannabinol (THC)	30

[a]In Europe and places where testing for PCP is not of interest, benzodiazepines (BZO) test with a cut-off concentration of 5 ng/mL is substituted for PCP.

The collection pad is made of polymeric material chosen for its rigidity under wet conditions and good liquid flow. Size of the collection pad is optimized to collect the minimal oral-fluid volume to accomplish the testing and confirmation processes so that the time required to complete these procedures can be reduced to 5 to 8 min. It is estimated that the total sample volume collected by the pad is 0.55 mL. About 0.3 mL will be used to complete the screen testing, and this will leave 0.25 mL for confirmation testing.

Because of the sensitivity requirement of the tests, the chemistries of the test strips originally designed for urine testing have to be modified to allow for the lower C.O. detection limits. Furthermore, because THC residue in oral fluid is even more absorptive ("sticky") to polymeric surfaces than its carboxylic acid metabolite in urine, the choice of buffers and surfactants to be used requires extensive studies. Evaluations of the currently commercially available antibodies showed that all of them are designed for the carboxyl derivative and do not have high affinity toward THC. Hence, a compromise on the sensitivity of THC test has to be made.

2.2. Oratect Test Principle

The Oratect test is based on the principle of competitive immunoassay, in which drug derivatives immobilized on a lateral-flow membrane compete with the drugs that may be present in oral fluids for limited antibody binding sites on colored colloidal gold antibody conjugates. In the absence of drugs in the oral fluids, the colloidal gold antibody conjugates will bind to the drug derivatives on the membrane and form red colored lines indicating negative results. Conversely, drugs present in the oral-fluid samples will bind to the colloidal fluid antibody conjugates and prevent them from binding to the drug derivatives on the membrane. Hence, the absence of a colored line at a specific test region indicates a positive result for that particular test.

2.3. Test Procedures

The Oratect is noninstrumental, with all necessary reagents incorporated into the one-piece device (Fig. 1). To run the test, rub the collection pad in a circular motion inside both cheeks and on top of and beneath the tongue until gold conjugate appears in the window. Cap the pad and check for the presence of line within 5 min. If the screening test indicates a positive result, the collection pad can be sent to a laboratory for gas chromatography (GC)-mass spectrometry (MS) confirmation analysis of the drugs retained in the collection pad. This is accomplished by pinching of the collection pad with the cap to detach it from the test device. The pad is stored in a buffered vial to be sent to the laboratory.

The collection procedure serves several functions. Moving the device inside the mouth cavity may stimulate oral-fluid production. Moreover, it is believed that THC residues are most abundant inside the mouth cavity around the inside of cheek. A circular motion may be the best way to recover these residues.

2.4. Test Line Intensity Over Time

To ensure that the test results are readable within 3 to 5 min, the line intensities of positive and negative results have to remain differentiable over a period of 2 to 5 min. Results of a study shown in Fig. 2 demonstrate substantial color line intensity differentiation between positive and negative results for amphetamine (AMP) and cocaine (COC) tests, while the color for the control line did not change. It also shows there was little variance from 2 to 5 min. Similar results were obtained for the THC, methamphetamine (MET), opiates (OPI), and phencyclidine (PCP) tests.

2.5. Precision Study

The precision of the Oratect device was evaluated using pooled negative oral fluids spiked with various concentrations of the seven drugs. Twenty samples were run for each concentration. The results obtained are shown in Table 2.

3. CORRELATION WITH OTHER ASSAYS

3.1. Correlation With Enzyme-Linked Immunosorbent Assay

In a report comparing oral-fluid enzyme-linked immunosorbent assay (ELISA) (Immunalysis Corporation, Pomona, CA) with Oratect *(6)*, aliquots of pooled negative oral fluids were spiked with five drugs (COC, OPI, AMP, MET, and PCP), and the drug concentrations in these aliquots were assayed by both tests. All together, 26 serial dilutions at concentrations ranging from 600% (6X) to 0% (0X) of the C.O. concentrations were tested in duplicates by Oratect and ELISA. Results are summarized in Table 3. It shows that all samples spiked at 1.5X C.O. concentrations and above were determined to be positive by both ELISA and Oratect. All samples spiked at or below 0.7X C.O. concentrations gave negative results on both assays.

3.2. Correlation With Urine Drug Screen and Confirmation by GC-MS

A total of 465 volunteer subjects at a drug rehabilitation program were tested with both urine drug screens and the Oratect device. In this experiment, urine specimens were collected under observed conditions and screened for five drugs using Monitect® PC11 drug screen (Branan Medical Corporation). The Oratect tests were performed immediately after the subject exited the restroom. Results from the two test methods were compared only at the end of the day. The collection pads from the positive Oratect test devices were sent for GC-MS confirmation tests at Scientific Testing Lab (Richmond, VA). The

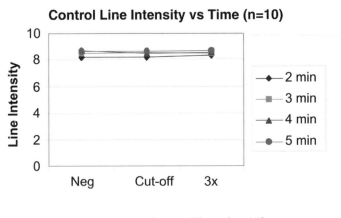

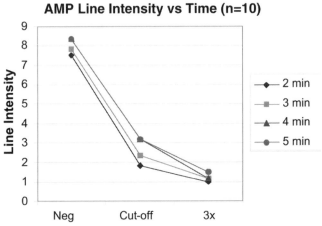

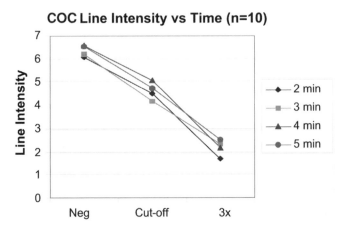

Fig. 2. Line intensity studies. Neg = negative; 3× = three times the cutoff concentration of that particular drug. The intensity of each line is assigned an arbitrary number from 1 to 10, with the number 10 showing the darkest line and 1 representing the total absence of a line. AMP, amphetamine; COC, cocaine.

Table 2
Precision Study on the Oratect®

Drug concentration as % cut-off	0%	25%	50%	75%	300%
COC	20–	20–	20–	18–/2+	20+
OPI	20–	20–	20–	18–/2+	20+
THC	20–	20–	18–/2+	18–/2+	1–/19+
AMP	20–	20–	20–	18–/2+	20+
MET	20–	20–	20–	18–/2+	20+
PCP	20–	20–	20–	18–/2+	20+
BZO	20–	20–	20–	18–/2+	20+

– indicates negative result and + indicates positive result.
COC, cocaine; OPI, opiates; THC, tetrahydrocannabinol; AMP, amphetamines; MET, methamphetamines; PCP, phencyclidine; BZO, benzodiazepines.

results are summarized in Table 4. None of the subjects tested positive for PCP. Subjects who tested positive by Oratect for COC and OPI were likely to be tested positive by the urine drug screen. Oratect appeared to detect AMP better than urine test, and all subjects tested MET positive by Oratect were tested positive by Monitect. Confirmation of Oratect results by GC-MS ranged from 85 to 100% for COC, MET, AMP, and OPI.

All the volunteer subjects tested at the drug rehabilitation program appeared to have a job, and the tests were undertaken in the afternoon. It was suggested that this situation allowed little time for the test subject to smoke a marijuana cigarette immediately prior to being tested. Because the Oratect device tests for THC residue in the mouth cavity and the concentration of THC decreases rapidly after marijuana cigarette smoking *(7)*, concentrations of THC might be too low to be detectable. The four samples that were detected positive by Oratect were all confirmed positive by GC-MS.

3.3. Correlation of Oratect Opiate Test With Oral-Fluid GC-MS and Urine Drug Screen

In another study *(4)*, 10 normal human subjects were each administered one dose of Prometh with Codeine Cough Syrup (Alpharma USPD, Inc., Baltimore, MD) containing 10 mg of codeine phosphate, and their oral fluids and urine were analyzed for opiate after 1 h, 4 h, and 6 h. The urine samples were tested with Monitect PC11 Multiple Urine Drug Screen Test, while the oral-fluid samples were analyzed with three methods: Oratect screening test, Oratect confirmation test by GC-MS, and a laboratory-based test—Intercept oral-fluids

Table 3
Comparison of Enzyme-Linked Immunosorbent Assay (ELISA) and Oratect® Test Results

Aliquot #	Drug level as multiple of C.O.	COC C.O. = 20 ng/mL		OPI C.O. = 20 ng/mL		PCP C.O. = 4 ng/mL		MET C.O. = 50 ng/mL		AMP C.O. = 50 ng/mL	
		ELISA	Oratect	ELISA	Oratect	ELISA	Oratect	ELISA	Oratect	ELISA	Oratect
1–11	6.0X to 1.5X	109–44	All +	79–35	All +	20–8	All +	171–75	All +	139–77	All +
12	1.3X	30	+,+	18	+,+	5	+,–	47	+,–	51	+,+
13	1.2X	25	+,–	24	+,+	5	–,–	45	+,+	45	–,+
14	1.1X	40	+,+	17	+,–	4	+,+	58	–,+	43	+,+
15	1.0X	40	+,–	28	+,+	4	–,–	40	+,+	52	+,+
16	0.8X	57	+,–	14	+,–	4	–,–	36	+,+	30	+,–
17–26	0.7X to 0X	23–0	All –	9–0	All –	3–0	All –	29–0	All –	24–0	All –

Oratect results are in duplicates. – indicates negative result, and + indicates positive result.
The ELISA results are the mean values of duplicate determinations and are expressed in ng/mL.
C.O., cut-off; COC, cocaine; OPI, opiates; PCP, phencyclidine; MET, methamphetamines; AMP, amphetamines.

152

Table 4
Correlation Study of Urine Drug Screen and Oratect®

Drug detected	# Monitect positive	# Oratect positive	# Both positive	# Monitect® positive/Oratect negative	Monitect negative/Oratect positive	% Oratect GC/MS confirmed
COC	36	34	32	4	2	90
MET	12	8	8	4	0	85
AMP	0	4	0	0	4	100
OPI	32	34	32	0	2	87
THC	28	4	4	24	0	100
PCP	0	0	0	0	0	N/A

GC-MS, gas chromatography-mass spectrometry; COC, cocaine; MET, methamphetamines; AMP, amphetamines; OPI, opiates; THC, tetrahydrocannabinol; PCP, phencyclidine.

confirmation test. The results as shown in Table 5 suggest that the Oratect device can detect the presence of codeine up to 6 h after the administration of a single 10-mg dose of codeine. It also confirms that GC-MS confirmatory testing using oral fluids collected with the Oratect device is a viable procedure and provides a correlation coefficient of 0.96 with the Intercept method.

4. EXTENSION OF ORATECT OPIATE DETECTION WINDOW

When the Oratect opiate C.O. concentration was lowered to 10 ng/mL *(6)*, the results (as shown in Table 6) suggested that the detection window can be extended twofold to 12 h. In this experiment, five healthy, normal subjects were each administered one dose of Prometh. Oratect test (with 10 ng/mL opiate C.O.) and Monitect urine drug screen were undertaken at 1, 6, 8, 10, 14, and 16 h after the administration of the dose.

5. DETECTION OF THC OVER TIME

Two men (subjects A and B) and one woman (subject C) were tested for THC after each of them smoked a single marijuana cigarette. Oratect drug screens and Intercept collections were performed at half-hour intervals. Both the Oratect collection pads and the Intecept devices were sent to Scientific Testing Laboratory for GC-MS analysis. The results as shown in Table 7 suggest that the Oratect can detect the presence of THC up to 2 h after use. Moreover, the Oractect GC-MS results correlate well with the Intercept GC-MS data.

6. DRUG INTERFERENCE STUDY

Drugs and metabolites that may potentially cross-react with the Oratect test were evaluated *(8)*, and the results are shown in Tables 8 and 9. Each

Table 5
Correlation of Oratect® Opiate Test With Oral-Fluid Gas Chromatography (GC)-Mass Spectrometry (MS) and Urine Drug Screen

Subj #	1 h				4 h				6 h			
	U	O	G	I	U	O	G	I	U	O	G	I
1	+	+	872	1084	+	+	30	28	+	+/−	18	18
2	+	+	192	200	+	+	20	34	+	+	ND	20
3	+	+	34	42	+	+	20	24	+	+/−	ND	ND
4	+	+	172	138	+	+	36	38	+	+	ND	ND
5	+	+	218	338	+	+	168	244	+	+	32	28
6	+	+	100	148	+	+	22	24	+	+	ND	18
7	+	+	104	154	+	+	24	42	+	+/−	16	20
8	+	+	64	78	+	+	28	26	+	+	16	22
9	+	+	84	106	+	+	38	60	+	+	30	28
10	+	+	196	554	+	+	50	84	+	−	12	38

U = Monitect® urine results; O = Oratect results; G = GC-MS confirmatory results using oral fluids collected with the Oratect device; I = GC-MS results using oral fluids collected with the Intercept device; ND = no drug detected.

Table 6
Oratect® Opiate Detection Window With Cut-Off at 10 ng/mL

#	1 h		6 h		8 h		10 h		12 h		14 h		16 h	
	U	O	U	O	U	O	U	O	U	O	U	O	U	O
1	+	+	+	+	+	+	+	+	+	+	+	−	−	−
2	+	+	+	+	+	+	+	+	+	+	+	+/−	−	−
3	+	+	+	+	+	+	+	+	+	+	+	+/−	−	−
4	+	+	+	+	+	+	+	+	+	+	+	−	−	−
5	+	+	+	+	+	+	+	+	+	+	+	+	−	−

U = urine result; O = Oratect result.

substance was dissolved in pooled normal negative saliva. Table 8 lists the drugs that do not interfere with Oratect results even at 100 µg/mL concentration. Interfering compounds with concentrations that would cause a positive result are summarized in Table 9.

7. POTENTIAL INTERFERENCE FROM NONDRUG SOURCES

Several studies have evaluated the potential interference from nondrug sources.

Table 7
Detection of Tetrahydrocannabinol Over Time

		Subject A	Subject B	Subject C
0 h	Oratect®	–	–	–
0.5 h	Oratect	+	+	+
	Oratect GC-MS	494	512	393
	Intercept™	253	322	211
1 h	Oratect	+	+	+
	Oratect GC-MS	94.5	100	91
	Intercept	NP	NP	NP
1.5 h	Oratect	+	+	+
	Oratect GC-MS	48	65	50
	Intercept	50	72	46
2 h	Oratect	+/–	+	+/–
	Oratect GC-MS	34	44	33
	Intercept	31	42	29
2.5 h	Oratect	–	+/–	–
	Oratect GC-MS	NP	25	NP
	Intercept	NP	28	NP

– indicates negative result; + indicates positive result; +/– indicates a borderline result; NP, test not performed; GC-MS, gas chromatography-mass spectrometry.

Table 8
Compounds That Do Not Cross-React at 100 µg/mL

Acetaminophen	1-ephedrine
Acetylsalicyclic acid	Imipramine
Amobarbital	Lidocaine
Aspartame	Methadone
Buprenorphine	Pentobarbital
Caffeine	Phenobarbital
Chlorpromazine	d,1-phenylpropanolamine
Chloroquine	Propoxyphene
Desipramine	d,1-pseudoephedrine
Dextromethorphan	Secobarbital

7.1. Ethnic Meals

Thirteen volunteers from three ethnic groups including Caucasians, Asians, and Hispanics were tested with Oratect drug screens 2 h after the consumption of a meal typical of their ethnicities. This was repeated for three

Table 9
Interfering Compounds

	ng/mL
Cocaine	
Benzoylecgonine	20
Ecgonine Methylester	>5000
Anhydroecgonine	>5000
Methamphetamines	
MDMA	200
Amphetamine	>5000
Ephredrine	>5000
Pseudoephredrine	>5000
MDA	>5000
Tetrahydrocannabinol	
11-nor-Δ9-Tetrahydrocannabinol-9-carboxylic acid	20
Δ8-Tetrahydrocannabinol	1000
Amphetamine	
MDA	100
Methmphetamine	>5,000
Ephredrine	>5,000
Pseudoephredrine	>5,000
MDMA	>5,000
Opiates	
Codeine	50
6-Acetyl morphine	50
Ethylmorphine	50
Hydrocodone	100
Oxycodone	10,000
Phencyclidine	
Phencyclidine	4
Benzodiazepines	
Temazepam	10
Triazolam	15
Oxazepam	20
Diazepam	25
Benzodiazepines	
Nitrazepam	30
Nordiazepam	40
Clobazam	100
Clonazepam	100
Flunitrazepam	150
Chlordiazepoxide	200
Prazepam	700

MDMA, methylenedioxymethamphetamine; MDA, methylenedioxyamphetamine.

different days. Each meal consisted of dishes favored by the particular individual. A total of 36 test devices were used and all gave negative results, suggesting that food intake does not give false-positive results.

7.2. Cosmetic and Hygienic Products

Eight volunteers were tested with Oratect 30 min after brushing their teeth. They were again tested 30 min after applying lipstick and 30 min after smoking a cigarette. All 24 tests showed negative results, demonstrating that toothpaste, lipstick, and cigarettes do not interfere with the Oratect results.

7.3. Beverages

Oral fluids from drug-free volunteers were collected and pooled. Aliquots of the pooled oral fluids were each spiked with 10% v/v of the following beverages: (a) Lipton® tea; (b) black coffee; (c) Pepsi® Cola soft drink; (d) Dr. Pepper® soft drink; and (e) reconstituted Minute Maid® orange juice. When these spiked samples were applied to Oratect drug-screen devices, the test results indicated that none of the beverages studied gave false-positive results.

7.4. Food Ingredients

Aliquots of drug-free oral fluids were spiked with: (a) 10% v/v of 1 mg/mL solution of citric acid; (b) sugar with the final concentration of 1 mg/mL; (c) table salt with the final concentration of 1 mg/mL; and (d) monosodium glutamate with the final concentration of 1 mg/mL. When these spiked samples were applied to Oratect drug-screen devices, the results were all negative.

8. ORATECTPLUS™: EXPANSION TO TEST FOR ALCOHOL

By incorporating into the Oratect device a dry reagent pad that accommodates the enzymatic reaction of alcohol oxidase and peroxidase, simultaneous determination of abused drugs and alcohol can be undertaken. This new configuration (Fig. 3), called the OratectPlus™ (9), uses the same procedure as the regular Oratect device except that the alcohol pad is read 2 min after the pink-purple flow appears in the test windows. The reported cut-off level was 0.04% blood-alcohol concentration, and the OratectPlus test results correlated well with an onsite alcohol test—AlcoScreen™ (Chematics, Inc. North Webster, IN).

9. CONCLUSIONS

The Oratect device has a simple design and an easy procedure for collection, testing, and confirmation sampling. Data presented here suggest that it

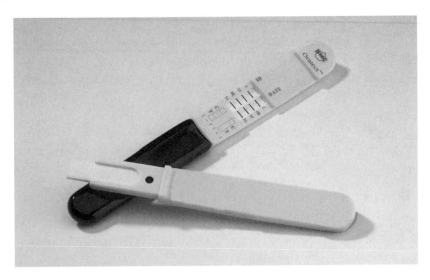

Fig. 3. OratectPlus® detecting abused drug and alcohol simultaneously.

can perform well and is a viable alternative to urine drug screen. To further the utility of the Oratect device platform, an alcohol pad has been incorporated so that drugs and alcohol can be detected simultaneously with the device. Such a development would further expand the use of Oratect.

REFERENCES

1. Huestis MA and Cone EJ. Alternative testing matrices, in Drug Abuse Handbook (Karch SB, ed), CRC, Boca Raton, FL: 1998; 799–813.
2. Caplan Y and Goldberger B. Alternative specimens for workplace drug testing. J Anal Toxicol 2001;25:396–399.
3. Wong R. The current status of drug testing in the U.S. workforce. American Clinical Laboratory 2002;21, 21–23.
4. Mandatory Guidelines for Federal Workplace Drug Testing Programs, April 13, 2004 (69 FR 19644).
5. Wong B, Wong R, Fan P, and Tran M. Detection of abused drugs in oral fluid by an on-site one-step drug screen—Oratect™. Clin Chem 2003;49:A125.
6. Wong R, Wong B, and Tran C. Opiate time course study with Oratect™. Presented at the 41st International Meeting of the International Association of Forensic Toxicologists, Melbourne, November 2003.
7. Huestis MA and Cone EJ. Relationship of δ^9-tetrahydrocannabinol concentrations in oral fluid and plasma after controlled administration of smoked cannabis. J Anal Toxicol 2004;28:394–399.

8. Wong R, Wong B, Tran C, and Fan P. Detection of benzodiazepines by a one step onsite oral fluid rapid drug screen—Oratect™. Presented at the 41st International Meeting of the International Association of Forensic Toxicologists, Melbourne, 2003.

9. Wong R, Sook J, and Zolteck R. Alcohol testing by an onsite one-step oral fluid alcohol and drug combination test device—OratectPlus™. Presented at TIAFT/ SOFT Joint Congress, Washington, DC, September 2004.

Chapter 10

Saliva and Sweat Testing With Drugwipe®

A Review

Franz Aberl and Robert VanDine

SUMMARY

Drugwipe® (Securetec Detektions-Systeme AG) is a pen-size detector for illegal drugs in saliva, in sweat, and on surfaces. It was first launched in 1995 to support drug law-enforcement police in their operations against smuggling and dealing of contraband. In 1996 the US Office for National Drug Control Policy (ONDCP) tested Drugwipe for its accuracy, sensitivity, and specificity in detecting invisible traces of narcotics on surfaces *(1)*. Since then, Drugwipe has been included in the technology transfer program of ONDCP.

With the increasing interest in saliva and sweat testing on the part of traffic police, the Drugwipe device has been significantly improved over the years. Today, Drugwipe is available for the detection of cocaine, opiates, cannabinoids, benzodiazepines, and amphetamines/methamphetamines ("ecstasy"). Drugwipe can be used to test oral fluids or sweat samples, or to detect invisible traces of narcotics. Commercially available Drugwipes include single, twin, and five-panel configurations. Drugwipe is especially designed for on-site applications and combines easy and rapid sampling with fast analysis. Drugwipe is used widely in Germany as a routine sweat or saliva test for roadside screening for driving under the influence of drugs (DUID). In the current Roadside Testing Assessment (ROSITA) II project, Drugwipe is under evaluation as a saliva test. The basic technology for analysis is lateral-flow immunoassay (see Chapters 3–6).

This chapter will first describe the technological basis of Drugwipe, including its major technical features. The second part will cover the various evaluation studies that

From: *Forensic Science and Medicine: Drugs of Abuse: Body Fluid Testing*
Edited by R. C. Wong and H. Y. Tse © Humana Press Inc., Totowa, NJ

have been performed using Drugwipe under controlled and general field conditions. Some of the data are not yet published.

Drugwipe can detect various benzodiazepines to as low as 5 ng/mL, and Δ9-tetrahydrocannabinol (THC) can be detected at 30 ng/mL. These sensitivities are currently unique for point-of-collection oral fluid/sweat test kits. The second part of this paper summarizes various published and unpublished data from trials and studies under controlled and general field conditions. Based on 1763 cases, a statistical evaluation by traffic police in Germany shows that more than 97% of all positive Drugwipe sweat tests are confirmed with positive blood results.

1. TECHNICAL DESCRIPTION OF DRUGWIPE

The product concept of Drugwipe is guided by user and operational requirements of law-enforcement units around the world. The testing procedures are similar to a laboratory process and consist of sampling, sample transfer, sample preparation, analysis, and output of the result. All of these procedures are integrated into a single-unit device. The sampling step is based on wiping. Wiping is fast, easy, and requires very little cooperation of the person under evaluation. Optimal sample transfer is guaranteed by the geometric design of the device. The lateral-flow immunoassay is specifically optimized to analyze various sample materials for the native drug. The signal output is simply visual and unambiguous.

1.1. Design of the Device

Figure 1 shows the major components of Drugwipe. The wiping element is designed for the collection of various types of samples. The collection step itself consists of a sequence of wipes. This sequence differs from specimen to specimen and is standardized according to the type of specimen. Next, the sample is transferred to a lateral-flow immunoassay strip sitting inside the detection element. The design of the wiping and the detection element guarantees automatic and efficient sample transfer.

Analysis of the sample starts with dipping of the Drugwipe absorbent pad into a small container of tap water for 15 s. The water container is part of the Drugwipe device and holds the correct amount of water to properly develop the test result. A positive test result develops within 2 to 5 min in the readout window, in the form of one line on a single-parameter strip and two red lines on a double-parameter strip. The time depends on the concentration and the type of drug to be analyzed, with high concentrations showing results quicker than low concentrations. In addition, a single red line has to appear in the internal control region. The appearance of only a control line indicates a negative result, confirming the correct usage of the device and the absence of interfering substances. A positive test result is shown as a second red line in the read-

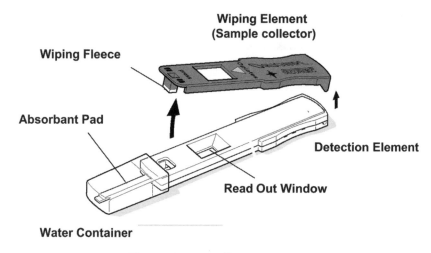

Fig. 1. Drugwipe® components.

out window. This form of presenting test results is unique in the area of lateral-flow assays for small molecules (e.g., drugs of abuse). The underlying principle is explained later.

1.2. Test Principle

Lateral-flow immunoassays utilize the recognition and binding capabilities of antibodies to differentiate between the presence and absence of a particular analyte. The detection limit is mainly influenced by the affinity of the selected antibodies for the target analyte. The Drugwipe immunoassay follows the general principles of other lateral-flow immunoassays for small molecules, with the major exception that a positive test result is correlated with the appearance of a test line. The Drugwipe lateral-flow immunoassay strip is schematically shown in Fig. 2.

Through the connection of the wiping element to the detection element, the sample medium (sweat, saliva) is automatically transferred into the sample application zone (area 2). This zone contains drug-specific antibodies coupled to colloidal gold particles. By means of the absorbent pad (area 1), water is drawn into the cassette and applied to the assay strip in a controlled process. The water supports the migration of the sample and the antibody conjugate along the strip. In the case of a sample containing drug molecules, the binding sites of the antibodies are saturated with the complementary hapten (drug) in the sample application zone. Downstream of the sample application zone, sample and antibody conjugate pass through a capture zone (area 3). This zone separates drug-saturated antibody-gold complexes from gold-antibody conjugates without the

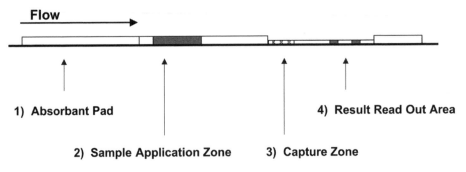

Fig. 2. Schematic drawing of the Drugwipe® lateral-flow immunoassay.

drug molecules. Only those gold conjugates that have been loaded with drug molecules are able to pass the capture zone and to migrate into the result readout area (area 4). In the result readout area, the gold conjugates are retained in a linear form on the strip in designated positions. Various design options for this area are possible. Figure 3 shows the test result for a five-panel Drugwipe test. The test is positive for all drugs.

1.3. Main Technical Features of the Drugwipe Device

Drugwipe provides detection capabilities for various drugs of abuse while maintaining maximum operational flexibility. Drugwipe is available in different test configurations:

- Single tests for cannabis, cocaine, opiates, amphetamines/methamphetamines, and benzodiazepines;
- Triple and twin test devices for amphetamines/methamphetamines/cannabis and cocaine/opiates;
- Five-panel device for cannabis, cocaine, opiates, amphetamines/methamphetamines (including "ecstasy").

Sweat or saliva samples can be analyzed according to the specimen available and operational needs. A sample volume of less than 10 µL is sufficient for analysis. The small sample volume is a critical feature for point-of-collection (POC) testing. A significant percentage of drug consumers abusing designer drugs or cannabis suffer from a dry-mouth syndrome and are not able to provide sufficient saliva for testing in conventional devices.

The cut-off values are identical for each test configuration and are given in Table 1.

All Drugwipe types are directed toward the native drugs that are the dominating compounds in sweat or saliva. The most sensitive assay is the Drugwipe

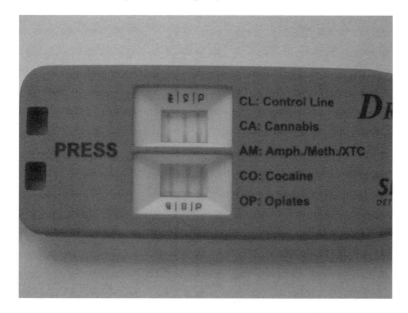

Fig. 3. A five-panel Drugwipe® test—positive for cannabis, amphetamines, methamphetamines, cocaine, and opiates.

test for benzodiazepines. Aminoflunitrazepam can be detected in oral fluid down to a concentration of 5 ng/mL. Characteristic of the amphetamine assay is its broad cross-reactivity, covering a range of five important amphetamines and methamphetamines.

1.4. Collection of Saliva Samples

Salivary glands continuously secrete a mucous, colorless fluid into the mouth. The composition of saliva is determined by the composition of the blood plasma and the physico-chemical properties of the plasma compounds. Drugs of abuse are excreted in higher or lower concentrations than present in plasma.

When testing with Drugwipe, saliva is taken from inside the cheek or directly from the tongue. The wiping fleece is firmly wiped three times over the mucus membrane on each side. The saliva volume is defined by the void volume of the wiping fleece.

1.5. Collection of Sweat Samples

Sweating is described as a continuous excretion of water and small molecules through the skin. Sweat is produced as the body's response to exercise

Table 1
Drugwipe® Cut-Off Values

		Cut-off in ng/mL
Cannabis	Δ-9-tetrahydrocannabinol	30
Cocaine	Cocaine	50
Opiates	Heroin	20
	Morphine	20
Amphetamines	d-Amphetamine	200
	Methylenedioxymethamphetamine	100
	d-Methamphetamine	100
	Methylenedioxyampthetamine	100
	Methylenedioxyethamphetamine	500
Benzodiazepines	Aminoflunitazepam	5
	Flunitrazepam	10
	Nitrazepam	10
	Temazepam	10
	Diazepam	10

or thermal stress. The water evaporates and low-volatile compounds like drugs
of abuse remain on the skin for a limited time. Sweat samples can be taken
from various parts of the body surface. The forehead is a compromise among
excretion characteristics, accessibility, and contamination risk. In earlier studies, Drugwipe was used to collect sweat from the armpit, but this sampling
location has operational disadvantages.

1.6. The Drugwipe Reader

A laptop-/palmtop-controlled reader is available for recording of the
Drugwipe result in an electronic format. Figure 4 is a picture of the reader,
which is marketed under the brand name DrugRead® (Securetec). DrugRead
is advantageous under poor light conditions or when the Drugwipe result
must be obtained independent of a visual interpretation. A further benefit is
that all test data are stored on a hard disk and can be further processed (e.g.,
mathematically interpreted) or printed. Calibration curves for the different
target drugs can be implemented and used to correlate the Drugwipe signal
with certain drug quantities. An example for a correlation curve is given in
Fig. 5.

The individual points in the calibration curve are mean values of 10 single
measurements. Drugwipe starts to show positive signals between 20 and 30 ng
of Δ-9-THC per mL of saliva.

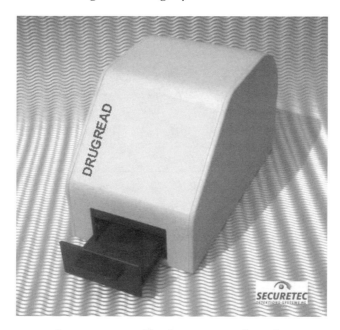

Fig. 4. DrugRead®—the Drugwipe® reader.

2. DRUGWIPE AS A SALIVA TEST

2.1. Roadside Drug Testing Assessment (ROSITA II): Confirmation of the Drugwipe Cut-Off Values (2,3)

In 2003, the Office of National Drug Control Policy (ONDCP) and the National Highway Traffic Safety Administration (NHTSA) sponsored an initial comparative laboratory evaluation of eight commercially available oral-fluid testing devices. Under supervision of the Walsh Group (TWG), the Center for Human Toxicology (CHT) of the University of Utah conducted the analytical evaluation at their laboratories in Salt Lake City, UT.

Human oral fluid was collected from drug-free individuals, pooled, and purified by freezing, thawing, and centrifugation. Standard solutions were prepared through the addition of known amounts of drugs to the purified saliva. The fortified solutions were assayed by gas chromatography (GC)-mass spectrometry (MS) or liquid chromatography (LC)-MS for the quantitative levels of spiked drugs. Drug-free saliva was used as negative control.

In the case of Drugwipe, 10 µL of each drug-saliva solution was added to the wiping fleece and the test was performed as described in the instructions for use *(4)*. The negative control experiments were repeated five times, and spiked

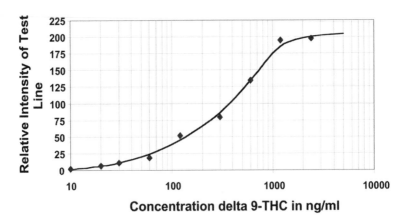

Fig. 5. DrugRead® calibration curve for Drugwipe® Cannabis. The relative intensity of the test line shown is dependent on the concentration of Δ9-tetrahydrocannabinol.

(positive) saliva samples were tested 10 times. The applied concentrations of drugs were selected in such a way that the cut-off values of Drugwipe were challenged. Three concentration levels of each drug were applied.

The Drugwipe evaluation results are summarized in Table 2.

For each Drugwipe type, the official Drugwipe cut-off level is also given in Table 2. The percentage of correct results represents the proportion of Drugwipe data that correctly identifies control vs drug-spiked samples. Drug-free and fortified saliva samples with drug concentrations below the official cut-off level of the device were scored as negatives. Saliva samples with drug concentrations above the cut-off level were expected positives. At the time of evaluation, the Drugwipe amphetamines testing device did detected the100-ng/mL concentration with low signal intensity. After this evaluation campaign, the manufacturer of Drugwipe lowered the official cut-off level for amphetamines to 200 µg/mL.

Overall, Drugwipe was 90% accurate in identifying positive saliva samples with drug concentrations above the cut-off levels and 100% accurate in identifying negative saliva samples without or spiked with drug concentrations below the cut-off levels. In this study, Drugwipe was the only instrument-free device that performed according to the specifications and was able to detect THC concentrations at the 50 ng/mL level. The 30 ng/mL level (THC cut-off) was not challenged. THC is the most prevalent drug in the driving population, and a low cut-off for THC is critical for roadside applications.

Table 2
Independent Evaluation of the Drugwipe® Cut-Off Values With Spiked Saliva Samples

Drugwipe type	Cannabis		Amphetamines		Methamphetamines		Cocaine		Opiates	
Cut-off value in ng/mL	30		200		100		50		20	
	Conc. in ng/mL	Correct results in %	Conc. in ng/mL	Correct results in %	Conc. in ng/mL	Correct results in %	Conc. in ng/mL	Correct results in %	Conc. in ng/mL	Correct results in %
Negative saliva	0	100	0	10	0	100	0	100	0	10
Positive saliva										
Level I	20	100	25	100	25	100	10	100	20	40
Level II	50	100	100	100*	100	100	40	100	100	90
Level III	100	100	500	100	500	100	200	100	500	100

*See text for explanation.

169

2.2. Testing Saliva With Drugwipe/Drugread: A Controlled Study With Methylenedioxymethamphetamine (5)

In 1999, the Instituto Municipal d'Investigació Mèdica (IMIM) in Barcelona, Spain, performed a controlled, double-blinded study with methylenedioxymethamphetamine (MDMA; "ecstasy") and eight volunteers. Each subject was orally administered a single dose of 100 mg MDMA or placebo. At time zero (0, predose) and at 1.5, 4, 6, 10, and 24 h after MDMA administration, a sample of saliva (1–2 mL) was collected by spitting into a plastic tube and immediately stored at –20°C. Samples were analyzed for MDMA and metabolites by GC-MS. In this study, 2 µL of each saliva sample were applied to the wiping fleece of Drugwipe Amphetamines (test kit for amphetamines), and the test was performed according to the instructions for use. Drugwipe results were measured with the DrugRead device and compared with the MDMA concentrations determined by GC-MS.

Figure 6 shows the concentration curve of MDMA in the saliva of one of the volunteers after oral administration of 100 mg of MDMA. The maximum in the concentration curve is reached after approx 2 h. The concentration of MDMA in saliva at this point is more than 3000 ng/mL. The window of detection with GC-MS is at least 24 h. The window of detection with Drugwipe/DrugRead is approx 10 to 12 h and can be adjusted by changing the cut-off value of the Drugwipe/DrugRead system. All subjects showed a similar concentration curve in saliva, and Drugwipe gave a positive result for all volunteers at 1.5 and 4 h after drug administration. After 6 h, only one out of eight subjects gave a negative result. This subject showed the lowest MDMA concentrations among all the volunteers at that time. At 10 h after MDMA administration, it was still possible to detect consumption in five of the eight subjects. For the three subjects who had negative test results, the concentrations of MDMA in their saliva as determined by GC-MS were below the cut-off levels of the Drugwipe device. At 24 h, no positive results were reported.

The concentration curve of the Drugwipe/DrugRead system correlated well with the concentration curve measured with GC-MS. Provided that the sample volume is thoroughly controlled and the Drugwipe/DrugRead system is calibrated to a specific drug, quantitative measurements can be performed. The apparent slower disappearance rate in the DrugRead signal was probably due more to a saturation effect in the Drugwipe test than to the contribution of MDMA metabolites. In fact, MDMA was reported as the principal analyte that could be detected in saliva, while its principal metabolites were found only in minute amounts. Overall, the Drugwipe/DrugRead system not only detects consumption but also recent use of MDMA.

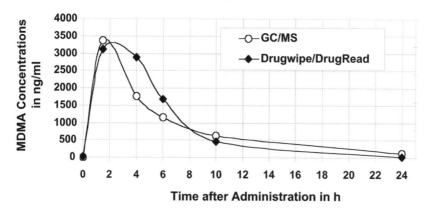

Fig. 6. Concentration curve of methylenedioxymethamphetamine (MDMA) in saliva measured with gas chromatography-mass spectrometry and with Drugwipe®/DrugRead® after a controlled oral administration of 100 mg MDMA.

2.3. Drugwipe Amphetamines: Sweat vs Saliva in a Driver Population

In the winter of 2003, Drugwipe Amphetamine was evaluated by the Institute for Legal Medicine at the University of Munich, Germany, for sensitivity, specificity, and accuracy. Traffic police in Munich selected drivers from the street who were suspected of DUID. Drivers were brought to the Institute for Legal Medicine for blood samples. At the same time, sweat from the forehead and from inside the palm, as well as saliva, were collected with the Drugwipe device. All Drugwipe tests were administered on a voluntary basis. All volunteers were tested three times (one saliva test and two sweat tests). In the final analysis, Drugwipe test results were correlated to those of the blood samples.

Table 3 summarizes the results of this comparative study with Drugwipe Amphetamines. *Accuracy* in the context of this study describes how reliable Drugwipe Amphetamines is in predicting the blood results of a suspected driver. *Sensitivity* refers to the percentage of positive blood samples, and *specificity* the percentage of negative blood samples corrected identified by Drugwipe. Between 76 and 80 persons were tested with Drugwipe and approx 30% were tested positive in the blood for amphetamines or ecstasy. Seventy percent were amphetamine free. The accuracy of Drugwipe Amphetamines was in the range of 92 to 97% depending on the specimen and the sampling location on the body. Specificity ranged between 89 and 96%, whereas sensitivity was always 100%. It was also noted that the best accuracy and specificity were achieved with sweat samples from inside the palm of the hand. Saliva samples and sweat

Table 3
Accuracy, Sensitivity, and Specificity of the Drugwipe® Results
in Relation to the Blood Status of Drivers Suspected
for Driving Under the Influence of Drugs

Specimen	Sampling location	Accuracy	Sensitivity	Specificity	Number of cases
Sweat/skin	Forehead	92%	100%	89%	80
	Inside the palm	97%	100%	96%	76
Saliva	Tongue	94%	10%	91%	78

taken from the forehead were comparable with each other in terms of accuracy and specificity but were obviously not as good as palm sweat. It appears that contaminants on the hand have no major influence on assay accuracy.

The findings of this study are in contrast with the work of other researchers, who claim that sweat is of less value for the detection of recent drug use. In this study, testing of sweat has been shown to be comparable to saliva testing in terms of assay accuracy, specificity, and sensitivity.

3. DRUGWIPE AS A SWEAT TEST

3.1. A Controlled Study With MDMA (6)

In this study, two male volunteers were given a single dose of 100 mg MDMA. MDMA was administered orally with 100 mL of tap water (two capsules each time). Subjects were swabbed in their armpit for 10 s at time zero (0, predose) and at 2, 6, 8, 12, 24, 36, and 48 h after MDMA administration. The sweat sample was collected with the wiping fleece of the test kit for amphetamines. The wiping fleece was moistened with tap water. The analysis of the sweat sample was performed in accordance with the instructions for use (3). Blood samples from the volunteers were also taken at 0 (predose), 2, 4, 6, 8, 12, and 24 h after drug administration. Blood was immediately centrifuged, and plasma was stored at −20°C until analysis. The plasma was analyzed for the presence of MDMA by GC-MS (6).

The major experimental findings with respect to the performance of Drugwipe are summarized in Fig. 7. The concentration curve shown in the diagram is the mean plasma concentration of both volunteers. The individual curves are only slightly different, and the data are published in Pacifici et al. (6). The maximum mean value was reached after 4 h and was approx 150 ng/mL. Drug-

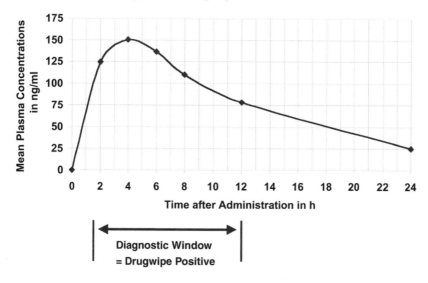

Fig 7. Mean plasma concentrations of two volunteers after administration of 100 mg of methylenedioxymethamphetamine (MDMA). The time window where Drugwipe® was positive is indicated as "diagnostic window."

wipe test results were positive between 2 and 12 h after drug administration. Later measurements were negative. It is notable that the 2-h time point corresponds to the time of maximal physiological and psychomotoric effects of MDMA. These effects last for at least 6 h unless there is a repeated administration. The results of this pilot study support sweat testing with Drugwipe for monitoring MDMA use in the early hours following drug administration.

3.2. Roadside Trial Study and Field Operation in Germany (7,8)

In 1998, the German government extended existing traffic regulations to include testing for drugs of abuse. Following these legislative changes, traffic police in Germany undertook an evaluation of Drugwipe as a sweat test for roadside applications. Selected traffic police units were equipped with and trained in the application of Drugwipe. At the same time, police officers were also trained in the recognition of driving impairments as an initial screen for drivers under the influence of drugs. Suspected drivers were subjected to Drugwipe sweat testing. Blood samples were also taken as the standard for comparison. All blood samples were analyzed with GC-MS.

Within the time frame of the trial, 96 individuals were tested for the following drugs: cocaine, opiates, and amphetamines/methamphetamines. Drugwipe detected 62 positive cases, whereas GC-MS test results from the blood

Table 4
Comparison of Drugwipe® Sweat Results With Gas Chromatography-Mass Spectrometry Blood Result in Roadside Testing

Drugwipe type	Cocaine	Opiates	Amphetamines	Total
Confirmed positives	5	8	45	58
Confirmed negatives	12	5	4	31
Unconfirmed positives	1	0	3	4
Unconfirmed negatives	1	2	0	3

samples indicated that 58 were positive. Of the 34 negatives indicated by Drugwipe, 31 were confirmed negatives by blood analysis. Table 4 shows a breakdown of the data for the three drugs tested. Because blood was the only reference specimen, Drugwipe results were grouped into confirmed or unconfirmed positives and negatives. Overall accuracy was 93%, diagnostic sensitivity 95%, and specificity 89%. The positive predictive value is 94%. Discrepancies between Drugwipe results and the results of the blood analysis could be a result of differential pharmacological distribution of drugs in sweat and blood. During the first 30 to 90 min, there is a diagnostic window in which drug concentrations present on the skin are not yet above the cut-off values detectable by Drugwipe. In general, the concentration curve for drugs in sweat tends to shift towards a longer time window indicating a longer distribution period. The findings of this field trial, together with previous laboratory studies under controlled conditions, clearly confirm the usefulness of Drugwipe as a sweat test for roadside operations.

As a result of this field trial, the majority of the German states have since introduced Drugwipe as a sweat test for routine roadside screening for DUID. Sweat testing is favored over that of saliva because it is less invasive and more hygienic, and can even be performed without cooperation of the driver suspects. Table 5 summarizes the overall data of a 6-mo field operation in Nordrhein-Westfahlen *(8)* starting in the summer of 2003. Of 1763 tests, accuracy and predictive values of Drugwipe ranged between 93 and 97%. In this operation, field officers were extensively trained in impairment recognition as well as general metabolic patterns of different drugs in different human testing specimens. Through this training, the police officers developed a thorough understanding of the advantages and disadvantages of various body fluids for roadside testing and the importance of their observations during the testing process.

Table 5
Overall Accuracy and Positive Predictive Values
for Drugwipe® Under Field Conditions

	Cannabis	Opiates	Amph./ methamph.	Cocaine	Total number
Quantity of Drugwipes used	950	220	445	148	1763
No. of Drugwipe tests positive in sweat	359	83	168	78	688
No. of tests not confirmed in blood	27	2	13	8	50
Overall accuracy	97%	99%	97%	95%	97%
Positive predictive value	92%	97%	92%	90%	93%

ACKNOWLEDGMENTS

Securetec greatly acknowledges the cooperation of the traffic police in Germany, especially in Baden-Würtemberg and Nordrhein-Westfahlen. A special thanks to the Institute for Legal Medicine in Munich (Dr. Hans Sachs and Dr. Santjohanser) for testing and scientific discussions.

REFERENCES

1. Report No. NDTA96-002A, Report on the Drugwipe evaluation study, ONDCP/ CTAC, 1966.
2. Walsh JM, Flegel R, Crouch DJ, Cangianelli L, and Baudys J. An evaluation of rapid point-of-collection oral fluid drug-testing devices. J Anal Toxicol 2003;27 (7):429–439.
3. Crouch DJ, Walsh JM, Flegel R, Cangianelli L, Baudys J, and Adkins R. An evaluation of selected rapid oral fluid point-of-collection drug-testing devices. J Anal Toxicol, submitted.
4. Securetec AG, Drugwipe—Instructions for Use, 2004.
5. Pichini S, Navarro M, Farré M, et al. On-site testing of MDMA ("Ecstasy") in saliva with Drugwipe® and Drugread®: a controlled study in recreational users. Clin Chem 2002;48(1):174–176.
6. Pacifici R, Farré M, Pichini S, et al. Sweat testing of MDMA with the Drugwipe analytical device: a controlled study with two volunteers. J Anal Toxicol 2001;25: 144–146.
7. Landespolizeidirektion Stuttgart I, in cooperation with the Institute for Legal Medicine, Munich. Internal Evaluation Report on the Performance of Drugwipe for Cannabis, Amphetamines, Opiates and Cocaine for Roadside Testing, Stuttgart, 1998.
8. Innenministerium Nordrhein-Westfahlen. Internal Evaluation Report on the Drugwipe: Results during the Introduction Period, 2004.

Chapter 11

Hair Analysis in Drugs-of-Abuse Testing

Michael I. Schaffer and Virginia A. Hill

SUMMARY

Compounds trapped in hair during growth collect and remain in the mature hair strand. Defined lengths of the hair strand can be analyzed to provide information on ingestion of a substance during the window of time corresponding to the growth period of the segment of hair analyzed. Both screening (immunoassay) and confirmation (liquid chromatography-tandem mass spectrometry, gas chromatography-mass spectrometry, gass chromatography-tandem mass spectrometry) methods for drugs in hair require methods of liquefaction and/or extraction of the solid hair fiber. Extensive washing of hair samples to remove external contamination and/or drugs from sweat prior to analysis is integral to a meaningful hair result, particularly to distinguish use from contamination and to utilize the hair's ability to reflect dose. Some results of drugs-of-abuse analysis in washed hair of proven drug users ranged (in ng/10 mg hair) from the cut-offs to 2270 (cocaine), 559 (morphine), 79 (methamphetamine), and 150 (phencyclidine). The metabolite of cannabis use, carboxy-tetrahydrocannabinol, was present in users' hair samples in amounts up to 76 pg/10 mg hair. Hair analysis for drugs of abuse is most widely used for pre-employment and workplace testing, but has also shown utility in criminal justice settings, for diagnostic and monitoring purposes in rehabilitation programs, in determining prenatal drug exposure, and other arenas.

1. INTRODUCTION

Over the past 25 yr, analysis of hair to examine retrospectively a subject's drug ingestion has become an accepted and even routine procedure. This

From: *Forensic Science and Medicine: Drugs of Abuse: Body Fluid Testing*
Edited by R. C. Wong and H. Y. Tse © Humana Press Inc., Totowa, NJ

acceptance is reflected in a bibliography of publications that includes over 750 citations worldwide from 1984 to 2002 *(1)*. Although the most common use of hair testing in the United States may be workplace testing, especially pre-employment testing for drugs of abuse, other applications include maternal prenatal testing, post-partum testing, epidemiology, criminal justice, drug reha-bilitation, and anthropological studies *(2)*.

Hair analysis is unique in that it contains retrospective information, as compared with point-in-time information provided by other body fluids or tis-sues. This stems from the unique property that trace amounts of a substance from blood circulation can be trapped in a segment of hair as it develops in the hair follicle—that is, once a hair segment emerges from the follicle and becomes keratinized, it carries with it the substance it has trapped in the hair follicle. This trapping allows analysis of a sample that may be of a few months' growth to detect ingestion of a substance back in time when this hair segment was still growing in the follicle *(3)*. In addition, relative to urine in workplace testing, hair has the advantages of ease of collection, the capacity for full obser-vation over the course of the process, and fewer privacy issues. Handling, ship-ping, and storage of samples require no special packaging, preservatives, or refrigeration. Whereas a urine or blood sample represents a single point in time that can never be re-sampled, a second hair sample taken some days later can produce results similar to the first. Furthermore, hair is not amenable to adul-teration, a common problem with urine.

With its inclusion in the 2004 Proposed Federal Workplace Testing Guide-lines *(4)*, hair testing has achieved recognition as a valid matrix for monitoring use of drugs of abuse. Advances have been made in many aspects of hair analy-sis, such as the mechanisms of substance incorporation, methods of dissolving and/or extracting substances from hair, and technologies for quick screening of large numbers of samples for the presence of substances. Improvement has also been made in chromatographic/mass spectrometric identification and quantita-tion of drugs at ever lower levels. It is also possible to distinguish external con-tamination from metabolically deposited drug.

2. HAIR STRUCTURE AND MECHANISMS OF DRUG INCORPORATION

Hair follicles are surrounded by a dense network of capillaries, which nourish the rapidly growing hair follicles and moderate body temperature. A hair strand consists of a root or bulb, which lies below the surface of the skin, and a keratinized hair shaft, which projects above the skin surface *(43)*. Drugs and their metabolites present in blood circulation diffuse into rapidly growing hair follicles during histogenesis, and are deposited into the hair follicle in keratin structures called microfibrils. Microfibrils are bundled and predominate in the cortex of the hair structure, surrounded by the cuticle. There are three phases of hair growth: anagen, the growth phase; catagen, the resting or transition stage; and telogen, the phase where the hair is readied for removal from the surface of the skin. This is followed by a return to anagen or active growth phase, during which time the dermal papilla forms the hair matrix, resulting in new hair growth. Hair growth rates differ at various body sites; in brief, head hair taken at the vertex grows about 0.51 in per month. Hair from the axilla grows at an average rate of 0.31 in per month, chest hair at an average of 0.47 in per month, and beard hair at an average rate of 0.31 in per month *(5)*. These variations, in addition to dormancy periods, may become significant when interpreting hair analysis results as they relate to a time period of drug use *(3,5)*.

3. COLLECTION AND HANDLING OF HAIR SAMPLES

When appropriate, as in all forensic testing including workplace drug testing, a hair sample is collected under a chain of custody. The preferred sample is one taken from the posterior vertex of the head, an anatomical site where the majority of the hair population is in the anagen growth phase, with fewer dormant hairs. Normally, the sample is cut with scissors, as close to the skin as possible. A sufficient sample is usually about 50 mg (about the thickness of a shoe-lace tip), depending on the capabilities of the laboratory. The sample is placed in a collection device with the root end identified. If desired, the collection procedure can be viewed by the donor using a mirror. In the laboratory, the strand of hair is cut to a desired length and the segment of interest weighed, as hair results are expressed as mass of drug per weight of hair.

Making a liquid sample of a hair specimen is a primary challenge of hair analysis. Three main approaches to sample preparation for screening assays as well as for chromatographic/mass spectrometric analyses have been described and are currently in use in hair-testing laboratories: enzymatic digestion *(6–8)*, treatment with acid *(9)* or strong base *(9–11)*, and organic solvent extraction, most often with methanol *(8,9,12)*. Enzymatic digestion has the advantages of dissolving the sample, releasing all of the drug from the hair, and allowing the melanin fraction to be removed by centrifugation. A solvent extraction method, if it is to be reliable, must be tested for equivalent efficiency and completeness, or at least for uniform results among different samples. This is especially critical at lower levels of drug, where incomplete extraction may result in misidentifying a sample containing drug as negative simply because the drug was not extracted.

4. PRELIMINARY SCREENING ASSAYS FOR DRUGS OF ABUSE IN HAIR

Performing a preliminary screening test is a practical necessity for laboratories that process a large volume of hair samples. In workplace testing, a confirmation test is initiated only after a positive screening test. Although instrumental methods such as ion spray liquid chromatography (LC)-tandem mass spectrometry (MS-MS) *(13)* and gas chromatography (GC)-mass spectrometry (MS)-electron ionization (EI) *(14,15)* have been utilized to test for a number of analytes simultaneously, immunoassays such as radioimmunoassay (RIA) or enzyme immunoassay (EIA) are the modality most amenable to high-volume screening *(16–21)*. The challenges of developing an immunoassay for hair samples involve solubilizing or extracting the samples, achieving the level of sensitivity required, managing possible matrix effects (nonspecific interference which, if unchecked, could cause both false-negatives and -positives), and minimizing cross-reactivities. All of these components will impact the sensitivity and specificity, precision, and accuracy of the test.

Analysis for the presence of the drug opiates in hair was performed using RIA as early as 1979 *(22)*. This was followed soon after with tests for phencyclidine (PCP) *(23)* and cocaine *(24)*. In fact, it was the availability of RIA as an ultrasensitive analytical tool that initially prompted the pioneering testing of drugs in hair. As enzyme immunoassays develop greater sensitivity, nonradioactive immunoassays are increasingly being used for hair testing. A review of the immunological methods for testing drugs in hair from the early period to the year 2000 has been presented by Spiehler *(25)*. MS confirmation methods took a few additional years to achieve the necessary sensitivities.

4.1. The Analytical Goal of a Drug-Screening Assay

The goal of a drugs-of-abuse screening immunoassay is simpler than that of a clinical assay, which must accurately quantify normal serum components or abnormal markers over a range of concentrations. In forensic drug testing, there is usually just one standard reference, which contains the cut-off concentration of drug. Samples containing less than the cut-off drug concentration are considered negative, with no further testing required. Certain issues, such as cross-reactivity with related drugs or metabolites, which would produce unacceptable error in diagnostic clinical assays, are tolerable for workplace or other forensic screening because a second and more specific confirmatory test will be performed on the sample.

In an immunoassay, the essential aspects of sensitivity, precision, and accuracy are all hinged on the absence or control of sample-matrix effects. Sample-matrix effects are related to (1) the nature of the antibody, (2) the precision of the signal measurement, and (3) the level of nonspecific binding. Because hair-testing laboratories often purchase well-characterized immunoassay kits from vendors, the selection of the antibody is usually not a factor. The job of the laboratory is to optimize the composition and amount of sample so that interference resulting from matrix and sample variability is minimized and accounted for. It is also important that the cut-off concentration be in the optimal response region of the assay. It should be noted that current US Food and Drug Administration (FDA) regulations require that testing intended for use outside of a medical setting (e.g., in the home, sports, or workplace) must use assays that have been cleared, approved, or otherwise recognized by the FDA as accurate and reliable for the specimen being tested (21 CFR 809; 21 CFR 864.326).

4.2. Sample Preparation and Matrix Effects

As discussed earlier, preparing a liquid sample of a hair specimen is the first step in hair analysis. Enzymatic digestion of samples for testing in biological assays, coupled with RIA assays of the hair digests for the drugs cocaine, opiates, PCP, methamphetamine/methylenedioxymethamphetamine (MDMA), and cannabinoids, have been cleared by the FDA and used by this laboratory since 1985 *(7,21)*.

Although solvent extraction methods might be expected to produce a sample more amenable to immunoassay than the digestion method, these methods can present serious challenges. A solvent extract of a hair sample will not contain keratin, for example, but it will contain a significant and likely variable amount of lipid. When the solvent is evaporated, which it must be because only a small amount is tolerated in any immunoassay, the lipid is left to be partially solubilized or suspended in an aqueous medium added to the dried extracts. Detergents can be added to the extract to aid in the solubilization of the lipid, but this must be carefully monitored and controlled to avoid damaging the antibodies or enzymes in the subsequent immunoassay. Too much detergent can affect primary or secondary antibody binding, or can cause detachment of antibody bound to solid phase such as in microtiter wells. Variations in amounts of lipid among different hair samples, and in micelle formation when reconstituting samples in aqueous medium, can cause great variability among negative samples. Such reconstitution issues can even cause large variability among replicate samples of the same hair specimen. Nonspecific matrix problems such as these can be a serious limitation to solvent extraction in achieving the analytical goals of the screening test, because they impact precision, accuracy, and sensitivity.

As an illustration of the matrix effects in an assay of enzymatically digested samples, Fig. 1 shows the distribution of a population of 100 different

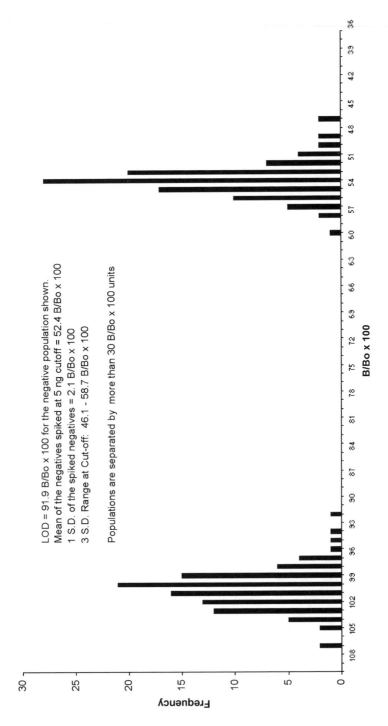

Fig. 1. Matrix effects among different samples and their impact on precision at the cutoff concentration in a screening assay for cocaine in hair.

LOD = 91.9 B/Bo x 100 for the negative population shown.
Mean of the negatives spiked at 5 ng cutoff = 52.4 B/Bo x 100
1 S.D. of the spiked negatives = 2.1 B/Bo x 100
3 S.D. Range at Cut-off: 46.1 - 58.7 B/Bo x 100

Populations are separated by more than 30 B/Bo x 100 units

Table 1
Intra-Assay Precision of a Radioimmunoassay (RIA) for Cocaine

% of Cutoff Concentrations	0	Minus 50	Minus 25	100	Plus 25	Plus 50
Cocaine (ng/10 mg hair)	Zero	2.5	3.75	5.0	6.25	7.5
RIA Response (% B/Bo)						
Mean	98.40	74.83	67.08	60.28	53.85	49.49
S.D.	1.74	1.18	1.88	1.31	0.99	0.98
%C.V.	1.8	1.6	2.8	2.2	1.8	2.0

hair samples with no drug and with drug at the cut-off concentration in a cocaine RIA used in the authors' laboratory. The distribution of 100 negatives is shown in the histogram nearest the y-axis, and the distribution of these same negatives spiked with cocaine at the cut-off concentration is shown to the right in the figure. If there is a great variability in the responses of the negative samples (termed the B_0, which is the amount of binding in the absence of nonradioactive drug), this variability will likely also occur at the cut-off, creating greater uncertainty in the correct identification of samples containing the cut-off concentration of cocaine. In this assay, the mean of the negatives shown was 99.1% B/B_0, with a standard deviation (SD) of 2.4. (% B/B_0 is the response of the unknown divided by the negative or B_0 reference, expressed as a percent). The spread of such a population of samples is a result not just of matrix effects, but also of the many factors that affect precision. One can estimate the contribution of matrix differences among different samples to this spread by comparing the precision of replicates of the same sample at zero and at the cut-off concentration of drug. In this case, the mean of 20 replicates of the same negative sample had a mean of 98.4% B/B_0 and a SD of 1.74 (Table 1), indicating that the matrix effects were quite small, because the precision among the 20 replicates of the same samples had nearly the same amount of error.

Figure 1 also illustrates another desirable feature of a screening assay (i.e., a clear separation between the negative population and the population at or beyond the cut-off). In this example, the lower edge of the negative 3 SD distribution of the zero-drug samples is a full 30% B/B_0 units above the upper edge of the 3 SD distribution of the samples at the cut-off. Note that at the cut-off there will always be one-half of the samples falling above and one-half falling below the cut-off. A sizable separation between the negatives (zero drug) and the cut-off must not be achieved, however, at the expense of operating in the optimal region of the assay. An assay usually has a working range for quantitation purposes of one to two orders of magnitude at best, with the optimum precision in the steeper part of the curve (in the case of a competitive RIA or EIA). Although assays using only a cut-off calibrator do not require a full dose-response curve, knowing the nature of such a curve is helpful in determining the optimum point for the cut-off. Placement of the cut-off in the most linear region of the curve facilitates achieving maximal precision at the cut-off and at points 25% and 50% above and below the cut-off.

Achieving acceptable statistical precision for samples containing drug at ±25% and ±50% of the cut-off has been a challenge for hair-screening assays. Controlling matrix effects, especially at the levels of sensitivity required, is likely the largest single factor in doing so.

5. ENVIRONMENTAL CONTAMINATION, WASHING, AND METABOLITE PRESENCE

Although there are circumstances in which the mere presence of a drug on the surface of the hair may provide significant information, the vast majority of situations require that external drug contamination be distinguished from presence of drug due to use. These environmental issues involve passive exposure of the hair surface to dust, aerosols, smoke, or powders. Although drugs in a subject's sweat may also deposit onto the hair, only a subject who uses drugs is likely to have drug-containing sweat, and thus sweat may affect quantitation but is less likely to cause an erroneous qualitative (i.e., false-positive) conclusions. This is not to imply that the need for removing sweat by washing is unimportant—in fact, its importance will be discussed further under Subheading 6. Removal of contamination has been attempted by various means, including multiple washes with organic and aqueous phases for various periods of time. For example, Koren *(26)* used extended washes with ethanol and was able to remove from hair all contamination due to cocaine free-base vapors. Wang et al. *(27)* were unable to remove cocaine contamination from hair using three 1-min methanol washes; their work was re-investigated and compared to extensive aqueous washing by Schaffer et al. *(28)*. Marsh et al. *(29)* compared three methods for removal of contaminating methadone on hair: four 15-min methanol washes at 37°C, two 15-min acetone washes followed by two water washes, and three 15-min washes with 1% dodecyl sulphate at 37°C followed by two water washes. The latter authors found, in most cases, greater than 90% removal of contaminating drug. Although adequate washing procedures can usually remove most contaminating drug *(2,30,31)*, it is critical also to identify those samples that may still exceed the cut-off as a result of the small percentage of contaminating drug that may not have been removed by the wash procedures. In the authors' laboratory, a very extensive wash schema includes 3.75 h of washing, and subsequent testing and evaluation of the last wash to better assess the effectiveness of the process. In this process the hair is washed at 37°C for 15 min in dry isopropanol to remove greasy contamination and loosely adhering drugs from the surface of the hair. This is then followed by three subsequent 30-min and two 60-min washes with phosphate buffer containing 0.1% bovine serum albumin (BSA), with all the washing done at 37°C and with vigorous shaking. From analysis of the last wash for cocaine, opiates, amphetamines, or PCP, the amount of drug in the last wash relative to the amount of drug remaining in the hair is used to calculate a wash criterion to distinguish between drug use and contamination *(31)*.

The necessity of an effective wash procedure, validated by testing on contaminated specimens and known positives, is generally recognized as a necessary precaution in determining drug use. Some laboratories, however, may attempt to skirt the requirement by reporting results indicating only the presence of drug, without interpretation regarding evidence of use, or relying on the presence of metabolites to indicate use. The presence of metabolites in the sample can sometimes constitute evidence of use in spite of contamination issues; however, without effective washing, this is true only if the metabolite is formed exclusively in vivo and is not found in the source or parent drug. For example, benzoylecgonine (BE), cocaethylene (CE), and norcocaine are all metabolites of cocaine, but only cocaethylene is a definitive marker of use, because it is formed only by simultaneous ingestion of cocaine and ethanol. An effective wash coupled with a metabolite profile and a judicious cutoff level are the requirements of an appropriately conservative approach to drug testing. Studies using extensive wash procedures have demonstrated that even in extreme exposure scenarios such as undercover narcotic officer's hair exposed directly to cocaine vapor and persons exposed in the room with users, contamination can still be distinguished from ingestion *(26,32)*.

6. THE INFLUENCES OF HAIR COLOR IN HAIR ANALYSIS

In spite of the serious flaws in studies purporting to indicate a color bias in hair analysis, the suggestion of such a bias in hair testing continues to receive attention. Some of the limitations in such studies are:

- Failing to adequately wash the hair before extraction to remove sweat and contamination as the source of the measured drug *(33–40)*;
- Extracting hair with sodium hydroxide (NaOH), a method that could never be used for workplace samples because it hydrolyzes 6-monoacetylmorphine and cocaine *(33–35,38,39)*;
- Use of in vitro models that mimic soaking/contamination but are not valid models of in vivo incorporation into the growing hair fiber within the hair follicle *(33,36,37)*;
- Use of animal models, which may not accurately reflect transport and biotransformation processes that occur in humans *(33,38–40)*;

- Extremely small data sets with low statistical significances *(41,42)*;
- Failure to use extraction methods that fully extract the drug from the hair matrix *(9,43)*;
- Failure to use a method that can exclude melanin from the extraction process itself *(34–41)*.

As pointed out earlier, an efficient extraction method, along with washing of the hair to remove sweat or environmentally deposited drug, is a major component of valid quantitative testing of ingested drug. Any study performed without aggressive washing of the hair samples cannot be interpreted to represent ingestion, much less to assess the presence of a color effect. In this regard, sweat is a complex variable. It is known that individuals vary greatly in the amount of sweat produced, depending on gender, exertion, stress, climate and season, hormonal status, clothing, nutritional and hydration states, and many other factors.

Sweat is produced by two types of glands—eccrine (generally distributed over the entire body) and apocrine (located in the axilla and pubic regions) *(3,52)*. Compounding the variations in sweat production, the kind and frequencies of shampoo and conditioner treatments used with different hairstyles also affect the amount of sweat residues left on hairs. In addition, the effects of an individual's sweat exposure on his/her own hair can vary greatly for different hair types. For example, porous hair may easily soak up hundreds of times more drug than nonporous hair, but such drug can also be removed with similar ease by effective washing procedures *(30)*. With these considerations, studies that purport to show hair-color effects but use inadequate or invalidated decontamination and/or extraction methodologies must be weighted accordingly. Analysis of a large amount of data obtained with washed hair dissolved by enzymatic digestion followed by extraction of the melanin-free component have indeed shown no evidence of color bias *(44–52)*.

7. EXTRACTION AND MASS-SPECTROMETRY ANALYSIS OF HAIR SAMPLES

7.1. Extraction Method Validation

Extraction methods for recovering drug from hair prior to MS analysis, as already discussed in previous sections, require extensive validation. One way to determine whether the drug is being completely extracted is to apply the selected solvent in sequential intervals and to observe the completeness of the extraction with time. It is also useful to compare the results of a solvent extraction method with the results obtained by a validated digestion method. Another analytical consideration is the equilibration of internal standard to assure equivalent recovery of internal standard and drug that is bound to the sample matrix. However, if the drug in question binds strongly to melanin and the melanin is not removed from the sample to be extracted, the distribution of the internal standard between melanin and the soluble fraction, and how this will affect quantitation, must be considered. An extraction method may also be evaluated by use of Standard Reference Materials (SRM) hair standards from the National Institute of Standards and Technology (NIST) program *(53)*. These standards are immensely important and should be used to evaluate the reliability of the extraction protocol that is under consideration. Finally, another method of validating a procedure is to participate in a hair proficiency testing program whereby the method may be compared with those of other laboratories.

7.2. Mass Spectrometry

Simple EI, a single-quadrupole mass analyzer, has been the cornerstone of identification in forensic urine drug-testing facilities. However, in most cases, this method is totally inadequate for determining the lower concentrations of drugs and their metabolites found in hair. Because of this fact and matrix effects seen with hair analysis, more sensitive and more specific MS technology has been developed. Psychemedics, the authors' laboratory and one which performs the most commercial hair analysis, presently uses the Finnigan TSQ 7000 MS analyzers operating in negative ion chemical ionization (NICI) GC-MS-MS for the determination of marijuana in drug samples, detecting the tetrahydrocannabinol (THC) metabolite carboxyTHC (cTHC), which is also the target analyte monitored in forensic urine drug testing. All confirmation procedures need to go through vigorous validation studies. Psychemedics also uses positive ion chemical ionization (PICI) LC-MS-MS for the determination of cocaine, amphetamine, and opiate in drug-positive samples. The instrument used is a Perkin Elmer Sciex API 2000 LC-MS-MS, which operates in the PICI mode and has an electrospray source. Chemical ionization (CI) techniques, which favor production of a protonated ion for characterization studies, have been used to help resolve problems in the identification process. The ability to determine the molecular weight of the compound under investigation is of paramount importance as the first step in identification. The proper use of CI coupled with MS-MS obviates intensive sample cleanup by suppressing the interfering fragment ions and resolving matrix effects as well. This technique has the sensitivity and specificity required in low-level or trace analysis measurements. This laboratory looks for traces of cocaine, BE, CE, and norcocaine in the cocaine analysis; amphetamine, methamphetamine, MDMA (ecstasy), methylenedioxyamphetamine (MDA), and methyledioxyethylamphetamine (MDEA, Eve) in the amphetamine assay; and codeine, 6-acetylmorphine, morphine, and oxycodone in the opiate analysis. PCP in hair can easily be measured by simple EI analysis, which in most cases is achieved by standard default monitoring of three ions and two ratios. We also perform a D & L enantiomer analysis for the separation of the isomers of methamphetamine, utilizing a special chiral column.

Figures 2 and 3 show typical printouts demonstrating the results of a calibration in an analysis for cocaine in hair, using a triple quad tandem mass spectrometer (LC-MS-MS). Cocaine, BE, CE, and norcocaine, and their deuterated internal standards, are monitored in the analysis. The instrument is set at unit resolution, and standard multiple reaction mode (MRM) transition analysis is performed. The first quad is set to monitor only the parent ions (M +1) of the four cocaine compounds and their respective deuterated internal standards. The second quad acts as a collision chamber, causing the breakdown of the parent compound into one main daughter/product ion, which is then sent on into the third quad for the final measurement. This system is much more sensitive and has greater specificity than a single-quad system. This is needed because of the matrix interference seen in hair analysis at these low trace levels, especially when monitoring the metabolites, which are often found at pg/mg levels.

Figure 4 shows a typical printout demonstrating the results of a calibration in an analysis for cTHC in a triple-quad tandem mass spectrometer (GC-MS-MS). As a result of the very low concentrations of cTHC observed in hair, single-quad MS is inadequate. The use of LC-MS-MS at the present time for marijuana analysis is also inadequate, because the levels found are below the limit of detection of this instrument. We currently use a Finnigan TSQ 7000 GC-MS-MS operating in the NICI mode. The distinct advantage of NICI lies in the greater sensitivity observed (low picogram range) over PICI, especially when electron-capturing derivatives of the target compound have been prepared using fluorine-containing material. Previously, we monitored two product ions produced from one parent, but because the concentration of second ion was so low as compared with the other, we looked for a better method and are now using a dual-derivative method, which measures two different compounds at two different retention times, and provides two distinct quantitative measurements for comparison purposes. This was modeled after work performed at the Cook County Medical Examiner's toxicology laboratory *(54)*. The majority of samples

---

Fig. 2. *(opposite page)* Liquid chromatography-tandem mass spectrometry positive ion chemical ionization calibrations for the determination of cocaine and benzoylecgonine at the respective cut-offs of 5 ng/10 mg hair and 0.5 ng/10 mg hair by isotope dilution. Precursor to product ion transitions and retention times are shown.

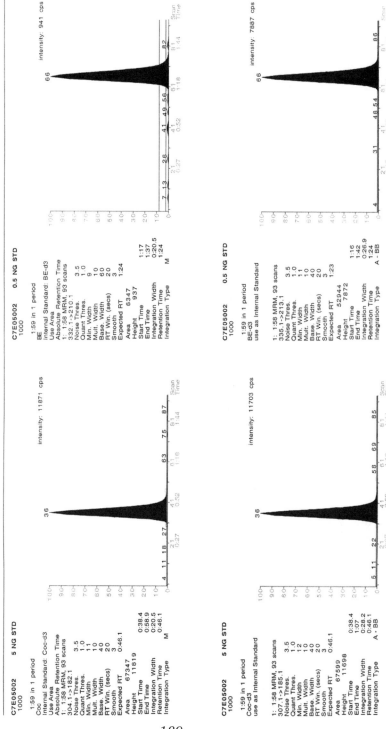

C7E05002   5 NG STD
1000

1:59 in 1 period
Coc
Internal Standard: Coc-d3
Use Area
Absolute Retention Time
1: 1:58 MRM, 93 scans
304.1->182.1
Noise Thres.   3.5
Quant Thres.   1.0
Min. Width   1.1
Mult. Width   1.0
Base. Width   4.0
RT Win. (secs)   2.0
Smooth   3
Expected RT   0:46.1
Area   67347
Height   11819
Start Time   0:38.4
End Time   0:58.9
Integration Width   0:20.5
Retention Time   0:46.1
Integration Type   M

intensity: 11871 cps

C7E05002   0.5 NG STD
1000

1:59 in 1 period
BE
Internal Standard: BE-d3
Use Area
Absolute Retention Time
1: 1:58 MRM, 93 scans
332.1->210.1
Noise Thres.   3.5
Quant Thres.   1.0
Min. Width   9
Mult. Width   1.0
Base. Width   60
RT Win. (secs)   20
Smooth   3
Expected RT   1:24
Area   6347
Height   937
Start Time   1:17
End Time   1:37
Integration Width   0:20.5
Retention Time   1:24
Integration Type   M

intensity: 941 cps

C7E05002   5 NG STD
1000

1:59 in 1 period
Coc-d3
use as Internal Standard

1: 1:58 MRM, 93 scans
307.1->185.1
Noise Thres.   3.5
Quant Thres.   1.0
Min. Width   1.2
Mult. Width   4.0
Base. Width   2.0
RT Win. (secs)   3
Smooth
Expected RT   0:46.1
Area   67599
Height   11698
Start Time   0:38.4
End Time   1:07
Integration Width   0:28.2
Retention Time   0:46.1
Integration Type   A - BB

intensity: 11703 cps

C7E05002   0.5 NG STD
1000

1:59 in 1 period
BE-d3
use as Internal Standard

1: 1:58 MRM, 93 scans
335.1->213.1
Noise Thres.   3.5
Quant Thres.   1.0
Min. Width   1.1
Mult. Width   1.0
Base. Width   4.0
RT Win. (secs)   2.0
Smooth   3
Expected RT   1:23
Area   52944
Height   7872
Start Time   1:16
End Time   1:42
Integration Width   0:26.9
Retention Time   1:24
Integration Type   A - BB

intensity: 7887 cps

189

MacQuan, version 1.6
Printed: Thu, Jul 15, 2004 16:22
Calibration File: MS.2004.07.14.005-API2000-1   Path: Macintosh HD: MassChrom 1.1:Cocaine data:COC2004:COC0704:MS.2004.07.14.005:
Comments: 5NG INTERNAL STD

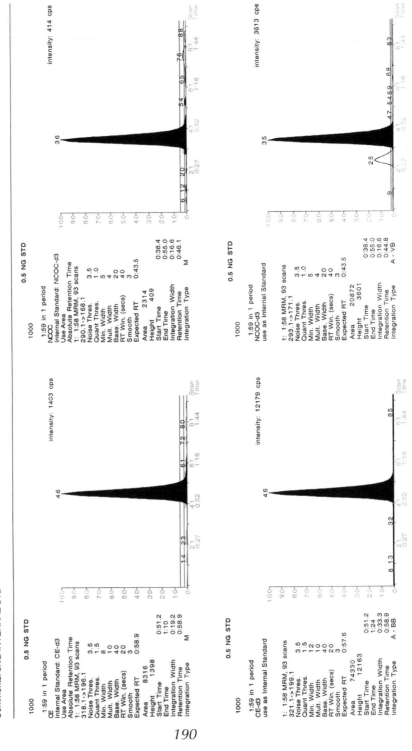

190

that screen positive by immunoassay fall in a range of 0.5 to 50 pg/10 mg hair, with occasional higher values (unpublished data).

8. CLINICAL AND FORENSIC ASPECTS

8.1. Expected Drug Levels in Hair of Proven Drug Users

The trapping of drugs in hair has been shown to be dose dependent *(55,56)*. Many variables, however, impact the use of hair results to indicate amount of drug use. These include biochemical individuality, effective washing, and cosmetic treatments. Severe cosmetic treatments can reduce the amount of some drugs in hair, whereas normal shampooing serves to decontaminate, although only partially in many cases.

Analyses of the hair from drug users who have tested positive in urinalysis provide a reference range of drug concentrations to be expected of such hair. Large studies of this nature have been performed by this laboratory for cocaine *(19)*, opiates *(21)*, methamphetamine *(20)*, and marijuana *(21)*. PCP was also studied, but with few users identified *(21)*. These studies also included negative control groups wherein hair samples from 60–80 nondrug-using subjects were collected and tested negative by both screening and confirmation analyses. In these studies, the cut-off levels (concentrations of the parent drugs in hair above which samples are considered positive) were 5 ng/10 mg hair for cocaine and methamphetamine, 2 ng/10 mg hair for morphine, 3 ng/10 mg hair for PCP, and 1 pg/10 mg hair for carboxy-THC, the metabolite found in hair as a result of marijuana use. All results of the studies were obtained by LC-MS-MS, GC-MS, or GC-MS-MS after application of our laboratory's wash procedures *(31)*.

8.1.1. Cocaine and Metabolites in Hair of Cocaine Users

In the case of cocaine, 70 urine cocaine-positive subjects had hair drug levels ranging from 6.5 to 2270 ng/10 mg hair, with 6 samples in the range of 5–20 ng/10 mg hair, 25 in the range of 21–200 ng/10 mg hair, and 39 greater than 200 ng/10 mg hair *(19)*. Three metabolites were analyzed in these samples: BE, CE, and norcocaine. CE is a definitive metabolite in that it can form only by the simultaneous ingestion of cocaine and ethanol. For this reason, CE is not present in all cocaine-user hair samples. BE, listed here as a percentage of cocaine, was found to range from 1.5 to 51%, with 3 samples less than 5%,

---

Fig. 3. *(facing page)* Liquid chromatography-tandem mass spectrometry positive ion chemical ionization calibrations for the determination of cocaethylene and norcocaine at the cut-off of 0.5 ng/10 mg hair by isotope dilution.

Carboxy-THC Analysis Report

Data File: T7A02X04
Sample Name: 1 PG STD   Barcode: 000002004
Vial: Tray01:4   ISTD Amt: 2.5 pg   **Dil Factor: 1.00**
 Data Path: D:\Xcalibur\Data   Acquisition Date:07/10/04 13:13:01
Comments: DB-XLB 30m x 0.25mm x 0.25um; Amm 5KmTorr; Ar 0.8mTorr @ 130C
Inst Method: C:\Xcalibur\methods\D9cthc.meth
Proc Method: C:\Xcalibur\methods\T7A02X04
Instrument   TSQ #5   Operator   HENRYS

Name	RT	Area	S/N	Calc. Amt. in pg/10mg
1_d9-CTHC(483)	4.86	327065	116.54	N/A
2_CTHC(474)	4.90	131720	48.00	1.000
3_d9-CTHC(533)	4.90	208893	100.57	N/A
4_CTHC(524)	4.94	102940	30.27	1.000

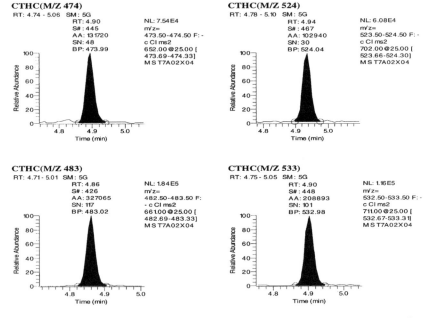

Fig. 4. Gas chromatography-tandem mass spectrometry negative ion chemical ionization calibration for the determination of carboxy-tetrahydrocannabinol in hair using the dual derivative and isotope dilution methodology. Precursor to product ion transitions, retention time, and both quantitations are shown.

22 samples between 5 and 10%, and 45 samples greater than 10%. Positive identification of BE in a test specimen in workplace testing is required to qualify the sample as cocaine positive. However, there is still uncertainty as to what levels of this metabolite are expected to be present in all cocaine users. Of those samples containing less than 5% BE relative to cocaine, one subject with 831 ng cocaine/10 mg hair and two positive urine tests showed a 1.5% BE content. Another subject with 80 ng cocaine/10 mg hair, a positive urine test, and 4.5 ng

CE/10 mg hair gave a 4.25% BE content. A third subject with 6.6 ng cocaine/ 10 mg hair and one positive urine test had a 4.5% BE content. The 25 subjects with BE between 5 and 10% were all proven cocaine users, some with two positive urine tests and many with CE as well. These results indicate that cocaine users at all levels of use can vary in the amounts of BE detected in the hair, and that a requirement for a minimum ratio of BE to cocaine can lead to an erroneous false-negative result on a confirmed, admitted cocaine user. In light of the above, the requirement that a positive sample contain BE in the amount of 5% of the cocaine value is a conservative policy in interpreting results.

Concentrations of CE greater than 0.5 ng/10 mg hair were present in about half of the samples with cocaine ≥5 ng/10 mg hair. The CE levels ranged from 0 to 127.9 ng, with 17 samples (24%) containing none, 17 (24%) containing less than 0.5 ng, 20 samples (28.6%) from 0.5 to 10 ng, and 16 samples (22.9%) greater than 10 ng, all in 10 mg of hair.

Norcocaine ranged from 0 to 55.6 ng/10 mg hair. Of 70 samples, 6 (8.6%) were less than 0.5 ng, 34 (49.3%) ranged from 0.5 to 10 ng, and 30 (43.5%) were greater than 10 ng, again all in 10 mg of hair.

8.1.2. Methamphetamine in Hair of Drug Users

Forty subjects provided hair samples in the study of methamphetamine users *(20)*. Hair samples had methamphetamine levels from 7.1 to 344 ng/ 10 mg hair, with 6 samples (15.4%) less than 20 ng/10 mg hair, 17 (43.6%) between 20 and 100 ng/10 mg hair, and 16 (41%) greater than 100 ng/10 mg hair. The levels of the metabolite amphetamine in these hair samples ranged from 0.1 to 44.6 ng/10 mg hair, with very low levels (<0.5 ng) in 4 samples with methamphetamine values from 7.1 to 78.9 ng/10 mg of hair.

8.1.3. Opiates in Hair of Heroin Users

Hair analysis offers distinct advantages relative to urinalysis in detecting heroin use, as it is not subject to positive results due to poppy-seed ingestion and it reliably shows the presence of the metabolite 6-monoacetylmorphine (6-MAM). In hair analysis for opiates, 6-MAM in a washed hair sample is a reliable indicator of heroin use. In a study of 68 subjects with urine morphine results above 2000 ng/mL by GC-MS, 37 were positive and 31 were negative for 6-MAM, whereas all the hair samples of these subjects contained 6-MAM, with the levels ranging from 0.8 to 527.2 ng/10 mg hair *(21)*. The morphine levels in these samples ranged from 3.1 to 558.8 ng/10 mg hair.

8.1.4. Carboxy-THC and PCP in Hair

PCP levels in hair range from the cut-off of 3 to as high as 150 ng/10 mg hair *(21)*. In head hair of 65 subjects shown positive in urine tests for marijuana use, carboxy-THC, the metabolite of cannabis, ranged from 0.3 to 76.3 pg/ 10 mg hair *(21)*.

8.2. Applications of Hair Analysis in Criminal Justice and Rehabilitation Settings

Mieczkowski et al. *(57)* have reported on use of hair testing as an objective measure of drug treatment outcome in a criminal justice diversionary treatment program for first-time, nonviolent offenders. Violations of the program conditions, including drug use, result in dismissal from the program. Hair samples were taken at intake to the program and at approx 2-mo intervals during the program, with random urine testing also being employed. Hair analysis at intake showed 50 of the 91 subjects positive for cocaine, 35 for marijuana, 3 for opiates, 1 for PCP, and none for amphetamines. Urinalysis done at the same time showed 12 positive for cocaine, 24 for marijuana, 1 for opiates, and none for PCP or amphetamines. These results highlight the diagnostic value of hair analysis in assessing the status of subjects as they enter a rehabilitation setting.

In another study, Mieczkowski and Newel *(44)* reported that hair analysis detected cocaine use at three times the incidence indicated by interviews. Similar results were obtained by Feucht et al. in a study by the Task Force on Violent Crime *(58)*, in which interviews, urinalysis, and hair analysis were performed. Hair results showed that 50 of 88 subjects (57%) had used cocaine, while urinalysis identified 8% as users, and interviews, 7.4%.

Magura et al. reported on the utility of hair analysis in determining the prevalence of cocaine use among criminally involved youth *(59)*. Interviews and hair samples were collected from 121 male youths, who were followed up in their communities after release from jail. Of the hair specimens, 67% were positive for cocaine, with only 23% of the hair-positive subjects admitting to cocaine use during the previous 3 mo. Associations were found between cocaine use and several behavioral variables: prior number of arrests, re-arrest after release from jail, not continuing education, and no legal employment.

The effectiveness of hair as a diagnostic tool in drug treatment has been discussed by Brewer *(60)*, who noted a good correlation between drug levels in hair and self reports of the amount of drug used. Perhaps owing to the evasion-resistant nature of a hair test, Brewer found that hair analysis was acceptable to both parties and resulted in an improved client-therapist relationship, frequently manifesting in more candid self-reporting of drug use prior to a scheduled hair test. Another contribution of hair testing to the therapeutic process is the ability to document improvement by segmental analysis or testing at regular intervals, a feature that only hair testing offers because of its ability to reflect dose over time.

8.3. Medical Applications of Hair Analysis

A number of investigators have applied hair testing to detect prenatal drug exposure *(61–70)*. The retrospective power of hair analysis allows, at the time of birth of an infant, an assessment of drug intake for as long a portion of the gestation period as the length of the mother's hair specimen permits. The first example of determining prenatal drug exposure by hair analysis, reported in 1987, was that of a mother who had ingested PCP during her pregnancy *(61)*. This study and that of Grant et al. *(66)* demonstrated that determining the pattern of drug usage over the term of the pregnancy by segmental hair analysis may be especially useful in evaluating effects on neurodevelopmental outcomes of varying levels of drug use during specific trimesters. Callahan et al. *(67)*, in comparing hair, meconium, and urine analyses for identifying cocaine use in mothers, found hair and meconium (when performed by GC-MS) to be about equivalent, whereas urine was about half as effective. The Hospital for Sick Children in Toronto has presented studies on hair analysis to determine fetal exposure to drugs of abuse *(69)* as well as to nicotine *(70)*. Sramek et al. reported on the use of hair testing to detect PCP use in newly admitted psychiatric patients *(71)*. The differentiation between toxic and nontoxic psychosis was facilitated by the detection of PCP in hair in patients where urine failed to detect PCP even at the level of 1 ng/mL.

9. THE PRESENT AND FUTURE OF HAIR TESTING

The unique characteristics of hair that allow estimation of dose and approximate dates of use, re-sampling and retesting, and other advantages make hair analysis of great value as either an alternative to other body fluids or as a complementary test. Effective washing of hair samples is a prerequisite for valid hair-testing results. There are additional benefits of hair analysis relative to the other body fluids in the case of specific analytes. For example, in analysis of opiates, hair does not produce a positive opiate result from consumption of even very high amounts of poppy seed *(21)*. Hair analysis of well-washed samples also allows distinction between heroin use and morphine use, as only heroin produces the metabolite 6-MAM, and significant amounts of morphine are not usually found in hair due to use of codeine. In the case of methamphetamine, the use of Vicks Inhalers has not produced false-positive results in washed hair samples. For some amphetamine-class substances such as MDMA and MDEA, recreational use on weekends often does not show up in urine analysis as a result of the low doses and urine's short detection window. Analysis of hair, on the other hand, detects these drugs even at low doses.

Applications of hair analysis in medical and pharmaceutical fields await serious exploration. For example, hair analysis can be applied to measure compliance with prescriptive medications or evaluating efficacy of the medications. Hair analysis can also be used to establish not only the intake of a drug under study, but also the effects of other medications, nutrients, or similar substances that may confound interpretation of study results.

REFERENCES

1. Society of Hair Testing. http://www.soht.org/html/Lit_Head.html.
2. Baumgartner WA and Hill VA. Hair analysis for organic analytes: methodology, reliability issues, and field studies, in Drug Testing in Hair (Kintz P, ed), CRC, New York, NY, 1996; pp. 223–265.
3. Pragst F, Rothe M, Spiegel K, and Sporkert F. Illegal and therapeutic drug concentrations in hair segments—a timetable of drug exposure? For Sci Rev 1998;10: 81–111.
4. Notice of Proposed Revisions to the Mandatory Guidelines for Federal Workplace Drug Testing Programs (69 FR 19673, April 13, 2004, FR Doc#04-7984) http://workplace.samhsa.gov/drugtesting/comments/comments.asp.
5. Saitoh M, Uzuka M, and Sakamoto M. Human hair cycle. J Invest Dermatol 1970; 51:65–81.
6. Baumgartner WA and Hill V. Hair analysis for drugs of abuse: sample preparation techniques. For Sci Int 1999;63:121–135.
7. Baumgartner WA. Ligand Assays of Enzymatic Hair Digests. U.S. Patent No. 5,324,642, 28 June 1994.
8. Sachs H. History of hair analysis. For Sci Int 1997;84:7–16.
9. Staub C. Analytical procedures for determination of opiates in hair: a review. For Sci Int 1995;70:111–123.
10. Kintz P, Trazcqui A, and Mangin P. Opiate concentrations in human head, axillary and pubic hair. J For Sci 1993;38:657–662.
11. Cone EJ. Testing human hair for drugs of abuse. I. Individual dose and time profiles of morphine and codeine in plasma, saliva, urine and beard compared to drug-induced effects on pupils and behavior. J Anal Toxicol 1990;14:1–7.
12. Eser H, Ptosch L, Skopp G, and Moeller MR. Influence of sample preparation on analytical results: drug analysis (GC/MS) on hair snippets versus hair powder using various extraction procedures. For Sci Int 1997;84:271–279.
13. Kronstrand R, Nystrom I, Druid H, and Strandberg J. Screening for drugs of abuse in hair with ion-spray LC-MS-MS. Presented at the Third European Meeting on Hair For Sci Int 2004;145:183–190.
14. Irgan D, Kuntz D, and Feldman M. The Simultaneous Analysis of Amphetamines, Cocaine, Phencyclidine and Opiates by GC/MS-EI. Presented at Society of Forensic Toxicology Annual Meeting 2003, Portland, OR, A23, 2003.
15. Wang L, Irvan D, Kuntz K, and Feldman M. Simultaneous Analysis of Morphine, Codeine, Oxymorphone, Hydromorphone, 6-Acetylmorphine, Oxycodone, Hydrocodone and Heroin in Hair and Oral Fluid, Presented at Society of Forensic Toxicology Annual Meeting 2003, Portland, OR, A27, 2003.

16. Cooper G, Baldwin D, and Hand C. Validation of the Cozart® Microplate ELISA for the Detection of Methadone in Hair. Presented at Society of Forensic Toxicology Annual Meeting 2003, Portland, OR, P17, 2003.

17. Cooper G, Wilson L, Reid C, Baldwin D, Hand C, and Spiehler V. Validation of the Cozart® Microplate ELISA for detection of opiates in hair. J Anal Toxicol 200327:581–586.

18. Setter C, Brown W, Kuntz D, and Feldman M. Comparison of Commercially Available ELISA kits for the Analysis of THC-COOH, Presented at Society of Forensic Toxicology Annual Meeting 2003, Portland, OR, A26, 2003.

19. Cairns T, Hill V, Schaffer M, and Thistle W. Levels of cocaine and its metabolites in washed hair of demonstrated amphetamine users, and workplace subjects. For Sci Int 2004;145:175–181.

20. Cairns T, Hill V, Schaffer M, and Thistle W. Levels of methamphetamine and amphetamine in washed hair of demonstrated amphetamine users and workplace subjects. For Sci Int 2004;145:137–142.

21. US Food and Drug Administration, Center for Devices and Radiological Health Http://accessdata.fda.gov/scripts/cdrh/cfdocs/cfPMN/PMN.cfm/.

22. Baumgartner A, Jones P, Baumgartner W, and Black C. Radioimmunoassay of hair for determining opiate abuse histories. J Nucl Med 1979;20:749–752.

23. Baumgartner A, Jones P, and Black C. Detection of phencyclidine in hair. J For Sci 1981;26:576–581.

24. Baumgartner W, Jones P, Black WC, and Blahd W. Radioimmunoassay of cocaine in hair. J Nucl Med 1982;20:790–792.

25. Spiehler V. Hair analysis by immunological methods from the beginning to 2000. For Sci Int 2000;107:249–259.

26. Koren G, Klein J, Forman R, and Graham K. Hair analysis of cocaine: differentiation between systemic exposure and external contamination J Clin Pharmacol 1992;32:671–675.

27. Wang WL and Cone E. Testing human hair for drugs of abuse. IV. Environmental cocaine contamination and washing effects. For Sci Int 1995;70:39–51.

28. Schaffer MI, Wang W-L, and Irving J. An evaluation of two wash procedures for the differentiation of external contamination versus ingestion in the analysis of human hair samples for cocaine. J Anal Toxicol 2002;26:485–488.

29. Marsh A and Evans M. Radioimmunoassay of drugs of abuse in hair. Part 1. Methadone in human hair, method adaptation and the evaluation of decontamination procedures. J Pharmaceutical and Biomedical Analysis 1994;12:1123–1130.

30. Baumgartner WA and Hill VA. Hair analysis for drugs of abuse: decontamination issues, in Recent Developments in Therapeutic Drug Monitoring and Clinical Toxicology (Sunshine I, ed), Marcel Dekker, New York, NY: 1992;pp. 577–597.

31. Cairns T, Hill V, Schaffer M, and Thistle W. Removing and identifying drug contamination in the analysis of human hair. For Sci Int 2004;145:97–108.

32. Mieczkowski T. Passive contamination of undercover narcotics officers by cocaine: an assessment of their exposure using hair analysis. Microgram 1995;28:193–198.

33. Hubbard DL, Wilkins DG, and Rollins DE. The incorporation of cocaine and metabolites into hair: effects of dose and hair pigmentation. Drug Metabolism and Disposition 2000;28:1464–1469.

34. Kronstrand R, Andersson MC, Ahlner J, and Larson G. Incorporation of selegiline metabolites into hair after oral selegiline intake. J Anal Toxicol 200125:594–601.

35. Claffey DJ, Stout PR, and Ruth J. 3H-nicotine, 3H -flunitrazepam, and ^{3}H-cocaine incorporation into melanin: a model for the examination of drug-melanin interactions. J Anal Toxicol 2001;25:607–611.

36. Reid RW, O'Connor FL, and Crayton JW. The in vitro differential binding of benzoylecgonine to pigmented hair samples. Clin Tox 1994;32:405–410.

37. Slawson MH, Wilkins DG, Foltz RL, and Rollins DE. Quantitative determination of phencyclidine in pigmented and nonpigmented hair by ion-trap mass spectrometry. J Anal Toxicol 1996;20:350–354.

38. Gygi SP, Wilkins DG, and Rollins DE. A comparison of phenobarbital and codeine incorporation into pigmented and nonpigmented rat hair. J Pharm Sci 1997;86: 209–213.

39. Slawson DE, Wilkins DG, and Rollins DE. The incorporation of drugs into hair: relationship of hair color and melanin concentration to phencyclidine incorporation. J Anal Toxicol 1998;22:406–413.

40. Wilkins DG, Mizuno A, Borges CR, Slawson MH, and Rollins DE. Ofloxacin as a reference marker in hair of various colors. J Anal Toxicol 2003;27:149–155.

41. Henderson GL, Harkey MR, Zhou C, Jones RT, and Jacob P. Incorporation of isotopically labeled cocaine into human hair: race as a factor. J Anal Toxicol 1998;22: 156–165.

42. Rollins DE, Wilkins DG, Krueger GG, Augsburger MP, and Mizuno A. The effect of hair color on the incorporation of codeine into human hair. J Anal Toxicol 2003;27:545–551.

43. Harding H and Rogers G. Physiology and growth of human hair, in: Forensic Examination of Hair (Robertson J, ed), Taylor & Francis, Philadelphia, PA: 1999; pp. 1–77.

44. Bradley KC, Day JE, Rollins DE, Andrenyak D, Ling W, and Wilkins D. G. Opiate recidivism in a drug treatment program: comparison of hair and urine data. J Anal Toxicol 2003;27:412–428.

45. Mieczkowski T and Newel R. An evaluation of patterns of racial bias in hair assays for cocaine: black and white arrestees compared. For Sci Int 1993;63: 85–98.

46. Mieczkowski T, Lersch T, and Kruger M. Police drug testing, hair analysis and the issue of race bias. Criminal Justice Rev 2002;27:124–139.

47. Mieczkowski T and Kruger M. Assessing the effect of hair color on cocaine positive outcomes in a large sample: a logistic regression on 56,445 cases using hair analysis. Bulletin of the International Association of Forensic Toxicologists 2000; 31:9–11.

48. Mieczkowski T and Newel R. An analysis of the racial bias controversy in the use of hair assays, in Drug Testing Technology (Mieczkowski T, ed), CRC, Boca Raton, FL: 1999; pp. 313–348.

49. Mieczkowski T. Effect of color and curvature on the concentration of morphine in hair analysis. Forensic Science Communications 2001;3:1–11.

50. Mieczkowski T. The further mismeasure: the curious use of racial categorizations in the interpretation of hair analysis. Int J Drug Testing 20002:1–20.

51. Mieczkowski T. Is a "color effect" demonstrated for hair analysis of carbamazepine? Life Sciences 2000;67:39–43.
52. Hoffman BH Analysis of race effects on drug test results. Business Health Management 1999;41:612–614.
53. Standards Reference Material Group, National Institute of Standards and Technology, 100 Bureau Drive, Stop 2322, Gaithersburg, MD 28899-2322 (srminfo @NIST.gov).
54. Chen NBW, Schaffer MI, Trojan C, Suero M, and Paul L. Simultaneous Qualitative and Quantitative Analysis of Dual Derivatives (HFIP-TFA and HFIP-PFP) of 9-Carboxy-11 Nor Delata-9-Tetrahydrocannabinol with Deuterated Internal Standards by Capillary Gas Chromatography/Mass Fragmentography. Presented at the 39th Annual Meeting of the American Academy of Forensic Sciences, San Diego, CA, 1987.
55. Baumgartner WA, Hill VA, and Kippenberger D. Workplace drug testing by hair analysis: advantages and issues, in Drug Testing Technology (Mieczkowski T, ed), CRC Press, Boca Raton, FL: 1999; pp. 283–311.
56. Baumgartner WA. and Hill VA. Hair analysis for drugs of abuse. J For Sci 1989; 34:1433–1453.
57. Mieczkowski T, Mumm R, and Connick HF. The use of hair analysis in a pretrial diversion program in New Orleans. Int J Offender Ther 1995;39:222–241.
58. Feucht T, Stephens RC, and Walker ML. Drug use among juvenile arrestees: a comparison of self-report, urinalysis and hair assay. J Drug Issues 1994;24: 99–116.
59. Magura S, Kang SY, and Shapiro JL. Measuring cocaine use by hair analysis among criminally-involved youth. J Drug Issues 1995;25:683–701.
60. Brewer C. Hair analysis as a tool for monitoring and managing patients on methadone maintenance: a discussion. For Sci Int 1993;63:277–283.
61. Parton L, Baumgartner WA, and Hill VA. Quantitation of fetal cocaine exposure by radioimmunoassay of hair. Pediatr Res 1987;21:A372.
62. Ostrea EM. Detection of prenatal drug exposure in the pregnant woman and her newborn infant. Clinics in Perinatology 1991;18:629–645.
63. Welch RA, Martier SS, Ager JW, Ostrea EM, and Sokol RJ. Radioimmunoassay of hair: a valid technique of determining maternal cocaine abuse. Substance Abuse 1990;11:214–217.
64. Ostrea EM, Knapp DK, Tannenbaum L, et al. Estimates of illlicit drug use during pregnancy by maternal interview, hair analysis and meconium analysis. J Pediatrics 2001;138:344–348.
65. Marques PR, Tippetts AS, and Branch DG. Cocaine in the hair of mother-infant pairs: quantitative analysis and correlations with urine measures and self report. Am J Drug Alcohol Abuse 1993;19:159–175.
66. Grant T, Brown Z, Callahan C, Barr H, and Streissguth AP. Cocaine exposure during pregnancy: improving assessment with radioimmunoassay of maternal hair. Obstet Gyneco 1984;83:524–531.
67. Callahan CM, Grant TM, Phipps P, Clark G, Novacek AH, and Streissguth AP. Measurement of gestational cocaine exposure: sensitivity of infants' hair, meconium, and urine. J Pediatr 1992;120:763–769.

68. Chasnoff IJ, Landress HJ, and Barrett ME. The prevalence of illicit drug or alcohol use during pregnancy and discrepancies in mandatory reporting in Pinellas County, Florida. N Engl J Med 1990;322:1202–1206.

69. Klein J, Karaskov T, and Koren G. Clinical applications of hair testing for drugs of abuse—the Canadian experience. For Sci Int 2000;107:281–288.

70. Chan D, Caprara D, Blanchette P, Klein J, and Koren G. Recent developments in meconium and hair testing methods for the confirmation of gestational exposures to alcohol and tobacco smoke. Clin Biochem 2004;37:429–438.

71. Sramek JJ, Baumgartner WA, Tallos J, Ahrens TN, Meiser JF, and Blahd WH. Hair analysis for detection of phencyclidine in newly admitted psychiatric patients. Am J Psychiatry 1995;142:950–953.

Chapter 12

Instrumented Urine Point-of-Collection Testing Using the eScreen® System

Murray Lappe

SUMMARY

New federal regulations proposed by the Department of Health and Human Services for drug testing of federal employees includes the addition of alternative specimens as well as the addition of alternative technologies for screening samples at the point of collection. Alternative technologies called point-of-collection tests (POCT) may use urine or oral fluids, and are either visually read or instrumented. eScreen® (eScreen, Inc.) is an instrumented urine POCT with an integrated SVT, adulteration assay, Web-based information management system, and paperless chain of custody form. eScreen's instrumented system eliminates many potential areas of concern when testing samples at the point of collection. Safeguards that are present in a laboratory-based drug-testing environment are duplicated in eScreen's decentralized point-of-collection drug-testing model. The key to eScreen's robust point-of-collection model lies in the use of an extensive installed base of Internet-enabled eReaders and Web tools.

1. INTRODUCTION

Drug testing is inherently an information science. Aside from the analytical aspects of the test, the purpose of drug testing is to accurately and efficiently deliver specific information to the customer regarding the presence or absence of drugs in a specimen. Since the introduction of drug testing more

From: *Forensic Science and Medicine: Drugs of Abuse: Body Fluid Testing*
Edited by R. C. Wong and H. Y. Tse © Humana Press Inc., Totowa, NJ

than 30 yr ago, service providers have struggled to deliver drug-test information more efficiently. The "proximal shift" of lateral-flow point-of-collection tests (POCT) with advancements in information technology has created a unique opportunity for the delivery of drug-test information and results remarkably more quickly and reliably than ever before. The eScreen® (eScreen, Inc.) system leverages the advancements in information technology with recent developments in near patient drugs-of-abuse (DOA) testing.

2. BENEFITS OF NEAR-PATIENT TESTING

With the introduction of urine dipsticks more than 40 yr ago for the rapid detection of glucose and other substances in urine, the benefits of immediate laboratory information became apparent *(1)*. The advantages in the clinical environment include changes to treatment plans while the patient is still in the doctor's office, cost improvements, and the elimination of specimen transportation and additional paperwork *(2–3)*.

By the early 1980s, pregnancy tests were available for near-patient, or point-of-collection use, but required multiple reagent mixing and positive and negative control comparisons. Within a few years, the lateral-flow pregnancy test was introduced. This eliminated the procedure of reagent handling and provided a visual indication of pregnancy by way of a color indicator utilizing colloidal gold. The benefits of this one-step pregnancy test were immediately apparent, and the simplicity of use allowed patients to be use the product in the home. Over time, the sensitivity and specificity of the antibody-β human chorionic gondaotropin (HCG) reaction improved to detect lower levels of βHCG, enabling the detection of pregnancy earlier in the cycle *(4–7)*.

3. COMPLICATIONS INTRODUCED BY POINT-OF-COLLECTION DRUG TESTS

By the early 1990s, pharmaceutical and diagnostic companies have been working on the antigen-antibody (Ag-Ab) pairs to DOA in urine. Lateral-flow methods utilized in pregnancy tests proved to be the most reliable and easiest to use, and both dipstick- and cassette-based lateral-flow DOA devices started to appear in the market. Cassettes hold the lateral-flow device in place within a plastic shell. The upper shell is configured with a well for the specimen to be placed over the absorbent pad, and a window for viewing the visual endpoint color-change reaction (*see* Chapters 3–5).

The introduction of these products, however, created special concerns in workplace DOA testing applications. Pregnancy tests, designed for home use by patients, were ideal in their design for self-collection, interpretation, and receipt of the test results in the privacy of the home *(8)*. For workplace DOA testing, there exist three distinct parties—a donor (employee), a collector (nurse or technician), and a customer (employer) who has ordered the tests and is the party authorized to receive the test results. Conventional POCT have missed, or ignored, this important distinction.

3.1. Concerns About Necessity of Specimen Aliquoting

Manually performed DOA tests introduce several complications to the standard model of laboratory-centric testing. The first complication in the process of testing for drugs at the point of collection is aliquoting the specimen. Although aliquoting the specimen is standard procedure in the laboratory, there are standard operating procedures (SOP) and supervisory controls to reduce the potential for contamination of the forensic specimens. In the decentralized, point-of-collection model of DOA testing, there is little standardization in the method and procedures for aliquoting or handling of the original specimen. The sealed specimen must have its tamper-evident seal broken, and the specimen exposed to allow for the introduction of the aliquoting device. The introduction of a foreign object, such as a pipet, to obtain the aliquot in an uncontrolled environment, creates a potential legal challenge to the integrity of the specimen. This concern led to the invention of the testing cup, with its integrated test strips. The most evolved designs of the testing cup contain an inherent aliquoting feature built into the cup, to allow for specimen aliquoting of the test strips without destruction of the tamper-evident seal.

3.2. Concerns About Accuracy of Analysis

Further complicating POCT is the shift in analysis from the laboratory to the point of collection. Decentralizing the analytical process of DOA testing places the burden of responsibility for analytical interpretation on the collector and potentially unskilled personnel. Visually read endpoints of test results, although quite simple in most pregnancy tests, is dramatically more complicated in DOA testing. Most DOA tests contain multiple analyses, testing for cannabinoid (tetrahydrocannabinol; THC), cocaine, amphetamine, morphine, and phencyclidine (PCP) on one or more lateral-flow strips. Included on each lateral-flow strip is a control, ensuring that the sample has migrated across the test area. A five-drug test will have one target zone for each drug analyte and one target control zone for each strip. Hence, a two-strip, five-drug panel will have a total of seven target zones. Most competitive binding assays produce a color indicator in the absence of the analyte. However, some tests produce a color reaction in the presence of the analyte. This can potentially confuse the collector into misinterpreting the test result, when using different products for different clients. Furthermore, the intensity of the color change varies with each drug-test target, often resulting in a mottled, nonuniform array of visual test lines. Several manufacturers indicate on the package insert that any presence of color change, no matter how faint it may appear, should be interpreted as a negative result. There is considerable subjectivity to the test-result interpretation, leading to potential false-negative and false-positive errors. Timing of the test is critical, and the interpreter must read the test result during the time indicated on the package insert, usually between 3 and 8 min. Improperly timed readings could potentially result in false-negative or false-positive results. Visual acuity, color vision, and lighting conditions may also play a role in the interpreter's accuracy in reading visually interpreted endpoints. Subjective interpretation, or translation of the analytical result from the test strip to the test result report, is of major concern in point-of-collection testing.

3.3. Concerns About Donor Anonymity

Laboratory-based DOA tests place considerable distance between the donor and the location of analysis. Anonymity of the donor is essential in the analytical process to remove any potential bias, specimen tampering, result tampering, and breaches in confidentiality. When the collector is also the point-of-collection test operator, there is no anonymity of the donor. This could result in potential abuses of bias, specimen tampering, and result tampering. One method of reducing this potential for error is to separate the functions of the collector from the analytical process, to allow for anonymity in the testing procedure. The POCT technician, who is not the collector of the specimen, would have a separate strand of the chain of custody, without the donor's name or identifying information, similar to the current laboratory model. The ultimate model of local analytical interpretation is to remove the technician altogether, and replace the technician with an instrumented interpretation. Instrumented tests eliminate operator bias and tampering, and preclude result disclosure to the collector and others who are not in a "need-to-know" capacity.

3.4. Concerns About Possible Transcription Errors

Experience in data management of corporate drug-testing programs has revealed that transcription errors, such as data entry errors, occur throughout the testing process. Once the test result is accurately determined, or translated from the lateral-flow test device, the information must be transcribed. The test result is translated from the visual endpoints to the test technician's mental interpretation. It is translated from a mental process to a written or verbal transmission of the test result *(9–11)*. A phone call to the employer may be requested with the test results. However, ultimately a written document demonstrating the final determination of the operator must be recorded. Errors in recording the test result are described as transcription errors. A written or verbal negative result when the test indicated the presence of drugs is a false-negative transcription error. Conversely, a written or verbal positive result when the test indicated the absence of drugs is a false-positive transcription error. Experience has shown that both error types occur in the use of visually read endpoint tests, where human translation and transcription are required to convey information to the customer *(12)*.

4. DECENTRALIZING LABORATORY SERVICES TO THE POINT OF COLLECTION

The laboratory has historically been demonstrated to be more effective and economical when centralized. One benefit of a centralized laboratory is that the handling and analysis of each specimen is identical. This high-volume production environment reduces the potential for errors through the efficient processing of thousands of specimens daily under strict controls and supervision. Decentralization of the analytical process to the point of collection, without proper standardization of procedures, instruments (point-of-collection devices), aliquoting methods, or translation and transcription methods, lends itself to a lack of consistency and control from location to location. Experience has shown that employers using multiple locations, especially large employers with hundreds or thousands of locations, are concerned about the lack of uniformity in the testing process from collection site to collection site.

In the laboratory-centric model of DOA testing, the testing process of negative and positive results is essentially indiscernible by all except those deeply engaged within the confirmation laboratory. Although the screening and confirmation laboratory are under one roof in a centralized laboratory facility, they are actually distinct in their objectives. The object of the screening laboratory is to identify which samples are negative (i.e., contain no drugs). The object of the confirmation laboratory is to identify which samples are positive (i.e., contain drugs). Nearly all laboratories utilize immunoassay testing, an inexpensive yet highly sensitive screening method capable of detecting nanogram quantities of drug analytes in a milliliter of urine. This highly sensitive method of screening, combined with automation and robotics in the laboratory, cost-effectively eliminates more than 93% of all specimens from further testing in normal workplace demographics. Criminal justice testing, with its inherently higher positive rates, would require more screened samples to go on for further testing, whereas certain workplace demographics (e.g., airline employees, federal workers, and so on, with inherently low positive rates) have seen negative screening rates as high as 99%. The importance of the negative screening rate cannot be overemphasized, because once a specimen screens negative it is discarded. It cannot be used again or retested, and has no further value to the laboratory or customer (employer). Only the screened positive samples are transferred to the confirmation laboratory for further testing. In the past 20 yr, data compiled on workplace drug-testing statistics indicated that the positive rates were falling annually, from a high of 25% in 1987, the first year such data were published, to about 7% in the past year. Improved awareness and increased use of drug education and testing methods may cause further declines in the positive rate over the coming years. As positive rates drop even further, it will no longer make sense economically or logistically to send 95% of samples to a laboratory only to find out that they were negative to begin with. Unbundling negative from positive samples at the point of collection and handling the processes separately was of significant importance to the marketplace.

The decentralization of laboratory services to the point of collection is made possible by the improved sensitivity and specificity of drug detection by lateral-flow DOA (LFDOA) testing devices. In the early 1990s, the sensitivity rate of LFDOA testing devices was approx 93% of the thresholds required for standardized workplace drug testing (then referred to as the National Institute of Drug Abuse [NIDA] cut-off levels). Tracking the progress of monoclonal techniques and antibody-antigen sensitivity and specificity demonstrated that overall, DOA sensitivity levels would improve at the rate of approx 1% annually. Beginning in 1993, it was expected that sensitivity rates for LFDOA devices would approach the sensitivity rate of laboratory-based immunoassays (then at 99%) by 1999. Once the sensitivity rate of LFDOA was equal to or better than laboratory-based immunoassays, one could easily argue for not sending negative samples to the laboratory.

5. CHANGEABLE BAR CODE: PRELUDE TO DIGITAL DRUG TESTING

When one examines the results at the target zone of a multi-drug lateral-flow testing device, it appears that the series of color lines and spaces are elements of bar coded symbols. Bar codes, a series of bars and spaces, are encoded data elements representing numbers and/or letters that can be decoded with the proper reader and decoder software. The configuration of the lateral-flow device with seven or more color lines and spaces may sometimes be confusing. The names of the drugs are marked on the cassette carrier adjacent to the target zone. If the drug names were removed from the cassette carrier, the interpreter would not know which drugs are being tested and which are the positive results. However, this should not matter because the collector is not privileged to know the test results, and consequently, if the test is presumptively positive, the nature of the drug detected is immaterial to the collector, because only the gas chromatography (GC)-mass spectrometry (MS) confirmation laboratory can positively identify the drug. Removing the drug names from the cassette means that if all the color lines are present, as is the case with most strips, no drugs are detected in the specimen (i.e., the result is negative). If one or more color lines are absent from the series, the result is presumptively positive. It does not matter which drug is detected, because in every case, the outcome is the same. The specimen must be sent to a confirmation laboratory for further testing. From the bar code prospective, this argument presents a unique opportunity to translate the lines and spaces on the LFDOA test strips into a digital code, or a series of 0s and 1s. Consider the presence of a target line as indicated by a 1 and a space by a 0, then a five-drug test with one control line would be translated by a barcode reader into 10101010101 (six lines and five spaces) when the sample is negative and all six lines appear. If, for example, the THC test in the second position is positive, and fails to produce a color change in the target zone, the outcome would be 10001010101. A cocaine positive test, in the third position, would produce 10100010101, and so on. In fact, any combination other than 10101010101 is an indication that the sample requires confirmation testing. Changing the position of the test target zones from lot to lot or from time to time sufficiently eliminates the possibility of learning the code configurations. Therefore, neither the donor nor the collector knows which drug is presumptively positive.

Drug testing by nature is inherently binary, because the outcome of a drug test for employment purposes is ultimately only positive or negative, pass/fail, qualified/unqualified, and so on, or qualitative in its result. In the information flow of drug testing, there exists a point where the analog processes become digital information. This point is referred to as the analog-to-digital conversion point (ADC). In the laboratory-centric model of drug testing, this point of conversion to digital information exists in the interface between the laboratory and the medical review officer (MRO). Improvements in efficiency of information transmission are realized as the ADC point shifts to the left, because little or no data entry or transcription is required into the drug test record after ADC. Digital conversion in the extreme case occurs when the data-entry process begins in the workplace as digital information.

6. THE ESCREEN SYSTEM

In view of the deficiencies associated with the conventional POCT and the perception that a digital drug test could be created, a system known as eScreen was developed. eScreen combines the benefits of point-of-collection specimen collection with recent advances in information technologies to create an instrumented POCT system. eScreen monitored the progress of LFDOA development closely. LFDOA clearly led the market as the analytical method of choice.

Easy-to-use, low-cost, highly sensitive lateral-flow test strips could do everything that the lab-based immunoassay could do. eScreen did not compete in the manufacturing of LFDOA devices, but realized that commoditization would likely develop as tests got better and cheaper. eScreen uses the current Federal drug testing standards as a starting point, extracts the immunoassay screening procedure from the centralized laboratory, and shifts it to the point of collection. It keeps in place many of the safeguards already built into the laboratory-centric model of testing, including the collection procedure and confirmation testing. This means that the chain of custody, collection procedures, specimen transportation, and confirmation processes were virtually unaffected. eScreen realized that what was desperately needed for the workplace was a method for implementing a sound POCT program that could effectively compete with the laboratory model for testing. eScreen designed a POCT method to wrap around the LFDOA test strip to closely mimic the laboratory model, with screening performed at the point of collection, and with the goal of eliminating the eight critical barriers to POCT (Table 1).

With the sensitivity and precision of the LFDOA test strips rapidly approaching laboratory-based immunoassay levels *(21–24)*, the next issue was to remove the subjective interpretation in POCT. eScreen knew that in order to remove the human subjectivity of interpretation, two essential elements of the LFDOA test had to change. First, it could not be readable by a human. This meant that the test result would have to be invisible to the naked eye, or be coded, or otherwise obscured from human interpretation. Secondly, it had to be decoded by an instrumented device, or reader. The transition from human vision to machine vision was inevitable.

By 1997, machine-vision systems were appearing in a variety of applications. Eyeball-type video cameras had dropped in price to unimaginable levels, and were appearing on every desktop, even though there were few applications for them, and less than adequate bandwidth to transmit quality video. Low-cost digital video charge-coupled device (CCD) processors were migrating into digital cameras, plant automation, and a myriad of machine-vision applications in medicine, logistics, inspection, quality systems, and robotics.

The task of removing human vision and interpretation at first seemed a fairly simple one. The practical application was much more difficult than first imagined. Strip characteristics, lighting, and lot-to-lot variability in strip manufacturing posed enormous obstacles. Precision application of target zones was necessary to allow the machine vision to focus on the areas of interest. Sharp demarcation between bars and spaces, an essential element in analog barcode readers, could not be achieved with lateral-flow devices. Background noise, in the form of conjugate streaking and carry-forward through the nitrocellulose membrane, had to be subtracted out using digital imaging, proprietary mathe-

Table 1
Eight Critical Barriers to Manual Point-of-Collection Tests (POCT)

Barriers	Proposed Solution
Sensitivity	The sensitivity of lateral-flow drugs-of-abuse testing must meet or exceed lab-based immunoassay sensitivity levels.
Aliquoting	Specimen must be aliquotted under tamper-evident seal.
Subjective interpretation (translation)	Machine-vision system or instrumented interpretation reader is required to interpret test result from lateral-flow device.
Bias	No human operator or opportunity to influence the test result.
Confidentiality	Result is unknown to donor, collector, or collection-site personnel.
Transcription	No result data entry or manual result reporting from collection-site personnel to employer.
Consistency	Each site uses identical operating procedure and standardized conditions for testing.
Endorsement	Adoption of the instrumented POCT system by large, national employers, or federal agencies, to drive standardization at local collection sites.

matical algorithms, and software logic. Solutions to these issues were built into the components of the eScreen system.

6.1. The eCup™

The eCup™ (eScreen) (Fig. 1) is a specimen-collecting device with an internal aliquoting pump to sequester an aliquot when the lid is closed onto the cup. The aliquot pump is a double-walled syringe designed to pump the sample aliquot up onto the two LFDOA test strips and adulteration strips. Adulteration strips (*see* Chapters 13 and 14), which contain tests for pH, creatinine, and nitrite, reside in the eCup lid in a third test-strip slot. The eCup has a unique patented lid label with an integrated tamper-evident seal. The label and seal are bar-coded with a unique specimen number. This is the specimen number used to create the electronic custody and control form, and to track the specimen and result throughout the testing process. Additional barcodes appear on the label to direct the eReader™ (eScreen) (discussed later) to decode certain coded information from the test-strip configurations, as well as lot numbers of cups and test strips. eCup test strips are integrated into the eCup lid. Cup designs that have test strips in the specimen collection container could

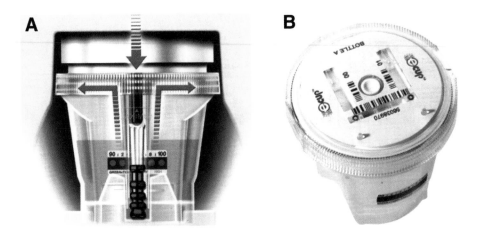

Fig. 1. (A) eCup™ in cross-section; **(B)** eCup lid.

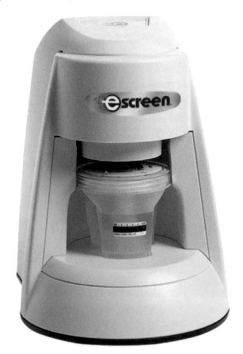

Fig. 2. eReader™.

result in donor tampering. eCup lids remain sealed until the donor returns with the specimen, when the lid is selected and opened in the presence of the donor and collector. The eCup collection container has guide rails on the lid and a banjo-shaped bottom to guide the cup into the reader base and eliminate rotation of the eCup in the reader.

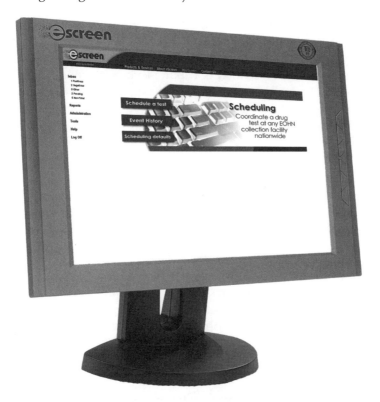

Fig. 3. eScreen123®.

6.2. The eScreen123® Software Runs the eScreen System

The eScreen system consists of a suite of hardware installed at the point of collection. The hardware suite consists of a Windows PC, monitor, eReader (Fig. 2), signature capture device, barcode reader, and laser printer. The PC is connected to the Internet, preferably via a broadband connection, and runs the eScreen123® (eScreen) software platform. The eScreen123 (Fig. 3) software is a Web-based application allowing each of the service providers—e.g., the collection site, laboratory, MRO, and administrator—to access their respective portion of the drug-testing record in real time throughout the drug-testing process. The collection site portal allows the collector to check in the donor, if not previously scheduled by the employer, based on a set of rules previously established by the system and embedded in the software. Collector screens guide the collector through the specimen-collection process, and require the completion of the custody and control form (CCF) elements. The date and time, collection site location, collector name, and so on are automatically filled in by the software. Failure to complete each step of the CCF is detected by the software, which prevents completion of the process until the required fields are completed. Once the collection is completed, the specimen is sealed and the barcode number of the specimen is captured via a barcode reader. No pre-printed paper CCFs are required for the eScreen system. The donor and collector sign via the digital signature pad, and the CCF is built "on the fly" and secured via a third-party verification system. This prevents changes or tampering with the CCF record.

The CCF document is now viewable online by each authorized party in real time, and the donor may be dismissed. The collection site does not have to fax or mail the MRO copy or employer copy. A copy can be printed at the collection site for the donor, and a second copy will accompany the specimen to the laboratory in the event of confirmation testing.

6.3. The eReader

Lighting conditions on the test strip are standardized and enhanced with white and green light-emitting diodes (LEDs) to improve the contrast between the background and test lines. Software was written to measure the optical activity of the CCD and produce a digital output in the form of translating the series of bars and spaces into 1s and 0s, as previously described. Thresholds were calibrated according to the strip manufacturer's specifications and the Substance Abuse and Mental Health Services Administration (SAMHSA) cut-off levels. The eReader has essentially only one moving part, the plunger mechanism. The plunger bracket is attached to an integrated light shield lowered onto the eCup lid to block ambient light from the camera. Once the eCup is inserted into the reader and the eScreen Web-based CCF is completed, an instruction is sent to the reader to begin the test. The plunger locks the eCup into the reader during the testing process and proceeds with the imaging and analysis in the background, which allows the collector to proceed with the next collection. An internal timing routine accurately measures the point in time that the plunger is activated, thereby wetting the test strips. Three minutes after the test strips are aliquoted, a series of images are taken and analyzed every 15 s until all test lines and control lines are imaged or until 8 min, when the test will end. Results considered perfect negatives, e.g., no drugs, or adulterants present and normal specimen validity, are reported instantly to the customer's myeScreen.com® Web site. The light shield and plunger mechanism are withdrawn, and the operator notified when the test is completed. Once complete, the reader automatically releases the specimen, and reports the result to the eScreen Web server. Customers pick up their test results on their portal.

6.4. The myeScreen.com Portal

In the eScreen model, the digital information record begins when the employer orders a drug test online, schedules the event at the collection site via the portal at myeScreen.com, and the collection site has the complete donor information "pre-accessioned."

The donor's failure to appear within the prescribed time frame, usually 24 h, results in an e-mail to the employer, and a flag on the collection site record to cancel the collection. If the collection proceeds as scheduled, the laboratory, MRO, administrator, and employer have pre-accessioned data of the eScreen drug test, and know whether they should expect a specimen or result in the coming days. Exception reports can be generated to alert the service providers that the specimen or result has not been received when expected, before the customer calls looking for a missing result.

myeScreen.com is a robust application service provider (ASP) software model, allowing employers to manage their drug-testing programs from beginning to end at their desktop. Report generators create standard and customized reports detailing turnaround times throughout the drug-testing process, results statistics, random selections, exception reports, CCF files, and background screening results.

6.5. Benefits of a Closed Information System

Historically, in the laboratory-centric model, drug testing has been an open information system. The MRO receives laboratory data when then lab completes the specimen testing. The MRO doesn't know what they will be receiving until they receive it. The same is true for the laboratory. The laboratory receives samples each day sent from the collection site, not knowing what they will be receiving. There is no feedback loop in an open system, and the result is a lack of anticipated information and an arduous task of tracking missing specimens or results, starting at the end of process and moving forward until the problem has been identified.

In the eScreen closed-loop information model, each of the parties to the transaction communicates via the Web to a common server. The donor, employer, collector, eReader, laboratory, and MRO each have access to the drug-test record in real time. Any party can access their respective portion of the record, sharing common file elements. Pre-accession data elements are available to downstream service providers. Clients and upstream service providers can track the progress of the record as it moves through the system.

7. CONCLUSIONS

The product of a drug test is information. Drug-testing laboratories have benefited from automation and information systems since they became practical to implement. Decentralization of the drug-testing laboratory, using the eScreen system, allows thousands of networked Internet readers to perform the immunoassay screen at the point of collection using lateral-flow drugs-of-abuse strips embedded in eScreen's eCup. The eScreen123 software platform allows each service provider real-time access to the drug-test record, creating a digital pathway of drug-test information from initiation of the drug-test order until the completion of the test, either at the point of collection or MRO service. myeScreen.com allows employers to schedule events and manage their drug-testing program at more than 1000 points of collection nationwide, each following a standardized method and standard operating procedures. The eReader removes subjective interpretation, bias, and transcription errors, and protects the donor's confidential information.

REFERENCES

1. Hohenberger EC. Urinalysis with test strips Roche Diagnostics: 2004; pp. 1–112.
2. Foster K, Despotis G, and Scott MG. Point-of-care testing. Cost issues and impact on hospital operations. Clin Lab Med 2001;21(2):269–284.
3. Delaney B, Wilson S, Fitzmaurice D, Hyde C, and Hobbs R. Near-patient tests in primary care: setting the standards for evaluation. J Health Serv Res Policy 2000; 5(1):37–41.
4. Daviaud J, Fournet D, Ballongue C, et al. Reliability and feasibility of pregnancy home-use tests: laboratory validation and diagnostic evaluation by 638 volunteers. Clin Chem 1993;39(1):53–59.
5. Alfthan H, Bjorses UM, Tiitinen A, and Stenman UH. Specificity and detection limit of ten pregnancy tests. Scand J Clin Lab Invest Suppl 1993;216:105–113.
6. O'Connor RE, Bibro CM, Pegg PJ, and Bouzoukis JK. The comparative sensitivity and specificity of serum and urine HCG determinations in the ED. Am J Emerg Med 1993;11(4):434–436.
7. Christensen H, Thyssen HH, Schebye O, and Berget A. Three highly sensitive "bedside" serum and urine tests for pregnancy compared. Clin Chem 1990;36(9):1686–1688.
8. Levy S, Van Hook S, and Knight J. A review of Internet-based home drug-testing products for parents. Pediatrics 2004;113(4):720–726.
9. Kost GJ. Knowledge optimization theory and application to point-of-care testing. Stud Health Technol Inform 1999;62:189–190.
10. Bissell M. Point-of-care testing at the millennium. Crit Care Nurs Q 2001;24(1): 39–43.
11. Gouget B, Barclay J, and Rakotoambinina B. Impact of emerging technologies and regulations on the role of POCT. Clin Chim Acta 2001;307(1–2):235–240.

12. Delaney B, Wilson S, Fitzmaurice D, Hyde C, and Hobbs R. Near-patient tests in primary care: setting the standards for evaluation. J Health Serv Res Policy 20005(1):37–41.
13. Jenkins AJ, Mills LC, Darwin WD, Huestis MA, Cone EJ, and Mitchell JM. Validity testing of the EZ-SCREEN cannabinoid test. J Anal Toxicol 1993;17(5):292–298.
14. Yang JM. Toxicology and drugs of abuse testing at the point of care. Clin Lab Med 2001;21(2):363–374, ix–x.
15. Kadehjian LJ. Performance of five non-instrumented urine drug-testing devices with challenging near-cutoff specimens. J Anal Toxicol 200125(8):670–679.
16. Caplan YH and Goldberger BA. Alternative specimens for workplace drug testing. J Anal Toxicol 2001;25(5):396–399.

Chapter 13

Adulteration of Drugs-of-Abuse Specimens

Amitava Dasgupta

SUMMARY

Persons abusing drugs attempt to adulterate urine specimens in order to beat drug testing. Dilution of urine in vivo by consuming excess fluid and various detoxifying agents available through the Internet is a common practice. Household chemicals such as bleach, acid, table salt, laundry detergent, toilet-bowl cleaner, vinegar, lemon juice, and Visine® (Pfizer) eye drops are also used for adulterating urine specimens. Most of these adulterants except Visine eye drops can be detected by routine specimen integrity tests (creatinine, pH, temperature, and specific gravity). However, certain adulterants, such as Klear™, Whizzies, Urine Luck™, and Stealth™, cannot be detected by using routine specimen integrity testing. These adulterants can successfully mask drug testing if the concentrations of certain abused drugs are moderate. Several spot tests have been described in the literature to detect the presence of such adulterants in urine. More recently, urine dipsticks are commercially available (AdultaCheck® 4 [Sciteck], Adulta-Check 6, Intect® 7 [Branan Medical Corporation]) for detecting the presence of such adulterants along with creatinine, pH, and specific gravity. Hair and saliva testing for abused drugs are gaining popularity because such specimens are collected directly from a person. Moreover, abused drugs can be detected for a longer time in hair. Recently, certain hair shampoo and saliva cleaning products have become available to beat drug testing involving hair or saliva specimens.

1. THE STATE OF DRUG ABUSE

Abuse of drugs is a critical problem in the United States and the rest of the world. Common drugs of abuse (DOA) include cocaine, cannabinoids,

From: *Forensic Science and Medicine: Drugs of Abuse: Body Fluid Testing*
Edited by R. C. Wong and H. Y. Tse © Humana Press Inc., Totowa, NJ

amphetamine, phencyclidine, and benzodiazepines. Recreational use of cocaine dates back to the Incas in South America 5000 yr ago. In the 1980s, cocaine was a popular DOA. Currently, in the United States, cocaine use is responsible for more emergency-room visits than any other drug. An estimated 25 million people between the ages of 26 and 34 yr have used cocaine at least once *(1)*. For centuries, marijuana has also been widely used as a recreational drug. This drug is very popular among young adults. Δ-9-Tetrahydrocannabinol (THC) is the principal active ingredient of *Cannabis sativa*, a hemp plant. Hashish, the resin extract from the tops of the flowering plants, may have a THC concentration of over 10%. Amphetamine, another popular DOA, was first synthesized in 1887 and was introduced into the United States in tablet forms in 1937 for the treatment of narcolepsy. During World War II, this drug was used to overcome battle fatigue among soldiers. Following World War II, there was an epidemic of amphetamine abuse. Today, the drug is still widely abused. Phencyclidine (PCP), also known as angel dust, is also popular on the street. The chemical name of PCP is 1-(1-phencyclohexyl) piperidine. It was discovered in 1956 by a pharmacologist at Parke-Davis. In addition, eleven benzodiazepines are currently available in the United States. For many years diazepam was the most prescribed drug in the United States. Lysergic acid diethylamide (LSD), a popular drug of the 1960s, is coming back on the illegal market. In recent years, designer drugs such as 3,4-methylenedioxy amphetamine (MDA) and 3.4-methylenedioxymethamphetamine (MDMA; "ecstasy") are commonly used in rave parties. Two notorious drugs, flunitrazepam (rohypnol) and γ-hydroxy butyric acid, have both gained publicity in date-rape situations. The window of detection for some of these drugs and their metabolites as well as the sensitivities of the screening immunoassays is given in Table 1.

A study of drug abuse among the Army and National Guards was conducted between 1991 and 2000. In fiscal year 2000, the positive drug-testing rate reached a 10-yr high of 1.04%, with marijuana (0.51%) and cocaine (0.19%) being among the most popular DOA *(2)*. It is interesting to note that, according to a recent survey of academic anesthesiology departments *(3)*, fentanyl was the most popular abused drug among university faculty members (1.0%) and medical residents (1.6%).

2. FEDERAL GUIDELINES FOR DRUGS-OF-ABUSE TESTING

Drug-testing programs in the United States can be classified as mandatory or nonmandatory. In the first group (e.g., Department of Transportation), a regulated employer is required by federal regulation to test their employees for drugs of abuse. In the second category, employers choose to test their employee for reasons other than the federal requirements. Private employers who are not

Table 1
Window of Detection and Detection Limit of Abused Drugs

Drug	Window	Screening cut-off	GC-MS confirmation cut-off
Amphetamine	2–3 d	1000 ng/mL	500 ng/mL
Methamphetamine	2–3 d	1000 ng/mL	500 ng/mL
Cocaine as	2–3 d	300 ng/mL	150 ng/mL
Benzoylecgonine		100 ng/mL for Military	
Marijuana metabolites	2 d–3 wk	20, 50–100 ng/mL	15 ng/mL
Opiate metabolites	2–3 d	2000 ng/mL*	2000 ng/mL*
6-monoacetylmorphine			10 ng/mL
Phencyclidine	8 d–3 wk	25 ng/mL	25 ng/mL
Benzodiazepines	3 or more d	300 ng/mL	300 ng/mL
Methadone	3 d	300 ng/mL	300 ng/mL
Methaqualone	2 wk	75 ng/mL	75 ng/mL

*The US Department of Health and Human Services has increased the cut-off for both screening and confirmation of opiates to 2000 ng/mL from 300 ng/mL in order to avoid false-positives caused by ingestion of food containing poppy seeds.
GC-MS, gas chromatography-mass spectrometry.

mandated to test under federal authority have instituted employee drug-testing programs in order to create a drug-free workplace. In fact, in 1986, President Reagan issued Executive Order No. 12564, directing all federal agencies to achieve a drug-free work environment. Guidelines for DOA testing were then developed by the Substance Abuse and Mental Health Services Administration (SAMHSA, formerly The National Institute on Drug Abuse [NIDA]) and became the gold standard for all drug-testing programs to follow. The overall testing process under mandatory testing consists of proper collection of specimen, initiation of chain of custody, and final analysis of specimen. Immunoassays are available for quick screening of abused drugs in urine. This must be performed with US Food and Drug Administration (FDA)-approved methods. Positive screening results must then be confirmed by a SAMHSA-certified laboratory using gas chromatography(GC)-mass spectrometry (MS). The cut-off values for DOA testing are included in Table 1.

3. SAMPLE ADULTERATION IN URINE DOA TESTING

The instant DOA testing procedures are instituted, opposing forces are at work to develop methods to avoid detection of drug use. Initially, common household chemicals such as laundry bleach, table salt, toilet-bowl cleaner, hand soap, and vinegar were used. More recently, a variety of products became commercially available, which can be ordered through Internet sites and toll-free telephone numbers. Commercially available adulteration products can be classified into two broad categories. The first category consists of specific fluids or tablets, which when taken along with plenty of water, serve to flush out drugs and metabolites, resulting in diluted urine and reduced concentrations of drugs or metabolites. Examples of products in this category include Absolute Detox XXL drink, Absolute Carbo Drinks, Ready Clean Drug Detox Drink, Fast Flush Capsules, and Ready Clean Gel Capsules. All products are available from Internet sites. Root Clean is a hair-cleansing system targeting drug tests involving hair specimens. It is claimed that using this shampoo will remove all "toxins" from hair within 10 min and the hair zone will be drug free up to 8 h.The second category consists of in vitro urinary adulterants, which are added to urine after collection in order to affect the results of a drug test. Stealth (containing peroxidase and peroxide), Klear (containing nitrite), Clean ADD-IT-ive™ (containing glutaraldehyde), and Urine Luck (containing pyridinium chlorochromate [PCC]) are urinary adulterants that are easily available through the Internet.

Another trick to avoid a positive drug test is to substitute a drug-positive urine sample with a drug-negative urine sample. Synthetic urine is commercial available and can be switched with the true sample in situations when sample collection is not supervised. For example, Quick Fix Synthetic Urine contains premixed laboratory urine having all the characteristics of natural urine, with correct pH, specific gravity and creatinine levels. The product can be heated in a microwave oven for up to 10 s to reach a temperature between 90 and 100°F. It can also be taped to a heater pad so that the temperature can be maintained for up to 6 h in a pocket.

3.1. Diluted Urine: A Simple Way to Beat Drug Tests

A negative result for the presence of abused drugs in a urine specimen does not necessarily mean that no drug is present. It is also possible that the amount of drug was below the cut-off values used in the drug-testing protocol. Diluting urine is a simple way to beat an otherwise positive drug test if the original concentrations of drugs in the urine are just slightly above the cut-off values. To counteract this strategy, creatinine analysis in urine is an effective method to detect diluted urine. Neeedleman and Porvaznik considered a creatinine value of less than 10 mg/dL as suggestive of replacement of urine specimen largely by water *(4)*. Beck et al. *(5)* reported that 11% of all urine specimens submitted to their laboratory for DOA testing were diluted. The SAMHSA program currently does not allow analysis of dilute urine specimens at lower screening and confirmation cut-offs. However, in Canada, the Correction Services of Canada (CSA) program incorporates the following lower drugs/metabolites screening and confirmation cut-offs for testing diluted urine specimens:

- Amphetamine—screening cut-off, 100 ng/mL; confirmation cut-off, 100 ng/mL;
- Benzoylecgonine (BE)—screening and confirmation cut-off, 15 ng/mL;
- Opiates—screening and confirmation cut-off, 120 ng/mL;
- Phencyclidine—screening and confirmation cut-off, 5 ng/mL;
- Cannabinoids—screening cut-off, 20 ng/mL; confirmation cut-off, 3 ng/mL.

Use of flushing and detoxification is frequently advertised as an effective means of passing drug tests. Cone et al. *(6)* evaluated the effect of excess fluid ingestion on false-negative marijuana and cocaine urine test results. These investigators studied the ability of Natural Clean Herbal Tea, goldenseal root, and hydrochlorothiazide to cause false-negative results. After 22 h of smoking marijuana cigarettes or intranasal administration of cocaine, volunteers drank 1 gal of either water, herbal tea, or hydrochlorothiazide, each in four doses over a 4-h period. It was found that within 2 h following these treatments, creatinine and specific gravity dropped to below 20 mg/dL and below 1.003, respectively. These levels were consistent with those of diluted specimens. In these experiments, marijuana and cocaine metabolite levels, as measured by enzyme-multiplied immunoassay technique (EMIT®, Dade-Behring), were also reduced significantly. It appeared that consumption of excess water was effective in diluting a urine specimen to cause false-negative results. However, consumption of herbal tea produced diluted urine faster than consumption of water alone.

In the sport scene, diuretics are used to flush out previously ingested banned substances by forced diuresis. The Medical Commission of the International Olympic Committee has banned the used of diuretics, and GC-MS is used to detect diuretics in urine. Deventer et al. *(7)* recently published a protocol to detect 18 common diuretics and probenecid in doping analysis using liquid chromatography and tandem mass spectrometry.

3.2. Household Chemicals as Urine Adulterants

Simple household chemicals are found to be effective adulterants of urine drug tests. These include table salt, vinegar, liquid laundry bleach, concentrated lemon juice, and Visine eye drops *(8,9)*. The effectiveness of these chemicals on specific drug tests is summarized below.

- Amphetamines: sodium chloride at a concentration of 75 gm/L of urine caused a false-negative drug test in a urine specimen containing 1420 ng/mL of amphetamine. Similarly, Drano® (bleach; SC Johnson & Son) at a concentration of 18 mL/L masked a urine specimen containing 1800 ng/mL of amphetamines by EMIT assay.
- Barbiturates: sodium chloride, liquid hand soap, and Drano all masked barbiturates with concentrations up to 1450 ng/mL.
- Benzodiazepines: Visine, hand soap, and Drano caused false-negative tests with benzodiazepines at concentrations less than 6500 ng/mL.
- Cocaine: Drano and sodium chloride can mask cocaine screens at BE concentrations up to 1180 ng/mL.
- Marijuana: sodium chloride, Drano, goldenseal root, soap, and vinegar all interfered with the marijuana immunoassay tests.
- Opiates: Drano and sodium chloride also interfered with the opiate assays. Urines with opiate up to 2700 ng/mL tested negative in the presence of 125 mL/L of Drano. Sodium chloride interfered only for drug concentrations below 780 ng/mL.

Although there are reports that adulterants interfere less with fluorescence polarization immune assay (FPIA) than with the EMIT assay, others have observed some interference. Sodium chloride caused negative interference with all drugs tested by EMIT and a slight decrease in measured concentrations of benzodiazepines by FPIA. Interestingly, sodium bicarbonate caused a false positive of opiate when assayed by EMIT and of PCP when assayed by FPIA. Hydrogen peroxide also caused a false-positive benzodiazepine result by FPIA *(9)*.

Schwarzhoff and Cody *(10)* systematically studied the effect of 16 different adulterating agents by FPIA analysis of urine for abused drugs. The authors tested these adulterating agents at 10% by volume concentration of urine. Out of six drugs tested (cocaine metabolite, amphetamines, opiates, phencyclidine, cannabinoid, and barbiturates), it was found that the cannabinoid test was the most susceptible to adulteration—approximately one-half of the agents (ascorbic acid, vinegar, bleach, lime solvent, Visine eye drops, goldenseal) tested caused false-negative results. Actual degradation of THC in the presence of the adulterants was observed by GC-MS analysis. The PCP and BE (the metabolite of cocaine) analyses were most affected by alkaline agents. Baiker et al. *(11)* also reported that hypochlorite (a common ingredient of household bleach) adulteration of urine caused decreased concentration of THC to be detected by GC-MS, FPIA, as well as Roche Abuscreen®.

In addition, Uebel and Wium *(12)* also studied the effect of common household chemicals such as Jik (a South African brand of bleach; sodium hypochlorite), Dettol (Reckitt Benckiser UK; chloroxylenol), G-cide Plus (JAST International; glutaraldehyde), Pearle Hand Soap, ethanol, isopropanol, and peroxide in causing false-negative results when used as adulterants in urine specimens. Most of these chemicals interfered with toxicological screening results using EMIT DOA urine-test reagents. Glutaraldehyde and Pearle Hand Soap had the greatest effect (false negative) on a methaqualone test. Chloroxylenol and Pearl Hand Soap also demonstrated maximum effect in causing a false negative in cannabis tests.

3.3. Pyridinium Chlorochromate As a Urine Adulterant

Besides simple household chemicals, more sophisticated substances are advertised commercially as adulterants for urine drug tests. Wu et al. *(13)* reported that the active ingredient of Urine Luck is 200 mmol/L of pyridinium chlorochromate (PCC). The authors reported that Urine Luck caused a decrease in response rate for all EMIT II drug screens and for the Abuscreen morphine and THC assays. In contrast, Abuscreen amphetamine assay produced a higher response rate, and no effect was observed on the results of BE and PCP. This adulteration of urine did not alter GC-MS confirmation of methamphetamine, BE, and PCP. However, apparent concentrations of opiates and THC were reduced.

3.4. Nitrites As Urine Adulterants

The commercial adulterant product Klear comes in two micro-tubes containing 500 mg of white crystalline material. This product readily dissolves in urine with no change in color or temperature of the urine. Klear may cause false-negative GC-MS confirmation of marijuana. ElSohly et al. *(14)* first reported this product as potassium nitrite and provided evidence that nitrite leads to decomposition of ions of Δ-9-THC and its internal standard. The authors reported that using a bisulfite step at the beginning of sample preparation could eliminate this interference. The group also investigated the effect of nitrite on immunoassay screening of other drugs. These drugs include cocaine metabolites, morphine, THC metabolites, amphetamine, and phencyclidine. Nitrite at a concentration of 1.0 M had no effect on the Abuscreen assay. At a higher nitrite concentration, the amphetamine assay becomes more sensitive and the THC assay becomes less sensitive. The GC-MS analyses of BE, morphine, amphetamine, and phencyclidine were not affected, whereas recovery of the THC metabolites was significantly reduced. Again, this interference could be eliminated by bisulfite treatment.

Nitrites also significantly affected the pH of urine samples, creating false-negative test results in immunoassays. Another important factor was the original drug concentration. However, for carboxyl-THC, regardless of the original drug concentration, all specimens with acidic pH showed negative immunoassay results using a SYVA EMIT dau or Roche Abuscreen OnLine® system or an onsite THC immunoassay (Roche OnTrak TesTstik™). Significant decreases in immunoassay results could be observed within 4 h of nitrite adulteration (15).

3.5. Peroxidase Activities in Urine Adulteration

Stealth is an adulterant advertised as an effective way to beat a urine drug test. Stealth consists of two vials, one containing a powder (peroxidase) and a second one containing a liquid (peroxide). Combining the contents of both vials results in a strong oxidizing potential capable of oxidizing several drugs and metabolites. Stealth can mask detection of marijuana metabolite, LSD, and opiate (morphine) at 125–150% of cut-off values assayed by Roche OnLine and Microgenic's CEDIA® immunoassay (16). Low concentration of morphine (2500 ng/mL) could be effectively masked by Stealth, but not higher concentrations (6000 ng/mL). Stealth also affects the GC-MS confirmation step. Cody et al. (17) reported that results of GC-MS analysis of Stealth-adulterated urine using standard procedures proved unsuccessful in several cases, and in 4 out of 12 cases, neither the drug nor the internal standard was recovered. Addition of sodium disulfite prior to extraction allowed recovery of both drugs and internal standard. However, concentrations of morphine and codeine were reduced by 17 to 30%.

3.6. Glutaraldehyde As a Urine Adulterant

Glutaraldehyde has also been used as an adulterant to mask urine drug tests (18). This product is available under the trade name of UrinAid. Each kit contains 4–5 mL solution of glutaraldehyde, which is to be added to 50–60 mL of urine.

Glutaraldehyde solutions are readily available in hospitals and clinics as a cleaning and sterilizing agent. A 10% solution of glutaraldehyde is also available from pharmacies as over-the-counter medication for treatment of warts. The addition of glutaraldehyde at a concentration of 0.75% volume to urine can lead to false-negative drug-screening results for cannabinoid tests using EMIT II immunoassays. Amphetamine, methadone, benzodiazepine, opiate, and cocaine metabolite tests can be affected at glutaraldehyde concentrations of between 1 and 2% using the EMIT screen. At a glutaraldehyde concentration of 2% by volume, Braithwaite *(18)* found that the assay of cocaine metabolite was significantly affected, with an apparent loss of 90% of assay sensitivity. A loss of 80% sensitivity was also observed with the benzodiazepine assay. Wu et al. *(19)* reported that glutaraldehyde also interfered with the CEDIA immunoassays for screening of abused drugs. Goldberger and Caplan *(20)* reported that glutaraldehyde caused false-negative results with EMIT but also caused false-positive phencyclidine results with the fluorescence polarization immunoassay (Abbott Laboratories) and the kinetic interaction of microparticles in a solution immunoassay (KIMS®, Roche Diagnostics); the Roche RIA assay was least affected.

4. ADULTERATION OF HAIR AND SALIVA SPECIMENS FOR DRUG TESTING

Hair and saliva specimens are alternatives to urine specimens for drug testing (*see* Chapter 11). Several products available through the Internet claim that washing hair with their shampoos can help pass a drug test. Clear Choice Hair Follicle Shampoo claims to remove all residues and toxins within 10 min of use. One application is sufficient for shoulder-length hair, and the effect can last for 8 h. Root Clean hair-cleansing system shampoo has also been commercially available. However, no systematic study has been reported to investigate the effect of using these products in a drug test. Saliva samples are also used for drug testing. The chances of adulteration of saliva specimen are very low to non-existent. However, the manufacturer of a commercially available mouthwash claims that by rinsing the mouth twice with this product, a person can beat saliva-based drug testing, which is a popular method of testing by insurance companies. The same company claims that its specially formulated shampoo cleans hair of any drugs or toxins. A product to clean fingernails to pass a drug test is also available.

5. SPECIMEN INTEGRITY CHECK

With the prevalent use of adulterants to mask known positive drug tests, a number of mechanisms have been developed to check potentially invalid specimens. The simplest adulterant-detection systems check urine samples that deviate from normal ranges of temperature, specific gravity, pH, and creatinine. The temperature for normal urine samples should be 90.5–98.9°F. The specific gravity should be 1.005–1.030, and pH should be 4.0–10.0. The creatinine concentration should be 20–400 mg/dL. Dilution of urine as a result of excess water consumption also lowers the concentration of creatinine in the urine. Adulteration with sodium chloride at a concentration necessary to produce a false-negative result always produces a specific gravity over 1.035. Household vinegar and concentrated lime juice cause urine to turn acidic.

5.1. Detection of Pyridinium Chlorochromate in Adulterated Urine

Wu et al. *(13)* have described a protocol for detection of PCC in urine using spot tests. The indicator solution contains 10 gm/L of 1,5-diphenylcarbazide in methanol. The indicator detects the presence of chromium ion and is colorless when prepared. Two drops of indicator solution is added to 1.0 mL of urine. If a reddish-purple color develops, the test is positive. Ferslew et al. *(21)* tested 36 urine specimens suspected of adulteration for the presence of chromate using a 1,5- diphenylcarbazide color test with detection of chromate ion using capillary ion electrophoretic analysis. The colorimetric chromate assay revealed a mean chromate concentration of 929 µg/mL, whereas the capillary ion electrophoresis showed a mean chromate concentration of 1009 µg/mL. The authors concluded that the colorimetric test could be used as a screening test, and the presence of chromate can be confirmed by using capillary electrophoresis.

Other simple and rapid spot tests have been described for detection of chromate in suspected adulterated urine *(22)*. Addition of four to five drops of 3% hydrogen peroxide in approx 200 µL of urine adulterated with PCC (approx six to seven drops from a transfer pipet) causes rapid formation of a dark brown color, and a dark brown precipitate appears on standing. In contrast, unadulterated urine turns colorless after addition of hydrogen peroxide. One percent potassium iodide in distilled water can also be used as an indicator solution for detection of chromate in urine. Addition of six to seven drops of urine adulterated with chromate to a few drop of 1% potassium iodide solution followed by adding a few drops of 2 *N* hydrochloric acid result in liberation of iodine from potassium iodide solution. Shaking this solution with *n*-butanol results in the transfer of iodine to the organic phase. If no chromate is present, the potassium iodide solution remained colorless. No interference was observed in these color tests from high glucose or ketone bodies.

5.2. *Detection of Excess Nitrite in Adulterated Urine*

Nitrite in urine may arise in vivo and is found in normal urine in low concentration. Patients receiving medications such as nitroglycerine, isosorbide dinitrate, nitroprusside, and ranitidine may have increased nitrite levels in their blood. However, concentrations of nitrite were below 36 µg/mL in specimens cultured positive for microorganisms, and nitrite concentrations were below 6 µg/mL in patients receiving medications that are metabolized to nitrite. On the other hand, nitrite concentrations were 1910–12,200 µg/mL in urine specimens adulterated with nitrite *(23)*. The authors analyzed nitrite concentrations in urine utilizing a Lachat QuickChem® AT automated continuous-flow analyzer (Lachat Instruments) using a protocol approved by the US Environmental Protection Agency.

Whizzies is another urine adulterant that contains potassium nitrite. The presence of nitrite in urine can be detected by a simple spot test using a standard solution of 2% potassium permanganate in distilled water and 2 *N* hydrochloric acid solution *(22)*. If nitrite is present in the urine sample, the pink permanganate solution turned colorless with effervescence immediately after addition of hydrochloric acid. This is because of reduction of heptavalent manganese ion of potassium permanganate by nitrite. The presence of very high glucose (>1000 mg/dL) and ketone bodies in urine may cause false positives. However, this may take approx 2–3 min for the solution to turn colorless, whereas if nitrite is present, the solution turns colorless immediately. The potassium iodide spot test, which is effective to detect the presence of chromate in urine, can also be used for detection of nitrite *(22)*. After addition of a few drops of 2 *N* hydrochloric acid, immediate release of iodine from the colorless potassium iodide solution is observed. As described earlier, shaking of this solution with *n*-butanol results in the transfer of iodine into the organic phase. If no nitrite is present, the potassium iodide solution remains colorless. No interference from high glucose or ketone bodies is observed if present in the urine.

5.3. *Detection of Peroxidase Activities in Adulterated Urine*

Valtier and Cody *(24)* described a rapid color test to detect the presence of the adulterant Stealth in urine. Addition of 10 µL of urine to 50 µL of tetramethylbenzidine (TMB) working solution followed by addition of 500 µL of 0.1-*M* phosphate buffer solution caused a dramatic color change of the specimen to dark brown. Peroxidase activity could also be monitored by using a spectrophotometer. Routine specimen integrity check using pH, creatinine, specific gravity and temperature did not detect the presence of Stealth in urine. If a urine specimen adulterated with Stealth is added to 1% potassium permanganate solution in water, the pink color of potassium permanganate turns colorless immediately after addition of a few drops of 2-*N* hydrochloric acid (Dasgupta et al., unpublished data).

5.4. Detection of Glutaraldehyde in Adulterated Urine

Although it is not possible to notice the presence of glutaraldehyde in urine as an adulterant by either color or smell of the specimen, concentrations of glutaraldehyde greater than 2% cause significant decrease in optical absorbance, and its presence can be detected indirectly based on final absorbance rate readings (dA/min) *(18)*. Although the presence of glutaraldehyde as an adulterant can also be detected by GC-MS, Wu et al. *(25)* described a simple fluorometric method for the detection of glutaraldehyde in urine. When 0.5 mL of urine was heated with 1 mL of 7.7 mmol/L potassium dihydrogen phosphate (pH 3.0) saturated with diethylthiobarbituric acid for 1 h at 96–98°C in a heating block, a yellow-green fluorophore developed if glutaldehyde was present. Shaking the specimen with *n*-butanol resulted in the transfer of this adduct to the organic layer, which can be viewed under long-wavelength ultraviolet light. Glutaraldehyde in urine can also be estimated using a fluorometer.

5.5. On-Site Adulteration Detection Devices for Urine Specimens

Recently, on-site adulterant detection devices have become commercially available. These devices offer an advantage over spot tests because an adulteration check can be performed at the collection site. Peace and Tarani *(26)* evaluated performance of three on-site devices—Intect 7, MASK™ Ultra Screen from Kacey, Inc., and AdultaCheck 4. Intect 7 simultaneously tests creatinine, nitrite, glutaraldehyde, pH, specific gravity, pyridinium chlorochromate (PCC), and bleach. Ultrascreen tests for creatinine, nitrite, pH, specific gravity, and oxidants. AdultaCheck 4 tests for creatinine, nitrite, glutaraldehyde, and pH. The authors adulterated urine specimens with Stealth, Urine Luck, Instant Clean ADD-IT-ive, and Klear according to the manufacturers' recommended procedures, and concluded that Intect 7 was the most sensitive and correctly identified the adulterants. AdultaCheck 4 did not detect Stealth, Urine Luck, or Instant Clean ADD-it-ive. Ultra Screen detected a broader range of adulterants than AdultaCheck 4. However, in practical terms, it only detected these adulterants at levels well above their optimum usage, making it less effective than Intect 7. However, King *(27)* has reported that AdultaCheck 4 is an excellent way to detect contamination in urine specimens.

AdultaCheck 6 test strips have recently become available, which can be used to detect creatinine, oxidants, nitrite, glutaraldehyde, pH, and chromate.

Intect 7 test strip for checking adulteration in urine is composed of seven different pads to test for creatinine, nitrite, glutaraldehyde, pH, specific gravity, bleach, and pyridinium chlorochromate (PCC). In our experience, both AdultaCheck 6 and Intect 7 effectively identified the presence of low and high concentrations of PCC in urine. For example, with a low PCC concentration (0.5 g/L), the Intect 7 test pad turned blue from colorless. In the presence of high PCC, the color changed to dark brown. For AdultaCheck 6, the color of the PCC pad turned to purple in the presence of low PCC, and a mustard-green color was observed if high concentrations of PCC were present in the specimen. AdultaCheck 6 and Intact 7 were superior to potassium iodide spot test in detecting the presence of small amounts of PCC in urine. The potassium iodide spot test was unable to detect a low PCC concentration of 0.5 g/L *(34)*. Intect 7 urine test strip has a pad for detecting the presence of bleach in urine. A positive response was observed even in the presence of only 5 µL of bleach per mL of urine. Such a small amount of bleach cannot be detected by AdultaCheck 6 test strip, because the test for the oxidant was still negative. No change of pH was observed. Moreover, no noticeable color change was observed in the potassium iodide solution after acidification. In the presence of 10 µL of bleach per mL of urine, the Intect 7 test pad for detecting bleach was strongly positive, along with the potassium iodide spot test *(28)*.

AdultaCheck 6 and Intect 7 test strips were effective for detecting the presence of glutaraldehyde in urine. When glutaraldehyde was present at a concentration of less than 0.4% by volume, neither AdultaCheck 6 nor Intect 7 showed the expected color change. However, at glutaraldehyde concentrations above 2% by volume both urine test strips showed the desired color change in the pad designed to detect the presence of glutaraldehyde.

AdultaCheck 6 has a test pad for determining the creatinine concentration in urine. The possible readings are 0, 10, 20, 50, 100, and 400 mg/dL. The Intect 7 test pad shows a reading of 0, 10, 20, 50, or 100 mg/dL, depending on color change of the test pad. AdultaCheck 6 or Intect 7 test strips can determine a range of creatinine value. The precise concentration of creatinine cannot be determined. Similarly, neither test strip can determine the precise pH of a urine specimen, but can only show the range. However, both AdultaCheck 6 and Intect 7 test strips successfully differentiated between abnormal values of creatinine and pH and normal values in urine as determined by precise measurement of creatinine using the Synchron LX 20 analyzer and pH using a pH meter. When acid or alkali was added to change the pH of urine, both AdultaCheck6 and Intect 7 urine test strips showed the correct trend of lower or higher pH (Table 2) *(28)*.

Table 2
Comparison of pH, Creatinine, and Specific Gravity Obtained by Direct Measurement and Urine Test Strips in 10 Urine Specimens

Specimen	pH			Specific gravity		Creatinine, mg/dL		
	Measured	AdultaCheck® 6	Intect® 7	Measured	Intect 7	Measured	AdultaCheck 6	Intect 7
1	7.2	9.0	10.0	1.016	1.015	102.7	100.0	100.0
2	6.4	9.0	5.0	1.011	1.005	85.3	100.0	100.0
3	7.1	9.0	10.0	1.015	1.005	101.6	100.0	100.0
4	6.8	9.0	10.0	1.002	1.003	22.1	20.0	20.0
5	7.0	9.0	10.0	1.004	1.005	22.4	20.0	20.0
6	6.6	5.0	5.0	1.013	1.005	18.7	20.0	20.0
7	6.5	5.0	5.0	1.015	1.015	93.7	100.0	100.0
8	4.9	5.0	5.0	1.013	1.015	57.0	50.0	50.0
9	6.4	9.0	10.0	1.009	1.005	60.1	50.0	50.0
10	5.5	5.0	5.0	1.010	1.005	72.1	100.0	100.0
11	6.5	9.0	10.0	1.005	1.005	27.0	20.0	20.0
11 (1:1 dil)	7.0	9.0	10.0	1.002	1.003	13.8	10.0	10.0
11 (Acidified)	2.8	3.0	3.0	1.002	1.003	26.8	20.0	20.0
11 (Alkali)	11.2	11.0	>11	1.002	1.003	27.9	20.0	20.0
12	5.9	5.0	5.0	1.005	1.005	20.9	20.0	20.0
12 (1:1 dil)	6.5	9.0	10.0	1.003	1.005	10.4	10.0	10.0
12 (Acidified)	3.1	3.0	3.0	1.002	1.003	21.1	20.0	20.0
12 (Alkali)	11.5	11	>11	1.001	1.000	21.3	20.0	20.0

Adapted from ref. 28.

6. CONCLUSIONS

Adulterants impose a new challenge in testing for abused drugs. Routine specimen integrity testing involving pH, creatinine, specific gravity, and temperature is not adequate to detect the presence of recently introduced adulterants such as Urine Luck, Klear, and Stealth. These agents can cause false negatives in immunoassay screening tests and may also affect the GC-MS confirmation tests. To counteract these effects, spot tests have been introduced, and several strip tests (AdultaCheck 4, AdultaCheck 6, Intect 7, and so on) are available for validation of specimen integrity. Studies are also needed to investigate effectiveness of hair shampoo in causing false negatives in a hair drug test and mouthwash products to invalidate saliva testing for abused drugs.

REFERENCES

1. Keller KB and Lemberg L. The cocaine abused heart. Am J Crit Care 2003;12: 562–566.
2. Bruins MR, Okano CK, Lyons TP, and Lukey BJ. Drug-positive rates for the army from fiscal year 1991 to 2000 and for National Guard from fiscal year 1997 to 2000. Mil Med 2002;167, 379–383.
3. Booth JV, Grossman D, Moore J, et al. Substance abuse among physicians: a survey of academic anesthesiology programs. Anesth Analg 2002;95:1024–1030.
4. Needleman SD. and Porvaznik M. Creatinine analysis in single collection urine specimens. J Forensic Sci 1992;37:1125–1133.
5. Beck O, Bohlin M, Bragd F, Bragd J, and Greitz O. Adulteration of urine drug testing-an exaggerated cause of concern [article in Swedish]. Lakartidningen 2000;97: 703–706.
6. Cone EJ, Lange R, and Darwin WD. In vivo adulteration: excess fluid ingestion cause false negative marijuana and cocaine urine test results. J Anal Toxicol 1998; 22:460–473.
7. Deventer K, Delbeke T, Roels K, and Van Eenoo P. Screening for 18 diuretics and probenecid in doping analysis by liquid chromatography-tandem mass spectrometry. Biomedical Chromatography 2002;16:529–535.
8. Mikkelsen SL and Ash O. Adulterants causing false negative in illicit drug test. Clin Chem 1988;34:2333–2336.
9. Warner A. Interference of household chemicals in immunoassay methods for drugs of abuse. Clin Chem 1989;35:648–651.
10. Schwarzhoff R and Cody JT. The effects of adulterating agents on FPIA analysis of urine for drugs of abuse. J Anal Toxicol 1993;17:14–17.
11. Baiker C, Serrano L, and Lindner B. Hypochlorite adulteration of urine causing decreased concentration of delta-9-THC-COOH by GC/MS. J Anal Toxicol 1994; 18:101–103.
12. Uebel RA and Wium CA. Toxicological screening for drugs of abuse in samples adulterated with household chemicals. S Afr Med J 2002;92:547–549.

13. Wu AH, Bristol B, Sexton K, Cassella-McLane G, Holtman V, and Hill DW. Adulteration of urine by Urine Luck. Clin. Chem. 1999;45:1051–1057.

14. ElSohly MA, Feng S, Kopycki WJ, et al. A procedure to overcome interferences caused by adulterant "Klear" in the GC-MS analysis of 11-nor-Δ9-THC-9-COOH. J Anal Toxicol 1997;20:240–242.

15. Tsai LS, ElSohly MA, Tsai SF, Murphy TP, Twarowska, B, and Salamone SJ. Investigation of nitrite adulteration on immunoassay and GC-MS analysis of cannabinoids in urine specimens. J Anal Toxicol 2000;24:708–714.

16. Cody JT and Valtier S. Effects of Stealth adulteration on immunoassay testing for drugs of abuse. J Anal Toxicol 2001;25:466–470.

17. Cody JT, Valtier S, and Kuhlman J. Analysis of morphine and codeine in samples adulterated with Stealth. J Anal Toxicol 2001;25:572–575.

18. George S and Braithwaite RA. The effect of glutaraldehyde adulteration of urine specimens on Syva EMIT II drugs of abuse assay. J Anal Toxicol 1996;20:195–196.

19. Wu AH, Forte E, Casella G, et al. CEDIA for screening drugs of abuse in urine and the effect of adulterants. J Foren Sci 1995;40:614–618.

20. Goldberger BA and Caplan YH. Effect of glutaraldehyde (UrinAid) on detection of abused drugs in urine by immunoassay [Letter]. Clin Chem 1994;40:1605–1606.

21. Ferslew KE, Nicolaides AN, and Robert TA. Determination of chromate adulteration of human urine by automated colorimetric and capillary ion electrophoretic analyses. J Anal Toxicol 2003;27:36–39.

22. Dasgupta A, Wahed A, and Well A. Rapid spot tests for detecting the presence of adulterants in urine specimens submitted for drug testing. Am J Clin Pathol. 2002; 117:325–329.

23. Urry F, Komaromy-Hiller G, Staley B, et al. Nitrite adulteration of workplace drug testing specimens: sources and associated concentrations of nitrite and distinction between natural sources and adulteration. J Anal Toxicol 1998;22:89–95.

24. Valtier S and Cody JT. A procedure for the detection of Stealth adulterant in urine samples. Clin Lab Sci 2002;15:111–115.

25. Wu A, Schmalz J, and Bennett W. Identification of Urin-Aid adulterated urine specimens by fluorometric analysis [Letter]. Clin Chem 1994;40:845–846.

26. Peace MR and Tarnai LD. Performance evaluation of three on-site adulteration detection devices for urine specimens. J Anal Toxicol 2002;26:464–470.

27. King EJ. Performance of AdultaCheck 4 test stripes for the detection of adulteration at the point of collection of urine specimens used for drugs of abuse testing. J Anal Toxicol 1999;23:72.

28. Dasgupta A, Chughtai O, Hannah C, Davis B, and Wells A. Comparison of spot tests with AdultaCheck 6 and Intect 7 urine test strips for detecting the presence of adulterants in urine specimens. Clin Chem Acta 2004;348(1–2):19–25.

Chapter 14

Adulteration Detection by Intect® 7

Raphael C. Wong and Harley Y. Tse

SUMMARY

The use of commercial adulterants with the aim of defeating urine drug tests has become a growing problem for the drug-testing industry. Such products are easily available and act by substitution, dilution, and chemical adulteration. Regulatory guidelines to detect the presence of adulteration have been established. Several on-site adulteration test products are available. One of the widely used devices is Intect® 7 (Branan Medical Corporation), which is a dipstick covered with seven dry reagent pads that tests for creatinine, specific gravity, pH, nitrite, glutaraldehyde, bleach, and pyridinium chlorochromate. Intect 7 has been shown to detect all currently available commercial adulterants. For two oxidizing adulterants that appear to dissipate within a short period of time, Intect 7 was shown to be useful in detecting their presence on site.

1. INTRODUCTION

A positive drug test result has important impact on one's life, which may include (a) loss of job, (b) extension or initiation of jail sentence, or (c) disqualification of participation privileges including school sports. Hence, the incentive to defeat a drug test is high. Furthermore, advocacy groups such as the National Organization for the Reform of Marijuana Laws (NORML) view drug testing as a violation of the Fourth Amendment to the US Constitution, which forbids unreasonable search and seizures.

Throughout the history of drug testing, masking the positive test result has been a serious problem, and this issue has been described in a number of

From: *Forensic Science and Medicine: Drugs of Abuse: Body Fluid Testing*
Edited by R. C. Wong and H. Y. Tse © Humana Press Inc., Totowa, NJ

publications *(1–3)*. An audit conducted at 66 certified laboratories in the National Laboratory Certification Program in 2001 identified a total of 6440 adulterated specimens and 2821 substituted specimens during a 2-yr period *(4)*. The semi-annual Drug Testing Index released by Quest Diagnostics, Inc. shows that adulteration rate (including the presence of oxidizing adulterants, abnormal acid and base range, and substituted samples) ranges from 2.67% of all positive samples (in 1999) to 1.10% (in 2003) *(5)*.

This chapter summarizes the current status of urine adulteration and describes an on-site device, Intect® 7 (Branan Medical Corporation), to detect such masking.

2. *Adulteration Techniques and Products*

Presently, the use of household products to defeat drug testing *(6)* has been mostly replaced by commercial products that are widely available via the Internet, mail-order through advertisements in such counter-culture, pro-marijuana-use magazines as *High Times* and *Cannabis Culture*, or purchase at head shops and the GNC vitamin store chain. To bypass the law, these products are frequently labeled as detoxification (detox) products and often come with a disclaimer that they are not intended for use on lawfully administered drug tests and are to be used in accordance with all federal and state laws.

The main techniques employed by these adulterants are substitution, dilution, and chemical adulteration.

2.1. Substitution

Substitution refers to the process of substituting a user's "dirty" urine with "clean" urine from another person or an animal, or with synthetic urine. Earlier substitution methods included collecting a "clean" person's or a pet's urine in a container and then dispensing it into the collection cup discreetly. However, the freshness of the urine became a problem. Further, it was difficult to constantly stash a volume of this urine in preparation for random testing. Recently, synthetic urine kits with long shelf life have become available. A typical kit consists of a pouch of liquid or lyophilized synthetic urine with temperature indicator, disposable heating pad, a strap to hold the pouch, and tubing with clamp to deliver the synthetic urine.

To prevent detection under observed collection, one company even markets a prosthetic delivery device shaped like a penis (named the Whizzinator™), which comes in five different colors that match the color of one's skin.

A modification of the substitution process is subjecting the "dirty" urine sample to a purification procedure to remove drug molecules. Products such as Zip N Flip™ and Bake-n-shake™ are kits with a zip-lock bag containing a resinous material like activated charcoal. The urine sample from the collection cup is poured into the bag and swished. The cleansed urine is then poured back into the cup. Such action, of course, can be performed only with unobserved collection.

2.2. Dilution

Dilution involves the process of lowering the concentration of the drugs in the urine by consumption of large amount of liquids *(7)*. The most common means is by water. Various commercial detox drinks, carbo drinks, or herbal teas are available. Most of these drinks contain diuretics supplemented with creatine and vitamin B. Use usually includes the consumption of up to 32 oz of water along with the commercial products.

2.3. Chemical Adulteration

Chemical adulteration is the process of adding exogenous chemicals to the urine sample to prevent proper identification of the drug. A wide range of commercial products is available. These adulterants, often comprised of corrosive and toxic chemicals, are advertised as being able to prevent laboratories from detecting drugs or their metabolites in urine. Usually, the product consists of one or two small vials, which can be easily hidden. During collection, the user would mix the vial content with the urine sample. Many of these products offer 200% money back guarantee if they fail to beat the drug tests. Although product formulations are frequently changed to foil detection, recently developed adulterants are mostly oxidants (examples include nitrite, pyridinium chlorochromate [PCC], hydrogen peroxide, and iodine). Brands like Urine Luck™, Stealth™, and ADD-It-ive™ are most popular.

3. MECHANISM OF ACTION OF CHEMICAL ADULTERATION

Chemical adulterants may act by destroying the drug moieties. In a study on the action of PCC, potassium chromate, and sodium chromate, Paul et al. found that the drug moiety was destroyed by these oxidants. The oxidative properties are shown to result from the chromate ions. PCC affected mainly 11-nor-Δ^9-tetrahydrocannabinol-9-carboxylic acid (THC-acid). PCC also affected morphine at very low pH *(8)*. Further study suggested that the effects of oxidizing agents depended on the reduction potential (E^0), pH, temperature, time of reaction, and urine constituents. Compounds like potassium chromate, sodium nitrite, potassium permanganate, periodic acid, potassium persulfate, Oxone®, hydrogen peroxide/ferrous ammonium sulfate, and sodium oxychloride destroyed THC-acid within 48 h *(9)*.

Chemical adulterants may also act by interfering with the extraction procedures in gas chromatography(GC)-mass spectrometry (MS). In a study on the effect of Stealth on morphine and codeine, Cody et al. found that the adulterant affects the extraction procedures in the GC-MS process *(10)*. Tsai et al. studied the effect of nitrite adulteration on immunoassays and GC-MS and found that nitrite has no significant effect on laboratory and on-site drug screens. However, it interferes with the GC-MS extraction of THC-acid so that adulterated samples that were tested THC-positive by screening tests would not be confirmed *(11)*.

Adulterants can also target the enzymatic assays of the laboratory drug screens. Wu et al. studied the effects of Urine Luck containing PCC and found that it decreased the response rates for several laboratory drug screens, leading to false-negative results partly as a result of the low pH induced by PCC *(12)*.

4. US Government Response to the Adulteration Problem

To counter the widespread use of adulterants and to preserve the integrity of drug testing, several states have enacted laws that bar the sale of adulterants. Currently, these states include Arkansas, Illinois, Kentucky, Oklahoma, New Jersey, and North and South Carolina. At the federal level, both the Substance Abuse and Mental Health Services Administration (SAMHSA) of the Department of Health and Human Services and the Department of Transportation (DOT) have established guidelines for specimen validity testing *(13,14)*. Table 1 summarizes the validation criteria from DOT and SAMHSA. Both these agencies utilize the paired criteria of creatinine and specific gravity to determine whether a sample is diluted or substituted. These criteria were validated in a study by Edgell et al. in which 56 subjects ingested at least 80 oz (2370 mL) of fluid over a 6-h period. Testing of the urine samples collected the next morning could not meet the paired substitution criteria of urine creatinine ≤5.0 mg/dL and specific gravity ≤1.001 or ≥1.020, suggesting that the established criteria would prevent false diluted or substituted results *(15)*.

5. Drug-Testing Industry Response
to the Adulteration Problem

5.1. Laboratory Adulteration Reagents

To prevent specimen adulteration, laboratories have instituted adulterant testing. Reagents for such use are available through companies such as Sciteck Diagnostics, Inc., and Axiom Diagnostics, Inc. Tests for pH, specific gravity, creatinine, glutaraldehyde, and various oxidants are available. However, not all the laboratories test for all the parameters routinely. Moreover, additional

Table 1
Department of Transportation (DOT) and Substance Abuse and Mental Health Services Administration (SAMHSA) Validation Criteria

Criteria	DOT			SAMHSA			
	Adulterated	Substituted	Diluted	Adulterated	Substituted	Diluted	Invalid
Creatinine		≤5 mg/dL	<20 mg/dL		<2 mg/dL	≥2 mg/dL and ≤20 mg/dL	Inconsistent result
Specific Gravity		≤1.001 or ≥1.020	<1.003		≤1.0010 or ≥1.0200	≥1.0010 but <1.0030	Inconsistent result
pH	≤3 or ≥11			<3 or ≥11			≥3 and <4.5; ≥9 and <11
Nitrite	≥500 µg/mL			≥500 µg/mL			≥200 µg/mL
Glutaraldehyde				Presence			Presence
Chromium (VI)				≥50 µg/mL			≥50 µg/mL
Pyridine				≥200 µg/mL Nitrite equivalent or ≥50 µg/mL Chromium (VI)-equivalent			
Halogen				Same as pyridine			Presence
Surfactant				≥100 µg/mL dodecylbenzene sulfonate-equivalent			Same as adulterated
Others							Oxidant presence, Immunoassay interference, equipment damage, appearance

charges are sometimes added to the cost of the drug tests for specimen validity testing, which further hinder widespread use.

5.2. On-Site Adulteration Test Strips

As a primary on-site screen for adulteration, test strips are available from several suppliers.

5.2.1. Urine Adulteration ID Test Strip

A lateral-flow device that detects substituted non-human urine called Urine ID™ is available from Applied Biotech, Inc. It uses a sandwich colloidal gold immunochromatographic dipstick to detect the presence of human immunoglobulin G in urine at a cut-off concentration of 0.5 μg/mL *(16)*.

5.2.2. Multi-Panel Adulteration Test Sticks

Urinalysis test strips such as Multistix® from Bayer Diagnostics and Combur-Test® from Roche Diagnostics were sometimes used as an on-site rapid test for sample adulteration. However, among the various panels of these urinalysis dipsticks, only three are related to specimen validity testing. These include specific gravity, pH, and nitrite. The pH and the nitrite panels, however, cover clinically significant ranges that are outside established specimen validity criteria. Moreover, the specific-gravity panel does not differentiate the levels between 1.000 and 1.005, rendering it useless as a detection tool for substitution and dilution.

Multi-panel dipsticks specifically developed to detect adulteration are available from several manufacturers. These include Adultacheck® from Sciteck Diagnostics, Inc., MASK™ Ultra Screen from Kacey, Inc., and Intect 7. Peace and Tarnai *(17)* evaluated the performance of several dipsticks for their ability to detect adulteration in urine contaminated with commercial and household adulterants; they found that Intect 7 can correctly detect all contaminated samples.

5.2.3. The Intect 7 Adulteration Detection Strip

Because of the continuous formulation changes of some commercial adulterants, the Intect adulteration dipstick product has been improved over time (Intect 6 I, Intect 6 II, Intect 6 III, Intect 7 ver. 1, and Intect 7 ver. 2) to meet the challenge. The following description is of the second generation of Intect 7 (Intect 7 ver. 2).

The Intect 7 ver. 2 test dipstick is a plastic strip covered with seven chemical-treated pads (Fig. 1). To run the test, the strip is dipped into the urine specimen, removed immediately, and blotted sidewise to remove excess

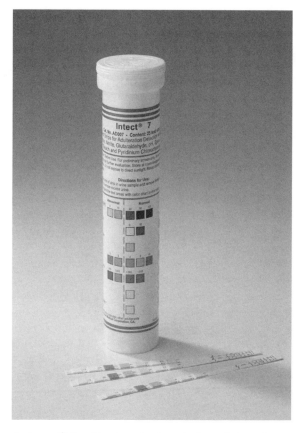

Fig. 1. Intect® 7 with chemical pads for adulteration tests.

urine. After 1 min, the color on each pad is read and compared with a color chart to determine whether the specimen shows abnormality on any of its pads. To aid correct interpretation, each pad is numbered and the orientation of the strip during the reading process is shown on the color chart. The pads provide qualitative results for the following criteria at the indicated levels: creatinine (Cr), 10 to100 mg/dL; nitrite (Ni), 10 to ≥50 mg/dL; glutaraldehyde (Gl), trace; pH, 2 to >11; specific gravity (SG), 1.000 to >1.020; bleach (Bl), trace; and pyridinium chlorochromate (PC), trace.

Test results of the Intect 7 strips on urine samples treated with various adulterants are shown in Table 2. All the adulterants were added to positive urine drug controls obtained from Biochemical Diagnostics, Inc., containing 150 ng/mL of THC-acid (THC), 900 ng/mL of benzoylecgonine (BE), 75 ng/mL of phencylidine (PCP), 900 ng/mL of morphine (MOR), and 3000 ng/mL of amphet-

Table 2

Effects of Adulterants on Abused Drugs and Intect® 7 Test Strips

Adulterant name (chemical composition)	On-site drug tests affected	Abnormal Intect 7 panels						
		Cr	Ni	GI	pH	SG	Bl	PC
Commercial products:								
ADD-IT-ive™	MOR, THC							X
Clear Choice™ᵃ	None						X	X
Instant Clean™ᵃ	THC, BE, PCP		X				X	X
Lucky Labs LL418™ᵃ (PCC)	All 5 drugs		X				X	X
Klear™ᵃ (nitrite)	None		X					
Krystal Kleen™ᵃ	None							
Purafyzit™ᵃ	None						X	X
Stealth™ Catalytic Purifierᵃ	None						X	X
Stealthᵃ(peroxidase and peroxide)	THC, BE, PCP		X				X	X
Urine Luck™ 5.3ᵃ(pyridine)	None						X	X
Urine Luck 6.3ᵃ (hydrofluoric acid)	THC, BE							X
Urine Luck 6.4ᵃ	THC							X
Urine Luck 6.5ᵃ (iodine)	THC, MOR						X	X
Urine Luck 6.7ᵃ	THC, MOR							X
UR'n Kleen™ᵃ	THC, BE, MOR, PCP					X		
Household products								
Chlorine bleachᵇ	All 5 drugs	X						
3% hydrogen peroxide solutionᵇ	None						X	X
Iodine tinctureᵇ	None				X	X		
Liquid drain cleaner (Drano®)ᶜ	MOR, AMP			X	X	X		
Vinegar (5% white distilled)ᵇ	AMP					X		
Chemicals								
Glutaraldehyde (50% liquid)ᵇ	None							
Pyridinium chlorochromateᶜ	All 5 drugs		X			X	X	X
Sodium Nitriteᶜ	None		X			X	X	X

ᵃUse per product instruction.
ᵇ10% volume/volume.
ᶜ10% weight/volume.
MOR, morphine; THC, tetrahydrocannabinol; BE, benzoylecgonine; PCP, phencyclidine; PCC, pyridinium chlorochromate.

amine (AMP). Commercial adulterants were added according to product instructions, and chemical and household adulterants were added according to the concentrations shown on the table. The effects of these adulterants on drugs were monitored by testing the adulterated urine samples on an on-site lateral-flow immunoassay drug-screen cassette, Monitect® PC11, from Branan Medical Corporation. Test results obtained after the urine controls were treated with adulterants for 5 min *(18,19)* showed that some adulterants were effective in masking the presence of some drugs, especially THC. The majority of these adulterants were oxidants. The results also confirmed that some adulterant manufacturers continue to modify their formulations to foil detection. There are also commercial adulterants that are not very effective in modifying the drug-test results. Chemicals used in some of the adulteration formulas have been reported. Available information on these formulas is also included in Table 2.

6. ADULTERANT EFFECTS ON POSITIVE DRUG SPECIMENS OVER TIME

The kinetics of adulterant effects were studied by Tse and Bogema *(20)*. In these experiments, urine controls containing two times the cut-off levels of THC, MOR, AMP, PCP, and cocaine (COC) were set up. The samples were divided into three groups. To the first group, Urine Luck Formula 6.3 was added according to the manufacturer's instructions. To the second group, Stealth was added. The third group served as positive control, with no adulterants added. Within 5 min after the addition of adulterants, samples from each group were taken and simultaneously tested for presence of drugs and adulterants. The tests were repeated at 30 min and at 1, 2, 3, 5, 8, 24, and 30 h after addition of adulterants. Detection of drugs was performed using Monitect, whereas adulterants were detected using Intect 7.

Results of the drug tests with Monitect were as expected. Urine Luck and Stealth were found to be potent adulterants for THC and MOR, but were only marginally effective for AMP, PCP, and COC. For adulterant testing with Intect 7, Urine Luck and Stealth did not provide any change in creatinine, glutaraldehyde, pH, and specific gravity in the drug-spiked urine samples. However, there were distinct changes when the samples were added to the nitrite, bleach, and PCC chemical pads (Table 3). The addition of Urine Luck (group 2) produced a dark blue coloration on the nitrite pad and a light blue coloration on the bleach and PCC pads. Addition of Stealth (groups 3) produced a very dark blue coloration on all three chemical pads. These color changes are regarded as highly abnormal, or abnormal in accordance with the expected color change in Intect 7 with unadulterated urine (group 1). The color change occurred imme-

Table 3
Kinetic Studies of Adulterant Detection in Adulterated Urine Control Samples Using Intect® 7 Testing Strips

Groups	Chemical pad	5 min	30 min	1 h	2 h	3 h	5 h	8 h	24 h	30 h
Group 1 (no adulterant added)	Nitrite	Normal (white to pink)	Normal	Normal	Normal	Normal	Normal	Normal	Normal	Normal
	Bleach	Normal (white)	Normal	Normal	Normal	Normal	Normal	Normal	Normal	Normal
	PCC	Normal (white)	Normal	Normal	Normal	Normal	Normal	Normal	Normal	Normal
Group 2 (Urine Luck™ added)	Nitrite	Abnormal (dark purple)	Abnormal (dark purple)	Abnormal (dark purple)	Abnormal (dark purple)	Abnormal (purple)	Abnormal (purple)	Normal (white to pink)	Normal (white to pink)	Normal (white to pink)
	Bleach	Abnormal (blue)	Abnormal (blue)	Abnormal (light blue)	Abnormal (blue)	Abnormal (light blue)	Abnormal (light blue)	Abnormal (lighter blue)	Abnormal (very light blue)	Normal (slight tint of blue)
	PCC	Abnormal (blue)	Abnormal (blue)	Abnormal (light blue)	Abnormal (light blue)	Abnormal (blue)	Abnormal (light blue)	Abnormal (light blue)	Normal (very light blue)	Normal (slight tint of blue)
Group 3 (Stealth™ added)	Nitrite	Abnormal (dark purple)	Abnormal (dark purple)	Abnormal (dark purple)	Abnormal (purple)	Normal (white to pink)	Normal (white to pink)	Normal (white to pink)	Normal (white to pink)	Normal (white to pink)
	Bleach	Abnormal (dark blue)	Abnormal (dark blue)	Abnormal (dark blue)	Abnormal (dark blue)	Abnormal (dark blue)	Abnormal (blue)	Abnormal (blue)	Abnormal (very light blue)	Normal (slight tint of blue)
	PCC	Abnormal (dark blue)	Abnormal (dark blue)	Abnormal (dark blue)	Abnormal (blue)	Abnormal (blue)	Abnormal (blue)	Abnormal (blue)	Abnormal (very light blue)	Normal (slight tint of blue)

Creatinine, Glutaraldehyde, pH and Specific Gravity were normal in all groups and are not listed in this table.
PCC, pyridinium chlorochromate.

diately after addition of the adulterants and lasted for at least 3–8 h. Thus, the presence of the adulterants Urine Luck and Stealth could be detected during the earlier time points. Unexpectedly, as the tests proceeded, the dark blue coloration in the nitrite tests became lighter and lighter, and exhibited normal coloration by 3 h in the Stealth group and by 8 h in the Urine Luck group. Similar color lightening was observed for the bleach and PCC tests, although the kinetic was much slower. Significantly, the lightening of color in these two tests continued, and by 24 h after addition, both adulterant groups showed only a very slight tint of blue to almost normal color levels. It was noteworthy that this discoloration process progressed more dramatically in the Stealth group than in the Urine Luck group. These results demonstrate that there is a built-in time limit for the detection of the adulterants Urine Luck and Stealth. Twenty-four hours after addition, these compounds appeared to have performed their adulteration functions and then faded away to almost undetectable levels. Such results underscore the importance of performing adulterant testing on site as soon as urine samples are collected. Delaying 24 to 48 h for testing runs the risk of not being able to detect them. Such observations were confirmed in a further study by Wong et al. *(21)*.

7. CONCLUSIONS

Adulteration will be a continuing problem for the drug-testing industry and scientific community. Manufacturers of adulterants have successfully developed innovative means and chemical formulas to mask positive drug results. Although banning the sales of these adulterants may prevent their availability in some areas, the Internet would always ensure their availability. Both governmental agencies and adulteration test manufacturers should constantly update their test criteria to combat the continuous formulation change strategy of the adulterant companies. Laboratory reagents and on-site dipsticks have proven to be effective in detecting their presence in adulterated urine specimens. For convenience, manufacturers of drug screens have started to produce devices that test for drug and screen for adulteration simultaneously. In this way, the integrity of the specimen is assured while the drug screen is being performed. Examples include Monitect PC11A, ToxCup® PT15A, and QuickTox® 51A from Branan Medical Corporation. However, the self-destructive nature of the new generation of adulterants suggests that testing for them should be performed as soon after collection as possible and preferably on-site. Presently, owing to economic pressure, adulteration testing is not always performed on all specimens. In these cases, false negatives may result and the value of drug testing is compromised.

REFERENCES

1. Winecker RE and Goldberger BA. Urine specimen suitability for drug testing, in Drug Abuse Handbook (Karch SB, ed), CRC, Boca Raton, FL: 1997; pp. 764–772.
2. Cody JT. Adulteration of urine specimens, in Handbook of Workplace Drug Testing (Liu RH and Goldberger BA, eds) AACC, Washington, D.C.: 1995; pp. 181–207.
3. Cody JT. Sample adulteration and on-site drug tests, in On-site Drug Testing (Jenkins AJ and Goldberger BA, eds), Humana, Totowa, NJ: 2002; pp. 253–264.
4. Mandatory Guidelines for Federal Workplace Drug Testing Programs, August 21, 2001 (66 FR 43876).
5. Quest Diagnostics, Inc. 2003 Drug Testing Index, July 22, 2004.
6. Warner A. Interference of common household chemicals in immunoassay methods for drugs of abuse. Clin Chem 1989;35:648–651.
7. Cone EJ, Lange R, and Darwin W. In vivo adulteration: excess fluid ingestion causes false-negative marijuana and cocaine urine test results. J Anal Toxicol 1998;22:460–473.
8. Paul BD, Martin KK, Maguilo J, and Smith ML. Effects of pyridinium chlorochromate adulterant (Urine Luck) on testing drugs of abuse and a method for quantitative detection of chromium (VI) in urine. J Anal Toxicol 2000;24: 233–237.
9. Buddha DP and Aaron J. Effects of oxidizing adulterants on detection of 11-nor-Δ^9-THC-9-carboxylic acid in urine. J Anal Toxicol 2002;26:460–463.
10. Cody J, Valtier S, and Kuhlman J. Analysis of morphine and codeine in samples adulterated with Stealth™. J Anal Toxicol 2001;25:572–575.
11. Tsai SC, ElSohly MA, Dubrovsky T, Twarowska B, Towt J, and Salamone SJ. Determination of five abused drugs in nitrite-adulterated urine by immunoassays and gas chromatography-mass spectrometry. J Anal Toxicol 1998;22: 474–480.
12. Wu A, Bristol B, Sexton K, Cassella-McLane G, Holtman V, and Hill D. Adulteration of urine by "Urine Luck." Clin Chem 1999;45:1051–1057.
13. Procedures for Transportation Workplace Drug and Alcohol Testing Programs, Dec. 19, 2000 (65 FR 79526).
14. Mandatory Guidelines for Federal Workplace Drug Testing Programs, April 13, 2004 (69 FR 19644).
15. Edgell K, Caplan Y, Glass L, and Cook JD. The defined HHS/DOT substituted urine criteria validated through a controlled hydration study. J Anal Toxicol 2002; 26:419–423.
16. Chang SH, Guo H, Nguyen T, Tung KK, and Wei YF. Identification of human urine for drug testing. US patent number 6,368,873, April 9, 2002.
17. Peace M and Tarnai L. Performance evaluation of three on-site adulterant detection devices for urine specimens. J Anal Toxicol 2002;26:464–470.
18. Wong R. The effect of adulterants on urine screen for drugs of abuse: detection by an on-site dipstick device. American Clinical Laboratory 2002;21:37–39.

19. Wong RC, Chien BP, Her C, and Johnson CM. Effects of urine adulterants on Intect™ 7 adulterant test strip and Monitect™ abused Drug Screen. Clin Chem 2001;47:A75.
20. Tse HY and Bogema S. Kinetic studies on the detection of adulterants and on their effectiveness in urine screens for drugs of abuse. Clin Chem 2002;48:A58.
21. Wong RC, Chien BP, Nguyen PT, and Tse H. Adulterants: Its Detection and Effects on Urine Drug Screens. Presented at the Society of Forensic Toxicologists Meeting, Michigan, October, 2002.

Chapter 15

Drug Testing and the Criminal Justice System
A Marriage Made in Court

John N. Marr

"The establishment of drug courts, coupled with their judicial leadership, constitutes one of the most monumental changes in social justice in this country since World War II."

> General Barry McCaffrey, Ret.,
> Director, Office of National Drug Control Policy *(1)*

SUMMARY

Since the development of specialized drug courts in 1989, the drug court movement in the United States has swept through the criminal justice system, revolutionizing the way many court systems process drug, domestic violence, driving under the influence (DUI)/driving while intoxicated (DWI), juvenile, re-entry, and mental health cases. The movement has grown from one experimental court in Miami, Florida, to more than 1000 specialty courts in operation and another 500 in some stage of planning. The federal government, through the Bureau of Justice Assistance, provided more than $45 million in direct funding for drug courts in the United States during 2003. The Office of Justice Programs initial funding proposal for drug courts during fiscal year 2004 was $68 million.

Why did they do this? Because drug courts work. Through the use of intensive therapy programs, court management of client participation, drug testing, and other measurable standards, drug courts provide an objective standard for success within a therapeutic system heretofore characterized by subjectivity and ambiguous outcome measures.

From: *Forensic Science and Medicine: Drugs of Abuse: Body Fluid Testing*
Edited by R. C. Wong and H. Y. Tse © Humana Press Inc., Totowa, NJ

1. NATURE OF DRUG COURT

Although every drug court has its own unique personality, there are a few things that most have in common. All drug courts are based on a highly structured, nonadversarial team approach. Participation in drug court is limited to criminal offenders whose antisocial behavior can be significantly attributed to the use, abuse, or addiction to controlled substances.

Prior to the development of specialty drug courts in the late 1980s, the various parties in the criminal justice system played very specific adversarial roles in drug-related cases. Prosecutors and defense attorneys entered into a dramatic debate in front of an independent judge, who then decided the fate of the defendant, who in most cases was not even allowed to address the court. If it was determined by court personnel that drug treatment was appropriate, the defendant was referred to an outside treatment agency and given a specified time within which to complete a prescribed course of treatment. At the end of the treatment episode, the defendant would return to court and some type of report from the agency would be presented. In most cases, this report would simply state whether the defendant had completed the prescribed course of treatment or not (Fig. 1).

In drug court, the scene is very different. All parties work together to determine client eligibility and appropriateness for treatment based on pre-established criteria. Eligible participants are then tested by a licensed treatment professional for appropriateness and matched with a treatment agency where their particular strengths can be augmented and their deficiencies strengthened. A multi-disciplinary treatment team manages every case individually, accepting input directly from all stakeholders. Whereas all key stakeholders participate in case management and processing, the lines of communication in the courtroom are directly between the defendant and the judge (Fig. 2). This direct interaction facilitates clients' responsibility for their successes and failures and establishes a process whereby the judge takes on a *parens patre* role that is recognized and accepted by the drug-court participants. A multi-disciplinary team coordinates the entire drug-court process from screening to aftercare and evaluation.

2. KEY STAKEHOLDERS OF DRUG COURTS

2.1. The Judge

A designated judge handles all cases referred to the court. While the judge leads the team and has the final say as to monitoring, incentives, and sanctions, the team avails itself of information presented by case managers, treatment providers, probation officers, and other ancillary service providers who may

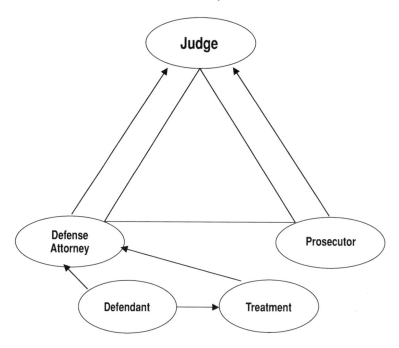

Fig. 1. Traditional legal system.

be working directly with the participant. Frequent status reviews before the judge are held throughout the duration of the drug-court program to provide immediate positive and negative consequences to participant behaviors.

2.2. Defense Attorney

Most drug courts utilize the services of the public defenders office to represent the participant in court and to ensure that their rights are protected. In a typical drug court, however, the participant is required to speak directly to the judge. The attorney, present as a part of the team, does not speak on behalf of the participant during the court proceeding. Defense attorneys in drug court adopt the principle that their clients are best served through a chance to face life drug-free and with the skills and opportunities necessary to be productive members of the community.

2.3. Prosecution

Prosecutors play a very vital role on the drug-court team. They represent the interests of the community and ensure that only eligible defendants are allowed into the program. In post-plea courts, they take a very supportive role

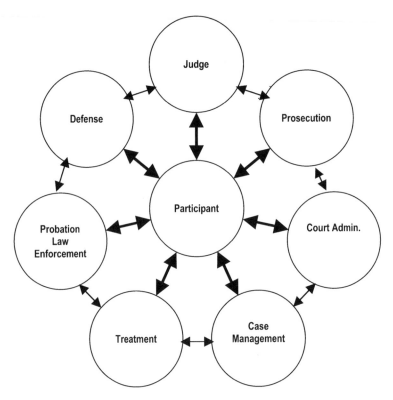

Fig. 2. Drug-court system.

and function according to the philosophy that a community is best protected and served through intervention in the downward spiral of an addict's life and through helping him or her become a productive and drug-free member of the community.

2.4. Court Administration

Because specialty drug-treatment courts have become an institutionalized part of the judicial system in most of the jurisdictions where they operate, these systems have found it expedient to provide a coordinator to oversee the administrative aspects of running a drug court. The coordinator tends to be responsible for process coordination, funding issues, and management of information flowing to and from the court. They also serve as a liaison between the judge and many of the ancillary service providers associated with the court.

2.5. Treatment

Depending on the jurisdiction, there may be one or several treatment providers serving the participants of the drug court. Unlike within the traditional model, treatment providers are active members of the team, participate in staffing of cases prior to the review hearings, recommend and enforce incentives and sanctions, share information concerning treatment compliance and drug-testing results with the court, and strive to educate the other members of the team on the basic aspects of addiction and how they affect the behavior of each participant.

2.6. Probation

Probation officers are an integral part of any post-plea drug court. Not only do they provide community supervision at a level not possible for other members of the team, but in many jurisdictions probation may also provide case management, house arrest, and/or drug testing. Probation also works with law enforcement to be the eyes and ears of the drug court when program participants are outside of the direct supervision of the other team members. Probation departments have learned that drug courts are a very cost-effective alternative to incarceration for persons found guilty of a technical violation of probation. This is especially true for those persons who test positive on probation-administered drug screens.

2.7. Law Enforcement

Local police participation on the oversight or policy team is important for the long-term stability of any drug court. Law enforcement is responsible for the arrest that places participants in the program. If law enforcement views drug court as a soft-on-crime, ineffective program, they will not only fail to support the program, but could even serve as a roadblock to a successful program. A strong linkage between drug court and law enforcement can bring an abundance of additional resources to the program.

2.8. Ancillary Services

Depending on the type of court and age of participants, a wide variety of ancillary service providers are involved in the operation of a successful drug court. Education, vocational training, public health, mental health, recreation, arts and leisure activities, transportation, public housing, social services, the faith community, all participate in the planning, oversight, and operation of the drug court. The more people involved in the process of servicing the needs of drug-court participants, the greater the odds of providing meaningful life change.

2.9. Evaluation

Every drug court needs to have an evaluation plan in place from the beginning of their program. Most courts utilize the services of outside evaluators, who are often from local colleges or universities. Ongoing evaluation and program enhancement is vital for successful outcomes and long-term funding.

3. FUNCTIONAL SIGNIFICANCE OF DRUG COURTS

Drug courts, through the cooperative efforts of all stakeholders, provide a comprehensive and efficient utilization of community resources and have proven very effective in reducing recidivism among program participants. According to a September 2003 report by the American University Drug Court Clearinghouse, the 1078 operational drug courts have collectively served more than 300,000 adults and 12,500 juveniles and graduated more than 73,000 adults and 4000 juveniles *(2)*. The report further states that 75,000 of these offenders had been sentenced to periods of incarceration prior to their entering drug court and that despite this fact, drug courts consistently retain over 70% of those who enroll. A 2001 Columbia University National Center on Addiction and Substance Abuse (CASA) study concluded that, even though drug-court participants receive significantly more comprehensive and closer supervision than offenders participating in other forms of community supervision, drug use and criminal behavior is significantly reduced among drug-court participants while they are in drug court *(3)*. The CASA report further concluded that the recidivism or re-arrest rate among drug-court graduates is less than 29%, whereas it exceeds 48% for drug offenders who have not completed a drug-court program.

4. KEY COMPONENTS OF DRUG COURTS

In 1996, twelve drug-court practitioners and ancillary experts began the process of establishing a set of guidelines upon which drug courts around the country could base their own unique programs. Recognizing the need for cultural and jurisdictional diversity, this group set out to identify the fundamental similarities and standards of the few operational drug courts at that time. What resulted was the publication of "Defining Drug Courts: The Key Components" *(4)*. The following is simply a listing of these 10 key components of a drug court:

1. *"Drug courts integrate alcohol and other drug treatment services with justice system case processing."* Drug courts serve as a true partnership between drug and alcohol treatment professionals and the court system. The treatment team, which is comprised of all major stakeholders, meets regularly to discuss each participant's progress and to determine incentives, sanctions, and the future direction of the case plan.

2. *"Using a non-adversarial approach, prosecution and defense counsel promote public safety while protecting participants' due process rights."* All members of

the drug-court team operate from the same philosophical basis—that what is in the best interest of both the community and the program participant is for the participant to be drug and alcohol free, working, taking care of family obligations, and not committing new offenses.

3. *"Eligible participants are identified early and promptly placed in the drug court program."* Drug courts are either pre- or post-plea programs. In pre-plea courts, where charges are held until program completion or failure, participants can be enrolled in drug court within a matter of hours or days from the time of their arrest. In post-conviction courts, this process takes longer. However, pre-set eligibility criteria allow persons to plead to the underlying offense and upon completion of drug court, withdraw the plea and either have the charges dismissed or plea to a lesser charge.

4. *"Drug courts provide access to a continuum of alcohol, drug, and other related treatment and rehabilitation services."* Drug courts bring available resources together in a comprehensive approach that addresses all identified issues supporting or hindering a person's road to recovery. No other system within the criminal justice arena has shown the ability to bring such diverse resources to the table consistently over time. Many communities that had limited resources available to serve their drug court population have developed their own treatment components, which, in turn, have provided greatly needed resources to non-drug court persons in the community.

5. *"Abstinence is monitored by frequent alcohol and other drug testing."* Drug testing is the objective measure of participant progress and program effectiveness. This issue will be discussed in greater detail in a later section.

6. *"A coordinated strategy governs drug court responses to participant's compliance."* A multi-disciplinary team establishes a system of incentives and sanctions for use within the drug-court system. Participants are rewarded when they make progress toward treatment and court goals, and receive graduated sanctions when they fail to comply with the expectations of the drug-court team. The treatment team meets prior to the scheduled status review hearing to discuss participant progress. This case review allows the team to agree on a course of action, ensuring consistency and fairness in the way the court responds to each participant.

7. *"Ongoing judicial interaction with each drug court participant is essential."* The primary factor that makes drug courts unique and effective is the regular status reviews before a designated drug-court judge. Drug-court judges are knowledgeable in addiction and recovery, and are able to support treatment-team recommendations using the full weight of the court. The drug-court judge serves as the director of the treatment drama as it unfolds in court, not only for the participant speaking to the judge, but also for those in the courtroom observing the interaction.

8. *"Monitoring and evaluation measure the achievement of program goals and gauge effectiveness."* Every drug court must have an evaluation program in place to monitor both process and outcome measures. Independent evaluators assist the court in monitoring what is done well and in identifying those areas that need improvement. The only way that a program can ensure that it is achieving its

goals and objectives is through the use of a formal evaluation process. Evaluations provide the accountability by which to justify future funding or even keeping a program operational.

9. *"Continuing interdisciplinary education promotes effective drug court planning, implementation, and operations."* Individual members of a drug-court team work hard to communicate their needs and expertise to other members of the team. Court personnel become very knowledgeable in areas of addiction and treatment, whereas social service and health care professionals learn about the limitations and requirements of the legal system. Only through learning about each other's world can the team truly function effectively.

10. *"Forging partnerships among drug courts, public agencies, and community-based organizations generates local support and enhances drug court effectiveness."* Drug courts are truly a community-wide effort assisting offenders in living drug- and crime-free lives. This partnership among all components of the criminal justice system, treatment and social service agencies, the faith community, law enforcement, civic organizations, educational institutions, and vocational programs is what places drug courts in a league of their own when it comes to effective intervention in the cycle of criminal and addictive behavior.

It has become apparent that the synergistic power of all 10 key components is what makes drug courts as successful as they are. However, the remainder of this chapter will deal specifically with component number five and its practical implication for monitoring participant and program effectiveness.

5. THE IMPORTANCE OF DRUG TESTING

Mental-health and alcohol-and-other-drug (AOD) treatment could both be considered "gray sciences." That is, they both operate within very subjective and fluid parameters. It is extremely difficult to monitor treatment effectiveness, as there are few measurable standards upon which to base a conclusion. Is a person less depressed today than they were last week or is their level of craving greater than a couple of days earlier? Because behavioral sciences are based upon interpretation of self-disclosure, there will always be a degree of opinion and even trial-and-error in dealing with people suffering from either of these afflictions.

The criminal justice system, on the other hand, is a very black-and-white segment of society. Either a person is guilty or they are not. It is not a segment of society that will accept subjective measures of guilt or innocence. How can these two very different philosophies thrive while working together in a drug court? Drug testing provides an objective measure of participant progress and allows the treatment team to make both clinical and legal decisions based upon concrete evidence. Participant progress, rewards, and sanctions are all based on the qualitative results of the drug-testing component of the program.

5.1. Drug-Court Testing Protocol

Each drug court is unique in how it operates based upon available resources, community and court expectations and limitations, demographics of participants, cultural requirements, and a myriad of other variables. However, there are guidelines that govern acceptable testing procedures, such as those established by the American Probation and Parole Association *(5)*, that are used in the development of policies and procedures used in drug court testing.

Owing to the impact of drug-test results in a drug-court system, it is imperative that the testing results be accurate and timely. Because cost is the major factor in the design of most drug court testing protocols, programs utilize the most comprehensive testing protocol possible based on available resources.

5.1.1. Minimum Standards

After a full panel test is run to establish a qualitative baseline, random tests are conducted not less than twice a week during the first 3–4 mo or until the participant demonstrates a prolonged (usually 3-mo) period of continuous sobriety. After this, random testing is conducted at least once a week for the duration of the program. Many programs test three times a week during the initial period of the program, twice per week during intermediate phases, and at least once per week during the later phases of the program. All participants must be tested for their primary and secondary drugs of choice, as determined on the baseline test and during the intake assessment. Full-panel screens are interspersed throughout the program to discourage drug-of-choice shifting. It is further suggested that samples be screened for adulterants and dilution, which further validates test results. All sample donations must be directly observed, their temperature monitored, and the chain of custody regulated. This is true for tests being sent to an outside laboratory as well as those being tested at the collection center.

Some drug-court participants go to great lengths in an attempt to continue using drugs while in the program. They will attempt to adulterate samples, dilute samples, bring in someone else's sample, have someone else donate samples for them, or just fail to give a urine sample.

Protocols are designed and followed to minimize these attempts to invalidate the drug-testing portion of the drug-court program.

A basic tenet of drug courts is the necessity of providing immediate responses to both negative and positive drug tests. Participants appear before the drug-court judge on a regular basis so that their progress in treatment can be reviewed, their compliance with other programs and community supervision conditions can be monitored, and their behavior can be rewarded or sanctioned.

Drug-test results are vital to this process. Research has shown consistently that rapid response is more effective than delayed response where any meaningful behavior change is the goal *(6)*. It is imperative that results be available to court and treatment personnel as soon after testing as possible. In many cases, as in open court, results must be available in minutes, not days. This need for rapid results has led many drug courts to utilize point-of-collection (POC) hand-held devices or to set up their own instrumented laboratories.

5.2. Drug-Testing Methodologies and Technology

As a result of the above-mentioned issues of cost and immediacy, drug courts have experimented with most of the testing methodologies in an effort to discover the most efficient means to achieve their testing agenda. Based upon the high concentration of drug metabolites present in urine, the basic ease of urine sample collection, the accuracy of urine testing, and the relatively low cost of testing a urine sample, urinalysis has become the primary choice of most drug courts. Drug courts have experimented with other matrices, such as hair, saliva, sweat, breath, and ocular scans. All of these methodologies have specific, limited value within a typical drug court. Because courts test multiple times per week and are concerned about new use, long-term methods such as sweat patches and hair testing have only minimal relevance in specific situations. Untimeliness of results, lack of long-term validity studies, and high cost have minimized the acceptance of saliva tests. Ocular scans have only recently become available to the general public consumer, so logistic and cost concerns have yet to allow this technology to enter the mainstream of drug court testing protocols. Breathalyzers are utilized by most drug courts for the testing of alcohol consumption. Ease of administration, immediacy of results, and the low cost per screen have made this a very valuable tool for drug court practitioners. As non-urine testing technologies become more efficient and cost-effective, they will undoubtedly gain greater acceptance and utilization within the drug-court environment.

It is established that the matrix of choice for most drug courts is urine. How the urine sample is tested varies from court to court. Cost factors into the decision to utilize lower-cost immunoassay screens over higher-cost chromatography tests like gas chromatography (GC)-mass spectrometry (MS). Courts that contract with an outside laboratory to conduct their testing usually include GC-MS confirmations of samples that test positive on the immunoassay screen. Courts that do their own screening using either noninstrumented or instrumented testing provide a confirmation option for participants who wish to challenge a positive test result. Because GC-MS confirmation screens can cost upward of $150, the participant is usually required to pay this extra cost unless the confirmation overturns the previous immunoassay results. Drug-court testing results are considered presumptive, and thus most drug courts do not confirm positive results unless the participant requests the confirmation test. The long-term duration of drug-court participation, the frequency of testing, and the graduated sanctions for positive test results all support this position of limited confirmation testing. Many drug-court participants will be tested more than 120 times during their drug-court experience. This fact does not minimize the need for accuracy, however, because testing is simply a part of a bigger picture. Drug testing is used to monitor participant progress in recovery, not to catch a participant using for the purpose of punishment. Drug courts realize that recovery and relapse are all a part of the process toward a lifetime of sobriety and socially appropriate behavior.

5.3. Drug-Testing Volume and Cost: A Mathematical Perspective

How important is drug testing to the overall drug-court experience? As stated earlier, drug testing provides the objective standard by which to measure a participant's progress and level of compliance. A December 2003 report by the Bureau of Justice Assistance Drug Court Clearinghouse at American University *(5)* stated that 1098 drug courts were operational at that time. A 2001 Drug Court Clearinghouse study *(6)* reported a moving total of nearly 80,000 active participants at any given time. Using the standard model of three drug tests per week during the first 3 mo in the program, two tests per week during the next 3 mo, and once per week during the final 6 mo, the average drug-court participant is drug tested 84 times during the first 12 mo in drug court. This does not take into account that many participants do not complete Pphase I in the minimum 3-mo period and that subsequent relapses result in a return to Phase I and its more frequent testing schedule. Length of stay in drug court actually ranges from 6 mo to 24 mo, resulting in an average testing volume of 120 tests per participant. Using the 80,000 participants figure, 9,600,000 drug panels were administered to drug-court participants during 2003. As the number of active drug courts increases and the costs associated with testing respond to competitive market conditions and decline, the volume of POC drug screens, instrumented tests, and tests using other methodologies should all increase.

6. THE FUTURE OF DRUG COURTS

The drug-court movement has experienced tremendous growth since 1989. With over 1200 active courts and approx 500 more in some stage of planning, there appears to be no end to the growth associated with this movement. In the mid- to late-1990s, the idea of therapeutic problem-solving courts began to expand into other specialty courts dealing with issues other than primary substance abuse. Domestic violence, mental health, driving under the influence (DUI), tribal, university campus, child support, and re-entry courts were added to the growing number of adult, juvenile, and family drug courts. With an ever-increasing volume of evaluation data supporting the efficacy of these intensive intervention strategies, the model promises to expand into other special-population areas. Early prison release, prostitution, property offenses, impulse-related violent offenses, and parole or probation violations are all viable arenas for specialty courts.

Even though most of these specialty courts do not deal with substance abuse as the primary issue, drug testing is still a very important component. Statistics shows that more than 80% of the crimes committed in the United States each year are drug-related *(6)*. That means either the defendant was under the influence of drugs or alcohol at the time of the offense, committed the offense in order to obtain drugs, or the crime included the manufacturing or distribution of illegal drugs. In each case, use of drugs or alcohol is at least a potential detriment to the long-term stability of any person involved in a therapeutic court. Drug testing, used in conjunction with a comprehensive continuum of treatment, case management, and community supervision, supported and coordinated by a caring and committed criminal justice system, provides the objective standard to support a wide range of specialty courts both today and into the future.

REFERENCES

1. NADCP News, Volume IV, No. 2, 1997.
2. OJP Drug Court Clearinghouse at American University: Implementation Status of Drug Court Programs. September 8, 2003.
3. Belenko S. Research on Drug Courts: A Critical Review 2001 Update, The National Center on Addiction and Substance Abuse at Columbia University, 2001.
4. National Association of Drug Court Professionals. Defining Drug Courts: The Key Components, January 1997.
5. BJA Drug Court Clearinghouse. Drug Court Activity Update: Composite Summary Information. American University, December 15, 2003.
6. OJP Drug Court Clearinghouse and Technical Assistance Project. Summary Information on All Drug Court Programs and Detailed Information on Adult Drug Courts. American University, June 25, 2001.

Chapter 16

Drugs-of-Abuse Testing
The European Perspective

Alex Yil Fai Wong

SUMMARY

Testing for drugs of abuse in Europe generally follows many of the trends that have been observed in the United States in recent times. However, adoption of drug testing in Europe as a whole is still considered to be around 10 yr behind that of the United States. Noticeably, there are vast differences within the individual countries in relation to end-users and legislation. In the health care arena, hospitals and treatment clinics are among the largest consumers of drug-testing kits. In the non-health care sector, criminal justice services and the workplace represent the high-volume end-users. At present, urine continues to be the most popular screening test matrix across Europe, with blood the preferred specimen for judicial and forensic confirmatory applications. Although more recently introduced matrices such as oral fluid and saliva have yet to gain widespread acceptance, they are expected to play an increasingly important role in the future.

1. INTRODUCTION

During the autumn of 2003, news of the possible use of "designer drugs" among athletes made headlines that rocked the UK sport scene *(1,2)*. As demonstrated by numerous debates appearing in newspaper columns and radio phone-ins, drug testing remained very much a poorly understood subject across Europe. These incidents afforded a prime opportunity to raise public awareness about the practice of drug testing and promote improved understanding of the discipline among a wider audience.

From: *Forensic Science and Medicine: Drugs of Abuse: Body Fluid Testing*
Edited by R. C. Wong and H. Y. Tse © Humana Press Inc., Totowa, NJ

Urine and blood have traditionally been the most commonly analyzed specimens in the field of drug testing in Europe. Over the past few years, the use of oral fluids in drug testing has aroused a considerable amount of interest in many European countries. Some experts believe that it is only a matter of time until oral fluid-based tests replace the conventional urine test, especially in the point-of-care (POC) environment.

This chapter aims at providing an overall view of the current status of drugs-of-abuse (DOA) testing in Europe.

2. MARKET VOLUME ACROSS EUROPE

In 2003, it had been estimated that the European market for drugs-of-abuse tests (DATs) was worth approx $85 million *(3,4)*. The top three markets, ranked in order of market revenues, were Germany, the United Kingdom, and Italy. Whereas the rates of market growth in Germany and Italy are likely to decline, demand in the United Kingdom and Ireland is expected to continue to rise. It is forecasted that demand for DATs across the rest of Europe (ROE) is likely to account for up to 30% of the total market by 2008. The three most significant markets, nevertheless, would still be responsible for the lion's share of DATs consumed. This is hardly surprising, given the fact that this trio represents some of the most heavily populated countries in Europe today.

In terms of market development and test utilities, the overall European market for DOA testing is still considered to be approx 10 yr behind the US market. It is believed that whereas certain European markets have been slow to accept DAT, others have shown much more enthusiasm *(3,4)*. Data indicate that there is a noticeable discrepancy in the level of test adoption in Europe in the form of a North–South divide, as illustrated in Fig. 1. Thus, cultural differences may be one of the factors responsible for holding back the development of the European DAT market *(4)*. Spain and France are the countries currently exhibiting the highest level of resistance to drug testing. In Spain, drug testing is viewed with caution, in both health care and non-health care environments *(4)*. Owing to the lack of legislation and national guidelines, doctors in Spain are reluctant to carry out a DAT, unless obligatory, for fear of being implicated in legal proceedings. In France, people involved in road accidents may be requested to provide a urine and/or blood sample under *la loi Gayssot*. Nevertheless, comprehensive roadside testing in France, as well as Spain, has yet to be fully approved. Furthermore, random screening of prisoners in France is still prohibited. As a result, the level of testing carried out in France continues to be extremely low.

In terms of rate of DAT usage, Germany, Italy, the Benelux region, and Denmark were ranked as medium-range users (Fig. 1). Whereas Belgium has

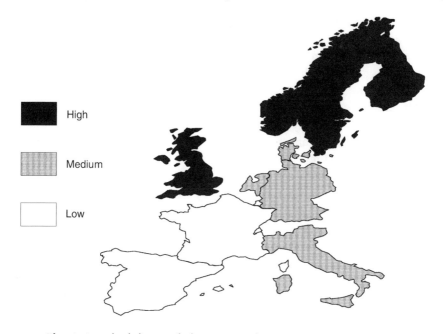

Fig. 1. Level of drugs-of-abuse test adoption in Europe (2003).

adopted a zero-tolerance policy, cracking down on drug abuse at all levels, the two other Benelux regions, along with Denmark, have yet to authorize roadside testing. In Luxembourg and the Netherlands, a stricter enforcement of existing laws has been suggested as an alternative to testing people suspected of driving under the influence of drugs *(5)*. Germany and Italy have traditionally been classified as high-volume consumers of diagnostic assays. This trend, however, does not apply to drug testing. In these two countries, workplace drug testing is prohibited by law. Further accounting for the low level of DAT usage, both Germany and Italy have recently experienced a reduction in healthcare spending, with Germany in particular suffering from a period of economic instability. Consequently, drug testing is now categorized as a low priority, especially in the health care sector. Although other consumers, such as the police, prisons, and the military, have expressed an interest in employing these tests to combat drug abuse, their use has been hindered by the current lack of regulatory guidelines.

In 2003, Scandinavian countries, with the exception of Denmark, were among the leading group of countries using high volumes of DATs within Europe *(3,4)*. Similarly to Belgium, both Sweden and Finland strictly oppose drug abuse in their societies. In order to implement and ensure the smooth operation of their respective drug strategies in the long term, Norway, Finland,

and Sweden have invested a combined total of approx $80 million to combat drug abuse. Consequently, over the next 5 yr, increasing volumes of DATs are likely to be employed in the Nordic regions. Criminal justice services and treatment centers, in particular, have been allocated substantial funds within the framework of the respective national drug policies.

On the total European level, the United Kingdom is currently the most advanced market. This is reflected in the requirement for mandatory testing of inmates in UK prisons and young persons' institutes, and by the increasing practice of workplace testing. Although the UK is widely considered to be the leading country in western Europe concerned with workplace drug testing (WPDT), more recent research conducted by Market & opinion Research International (MORI) *(5)* in 2003 indicated that only approx 4% of UK companies were testing their present and future staff for substance abuse. On this issue, there are several pieces of legislation supporting workplace testing, but over all, WPDT is still poorly understood in Europe. The Health and Safety at Work Act and the Transport and Works Act mandate that being under the influence of DOA represents a criminal offense, not only for the employees but also for employers who knowingly allow staff members to perform under the influence.

3. DRUG TARGETS

In Europe today, routinely tested DOA are shown in Table 1. In a typical screening assay, it is quite common to see combinations of these drugs being tested. At roadside screening, it has been reported that cannabis, opiates, cocaine, amphetamines (including methamphetamines), and benzodiazepines represent the most regularly tested DOA *(6,7)*. Codeine, cotinine, salicylate, and tricyclic antidepressants may also be present in test panels. Phencyclidine (PCP), regularly included in the Substance Abuse and Mental Health Services Administration (SAMHSA)-5 panel of drugs in the United States, is rarely included in European DATs, especially on the POC format. Commonly abused in the United States, PCP is consumed at much lower levels in Europe.

The European Monitoring Centre for Drugs and Drug Addiction (EMCDDA) recently reported that opiates are the class of drugs for which most people seek treatment *(8)*. In methadone clinics, the main drug being tested is heroin, as opposed to the less harmful substitute of methadone. In rehabilitation centers, POC assays also mainly test for heroin.

4. END-USERS OF DRUG TESTING

The main end-users of DATs in Europe in 2003 are listed in Table 2, categorized into health care and non-health care sectors.

Table 1
Drugs Most Commonly Included in Drugs-of-Abuse Tests
(Europe, 2003)

Amphetamine (AMP)	Methadone (MTD)
Barbiturate (BAR)	Methamphetamine (MET)
Benzodiazepine (BZO)	Morphine (MOR)
Cannabis (THC)	Opiates (OPI) / Heroin (HER)
Cocaine (COC)	

Table 2
Main End-Users of Drugs-of-Abuse Tests (Europe, 2003)

Health care	Non-health care
Hospital arena	Criminal justice services
• Central laboratories	• Police
• Emergency room (ER)	• Prisons
• Intensive care unit (ICU)	• Probation
• Private laboratories	Workplace
• Psychiatric laboratories	• Business risk (non-safety-sensitive/ business-sensitive)
• Toxicology laboratories	• Occupational health (safety-sensitive)
	Others
Primary care	• Customs and excise / border guards
• Doctors' offices	• Education
• Rehabilitation clinics	• Military (including coast guards)

4.1. Prisons

Interventions such as drug testing are thought to have a positive effect in the reduction of drug-related crime. As a result, DATs have become an increasingly important weapon at all levels of the criminal justice systems, particularly across northern Europe. DATs are not restricted to offenders; officers may also be randomly tested for drug abuse owing to their potential contact with drugs. As a result, prospective candidates looking to join the prison service or police force may also be subjected to a drug screen as part of their pre-employment assessment.

Just as drugs are easily obtainable in the community, drugs are also readily available in prisons. Being in prison or in young-offender institutes has never equated to the total cessation of drug abuse. According to recent EMCDDA data *(8)*, approximately one-third of the entire European inmate population in 2002 had admitted to consuming drugs while in prison. Prisons in Germany and Spain were believed to have the highest rates of drug abuse. In contrast, in countries like the United Kingdom, where mandatory drug testing (MDT) is carried out in conjunction with cell searches, a significantly lower rate of drug abuse has been recorded. Nevertheless, detecting drug abuse among inmates remains difficult and time-consuming.

4.2. Police

It has been estimated that driving under the influence of drugs (DUID) is responsible for at least 4500 deaths and up to 250,000 serious injuries per year in Europe (9). In the zero-tolerant countries of Sweden, Germany, and Belgium, DATs are regularly employed by traffic police to combat DUID. In other countries, such as Finland, Sweden, and Germany, the assessment of blood and urine samples has already been included in their general codes of judicial procedure. In contrast, roadside screening devices for drug abuse, based on sweat, oral fluid, and saliva, are still being evaluated in the United Kingdom, Italy, and France. In these regions, the arrival of the equivalent of a drunk-driving breathalyzer is eagerly awaited.

Of the countries participating in the Roadside Testing Assessment (ROSITA) study (*see* Chapter 17), only Belgium and Germany have actually implemented routine drug testing at the roadside (6,7). Other regions have adopted a more cautious approach to this practice, especially in light of recent problems experienced in Belgium, such as the difficulty in obtaining urine or sweat samples from drivers. In countries such as the United Kingdom, individuals are tested for drugs only when they are formally charged with an offense or are suspected of DUID (4). Numerous studies in the United Kingdom have demonstrated that DUID is linked to serious accidents (10). As a result, DUID is classified as a criminal offense in the majority of European countries. Whereas normal punishment may entail treatment and a driving suspension, in more serious cases, a fine and/or imprisonment may be imposed.

4.3. Probation

A variety of sanctions may may be imposed on offenders serving a conditional period of parole who test positive for the consumption of drugs. Such penalties may range from the revocation of probation to immediate return to prison. In many parts of Europe, offenders must make themselves available for assessment as well as take up a prescribed treatment regime over an agreed-upon length of time, which can range from months to years.

4.4. Workplace

The practice of WPDT is much more common in the United States than in Europe. Since its introduction over two decades ago, drug testing has now become commonplace in the United States. Indeed, some experts believe that certain European regions are at least 10 yr away from the adoption of routine WPDT *(4)*. This is reflected in the statistics that fewer than 1 in 10 companies are currently conducting drug testing in the United Kingdom, which is widely perceived as the leading market in Europe in terms of WPDT. Apart from the United Kingdom, some companies in countries such as Belgium, Ireland, Sweden, and—to a lesser extent—Germany, have begun to introduce WPDT policies. Meanwhile, the rest of Europe, particularly the Mediterranean region, remains highly skeptical of this practice owing to the dearth of evidence supporting the value of WPDT in producing a safer working environment.

Screening policies, as observed in northern European regions, may be applied as part of a selection process for job applicants, or for regular, occasional, voluntary, or random testing of the workforce. These tests are also valuable in circumstances such as after-accident or posttreatment. Initially, end-users of drug testing in Europe are mostly confined to safety-sensitive industries, with the aim of minimizing any potential risk to the health, safety, and welfare of staff. Over the past decade, the evolution of WPDT in Europe has started to penetrate non-safety-sensitive professions, such as banking and stock brokerages (Table 3). This latest trend is most noticeable in the United Kingdom. According to research carried out at Frost & Sullivan *(4)*, the demand for WPDT in Europe is expected to continue to rise over the next 5 yr, largely as a result of the sustained development of the UK market. However, there are reports that in a minority of cases, WPDT is being performed in the absence of quality control, chain of custody, adulteration testing, or confirmation of positive test results. This is in spite of the introduction in 2002 of guidelines for legally defensible workplace drug testing prepared by the European Workplace Drug Testing Society (EWDTS).

4.5. Hospitals

The use of DATs in the hospital sector has remained relatively steady over the last 5 yr. Hospital central laboratories were among the first sites where urine-based DATs were performed in Europe. Subsequently, the demand for DATs also emerged from more specialized clinical and toxicology laboratories, psychiatric units, and small, decentralized laboratories. Interestingly, usage in the emergency room (ER) accounts for the majority of point-of-collection DATs, owing to the need for instant results. In the primary-care domain, in

Table 3
Main Workplace Sectors Performing Drug Testing (Europe, 2003)

Banking	Petro-chemical
Construction	Printing
Energy	Airlines
Insurance	Maritime transport
Manufacturing	Railways
Mining	Road transport: buses, coaches, long-haul deliveries

addition to sending samples for laboratory analysis, rehabilitation clinics and doctors' offices often prefer to use urine-based POC DATs for their rapid results and ease of use. However, the use of POC DATs is likely to remain minimal in the health care sector because of current budget cuts across Europe. As a result, the majority of DATs are being sent for laboratory analysis *(3)*.

4.6. Other Applications

In 2003, lower-volume consumption of drug testing occurred within the military, at customs and excise services, at border crossings, airports, and docks. In such circumstances, urine assays and sweat-based tests are employed.

5. TESTING DEVICES

Similarly to the US system, testing for DOA relies on a two-tier system for screening and confirmation. The initial screening phase may be realized either on the POC format (small desktop instrument, hand-held devices, cassettes, strips, swabs) or on a laboratory platform. Confirmation analysis, if required, is typically performed in the laboratory using the gas chromatography (GC)-mass spectrometry (MS) technique, widely considered as the "gold standard." Alternative methods such as high-performance liquid chromatography (HPLC) and GC may also be employed (*see* Chapter 3). Currently, laboratory analysis is still the method of choice for DOA screening throughout Europe. This is unlikely to change in the near future, because laboratory assays are preferred as a result of their standardized quality control and high-throughput capabilities. High levels of sensitivity and specificity and low costs are also important determining factors. Despite these advantages, laboratory operation often requires skilled technicians, whereby the delivery of results takes days rather than minutes, in stark contrast with the convenience of disposable or re-usable POC tests *(11)*. Single-parameter, multi-parameter, and customized panels, on both the laboratory and POC formats, may be easily procured either through a known supplier or via the

Internet. Multi-panel POC assays are often preferred, since they give a more complete profile of a person's recent drug-consumption tendencies. Methadone clinics, on the other hand, may choose a more specific and cheaper test detecting only the consumption of heroin.

6. AVAILABLE MATRICES

In addition to the traditional specimens of blood and urine, a variety of alternative matrices, such as oral fluid, saliva, sweat, and hair, are available in Europe. However, until the accuracy and applicability of these matrices are established, urine and blood are likely to remain the most highly demanded DATs in the near future.

6.1. Urine Tests

During the past decade, urine-based DATs have been the most commonly used screening assays in both health care and non-health care sectors across Europe. Whereas the majority of urine samples continue to be performed on the laboratory platform, the popularity of urine POC tests is steadily growing. Urine tests are currently preferred because of their noninvasive nature and the ease with which large-volume specimens may be obtained and DOA detected *(4,12)*. At present, the urine test's low cost compared with other test matrices is still the overriding factor and ensures its high utility rate in Europe. POC urine tests are available in the form of dipsticks, test strips, test cassettes, and test cups. A test cup serves not only as a test device, but also as a collection tool. However, as demonstrated in the Belgian part of the ROSITA study *(6,7)*, urine collection at roadside is deemed impractical.

6.2. Blood Tests

Blood tests generally exhibit the best correlation with drug intoxication and impairment *(6,7)*. In the complex European field of litigation, results from blood tests are often the only ones that are acceptable in a court of law. Consequently, it is likely that the demand for blood tests will remain high. In contrast with urine and other matrices, there is a legal requirement in many countries for a medically qualified person to oversee the collection of blood samples. In Germany and Italy, both urine and blood samples are required when people are suspected of driving under the influence of drugs. This situation highlights the impracticality associated with blood testing. Highly invasive, time-consuming, and expensive, the analysis of blood is almost exclusively performed in the laboratory, in specialized toxicology facilities.

6.3. Oral-Fluid and Saliva Tests

In the 2003 European Workplace Drug Testing Society (EWDTS) Symposium, held in Barcelona, the merits of oral fluid, oral mucosal transudate, and saliva as DAT matrices were debated. Although the use of oral fluid-based assays remains low, their demand is definitely on the increase in Europe *(4)*. For example, the original British Rail Alcohol and Drug Policy recommended use of urine tests for standard DOA screening. However, at least one rail operator has already switched to using oral fluids instead, because it is more acceptable among its staff. Less invasive and intrusive than either blood or urine, testing of oral fluid may be performed under direct visual supervision. Furthermore, by eliminating the need to send the sample for laboratory analysis, less time is taken to obtain the results *(12)*. Presence of DOA in oral-fluid samples is also more indicative of recent consumption. At present, however, the levels of sensitivity and specificity of the current generation of oral-fluid tests are still questionable *(6,7)*. Although studies such as the ROSITA II project and the UK Home office custody suite project are still underway, oral-fluid DATs are soon expected to be adopted by other rail companies and police forces in the United Kingdom. In this scenario, oral fluid will quickly become the third most common specimen requested for DOA analysis across Europe.

6.4. Sweat Tests

Of all the test specimens discussed in this chapter, sweat remains the least employed in Europe *(4)*. For now, Germany and the United Kingdom represent the most advanced markets in Europe for sweat-based DATs. In Germany, the main end-users are the non-health care sectors, including customs officers, traffic police, and prison officers. Similarly to oral fluid-based tests, collection of sweat specimens on site avoids the necessity of a public toilet or hospital. Although sweat patches are known to be in use in the United States, sweat samples in Europe are mainly collected by swab-POC devices. Despite the fact that they are cheaper than oral-fluid tests *(4)*, it is believed that utility of these DATs will remain minimal over the near future, even in Germany and the United Kingdom. This is mainly because sweat tests exhibit only a weak correlation with impairment *(6,7)* and have limited exposure in the media.

6.5. Hair Tests

Hair testing, along with blood analysis, is principally associated with forensic science in Europe. Capable of providing a profile of a person's drug-abuse history, often measured in months rather than days, hair testing is becoming increasingly noticeable for its use in pre-employment screening.

Similarly to that of blood, the complex analysis of hair must be performed in a specialized laboratory *(12)*. Thus, it is a costly process in terms of both time and money.

7. REGULATORY MECHANISMS

The legal and regulatory aspect of drug testing across the various regions of Europe is highly complex. Countries such as France, the Netherlands, Germany, and the United Kingdom all have accreditation programs in place *(6)*. In the United Kingdom, the following pieces of legislation are known to have played an important role in the development of the DAT market, especially in the workplace:

1. Misuse of Drugs Act 1971
2. Health and Safety at Work Act 1974
3. Road Traffic Act 1988
4. Transport and Works Act 1992
5. Management of Health and Safety at Work Regulations 1992

In accordance with such laws, routine screening in the workplace must be carried out so as to protect the health, safety, and welfare of all employees as much as possible. Employers in Europe are becoming increasingly aware of the possibility of being held liable for the actions of their drug-impaired staff. Currently, WPDT in Europe is limited to safety-critical industries such as petrochemical, construction, and public transport. On the other hand, utility of WPDT in non-safety-critical industries remains low, even in the more advanced markets of the United Kingdom and Germany. This is the result of a general lack of enforcement of legislation demanding obligatory testing of staff in these sectors. This is even more apparent in southern European countries, where employees place a high value on their rights to privacy and family life, as permitted under Article 8 of the European Convention on Human Rights of 1998. Drug testing at the roadside in Europe is still not uniformly applied. For the time being, drivers suspected of DUID are tested only in Belgium and Switzerland *(6,7)*. Just before the year 2000, *per se*-type laws were implemented in both Germany and Sweden, whereby driving is prohibited if certain drugs are detectable in the blood. In the United Kingdom, police forces are currently being trained to recognize symptoms of DUID as part of a large-scale evaluation of roadside DATs. Nevertheless, no legislation has yet been established.

ACKNOWLEDGMENTS

This project was supported by Frost & Sullivan. Amanda Weaver provided expert editorial assistance.

REFERENCES

1. Kelso P. We've no idea how big the problem is. Guardian Unlimited. 2003;http://sport.guardian.co.uk/athletics/story/0,10082,1070015,00.html.
2. Dickinson M. FA to alter drugs rules after trying Ferdinand. Times online, 2003;http://www.timesonline.co.uk/article/0,,277-873357,00.html.
3. Frost & Sullivan. European Drugs of Abuse Testing: Healthcare Markets. 2003; www.frost.com.
4. Frost & Sullivan. European Drugs of Abuse Testing: Non-Healthcare Markets. 2003; www.frost.com.
5. Independent Inquiry into Drug Testing at Work. Final Topline Results. 2003;http://www.drugscope.org.uk/uploads/goodpractice/documents/MORI%20%20top%2oline%results.pdf.
6. Moeller M, Steinmeyer S, and Aberl F. Operational, User and Legal Requirements across EU Member States for Roadside Drug Testing Equipment. 1999; ROSITA Contract DG VII PL98-3032.
7. Verstraete A and Puddu M. General Conclusions and Recommendations, Deliverable D5 of the ROSITA Project. 2000;www.ROSITA.org.
8. European Monitoring Centre for Drugs and Drug Addiction. Annual report 2003: the state of the drugs problem in the European Union and Norway. 2003;http://annualreport.emcdda.eu.int/en/home-en.html
9. De Gier JJ. Drugs other than alcohol and driving in the European Union. Institute for Human Psychopharmacology, University of Limburg, Maastricht, The Netherlands, Tech Report IHP 95-54, 1995.
10. British Medical Association. Driving Under the Influence of Drugs, 2003.
11. Wong A. (2003). Trends in point-of-care testing for drugs of abuse. European Clinical Laboratory 2003;22:12--14.
12. Wong A. (2003). Boosting the drug abuse testing market. Global Discovery & Development 2004; pp. 6–7.

Chapter 17

The Results of the Roadside Drug Testing Assessment Project

Alain G. Verstraete

SUMMARY

The 21-mo Roadside Testing Assessment (ROSITA) project started in January 1999 and included a literature survey of drugs and medicines that have detrimental impacts on road users' performance, an inventory of the available roadside drug-testing equipment for urine, oral fluid, and sweat, an evaluation of the operational, user, and legal requirements for roadside testing equipment in the different European Union countries, and an extensive evaluation of several devices in eight countries. On-site immunoassays were used for the detection of drugs in urine, oral fluid, and/or sweat in 2968 subjects. Police officers liked having the tools to detect drivers under the influence of drugs, and they were very creative in finding solutions to the practical and operational problems they encountered. On-site drug testing gave the police confidence, and saved time and money. Police officers had no major objections to collecting specimens of body fluids. In the majority of the participating countries, oral fluid was the preferred specimen. Some on-site urine tests (Rapid Drug Screen® [American Bio Medica], Syva® RapidTest™ [Dade Behring], Dipro Drugscreen 5 [Dipro Diagnostics], Triage [Biosite Diagnostics]) yielded good results (accuracy >95%, sensitivity and specificity >90% compared with reference methods), but none had good results for all assays.

The sampling of oral-fluid or sweat specimens was well accepted by drivers. The on-site tests evaluated—Drugwipe® (Securetec Detektions-Systeme AG), Cozart Rapiscan (Cozart Bioscience Ltd.), and ORALscreen™ (Avitar Inc.)—were not sufficiently reliable (accuracy between 50 and 81% in comparison with blood results).

From: *Forensic Science and Medicine: Drugs of Abuse: Body Fluid Testing*
Edited by R. C. Wong and H. Y. Tse © Humana Press Inc., Totowa, NJ

Progress is needed for sampling, duration of the test, sample volume, and reliability. From 2003 to 2005, the ROSITA-II project will evaluate the newer on-site oral-fluid devices in six European countries and five US states.

1. INTRODUCTION

Road accidents account for approx 40,000 deaths and 1,700,000 injured in the European Union (EU) per year *(1)*. The costs resulting from road traffic accidents amount to approx €160 billion annually, or 2% of gross national product. Whereas the number of accidents in which alcohol is involved seems to be diminishing, increasing drug abuse and driving under the influence of drugs (DUID) are reasons for concern. Between 1999 and 2003, five European countries adopted *per se* laws for DUID: Germany, Belgium, Sweden, Finland, and France. Several other countries have adopted laws that allow taking samples of body fluids when DUID is suspected. The increased attention to DUID is illustrated by the adoption of a resolution by the European Council in November 2003 on combating the impact of psychoactive substance use on road accidents. This resolution invites the European Commission to follow up with timely and effective measures in accordance with the European Action Programme on Road Safety *(2)*, and in particular:

- To carry out a study on the effectiveness of neuro-behavioral and toxicological tests assessing the intake and influence of psychoactive substances on driving ability and, based on the outcome of such a study, to propose procedures or guidelines for conducting the above tests at the European level in order to ensure that the results are reliable and comparable.
- To propose guidelines, based on the best practices identified in the EU, for the management of psychoactive substances-related driving cases.
- To recommend guidelines, at the European level, for training of police officers and health professionals in cases of DUID.
- To consider introduction of appropriate harmonised pictograms on medical packaging.
- To consider proposals for appropriate levels of control on professional drivers.
- To establish a European Road Safety Observatory within the European Commission.

Reliable roadside screening tests are urgently needed to aid police in determining which drivers must provide a blood sample or in taking immediate administrative measures such as confiscating the driver's license or impounding the vehicle. However, because illegal drugs are not released in measurable amounts in the breath, roadside drug testing must be based on other specimens that are relatively easy to obtain, such as urine, oral fluid, and sweat. Roadside drug-test results are regarded only as preliminary and must be confirmed before they are admissible in court.

Table 1

Official Partners of the Roadside Testing Assessment (ROSITA) Project

No.	Name	Countries
1.	University of Gent (Project Management)	Belgium
2.	National Public Health Institute, KTL	Finland
3.	University of Glasgow, Forensic Medicine and Science	United Kingdom
4.	Institute of Legal Medicine, Homburg	Germany
5.	National Institute of Forensic Sciences, NICC, Brussels	Belgium
6.	National Institute of Forensic Toxicology, NIFT, Oslo Present name: Norwegian Institute of Public Health, Division of Forensic Toxicology and Drug Abuse	Norway
7.	Institute of Legal Medicine, University of Santiago de Compostela	Spain
8.	Institute of Legal Medicine, University of Strasbourg	France
9.	Centre of Behavioural and Forensic Toxicology, University of Padova Present name: Dipartimento di Medicina Ambientale e Sanità Pubblica	Italy
10.	Roche Diagnostics	Belgium; Germany
11.	Securetec Detektions-Systeme AG	Germany
12.	Dade-Behring GmbH	Germany

2. *The Roadside Testing Assessment Consortium*

During 1999 and 2000, the European Commission (Directorate-General Transport) funded a Roadside Testing Assessment (ROSITA) project in the fourth framework program in eight European countries. A total of nine European Institutes for Legal Medicine and Toxicology and three companies worked together on the five different project targets. The official ROSITA Partners are listed in Table 1.

The ROSITA study was divided into five working packages, which generally covered the following questions:

1. What are the drugs and medicines that have detrimental impacts on drivers' performance?
2. What are the state-of-the-art roadside testing devices for urine, sweat, and oral-fluid matrices? Are there other tests that can be used at the roadside to evaluate the impairment of drivers?
3. What kind of operational, user, and legal requirements exist across member states of the EU for roadside testing equipment?
4. What are the usability (practicability), sensitivity, specificity, and accuracy levels of available roadside test devices?
5. What equipment can be recommended for the use of roadside testing in Europe?

3. RESULTS OF THE ROSITA PROJECT

3.1. Survey of Drugs and Medicines That Have Detrimental Impacts on Drivers' Performance

A literature survey of drugs and medicines that have detrimental impacts on drivers' performance *(3)* focused on studies related to the effects of drugs on driving. Information was compiled in table form categorizing the available medicinal drugs according to their influence on driving in different systems in different countries. Driving is a complex task whereby the driver constantly receives information, analyzes it, and reacts to it. Substances that have an influence on brain functions or on mental processes involved in driving will clearly affect driving performance. Stimulant drugs, such as amphetamines, methylenedioxymethamphetamine (MDMA; "ecstasy") and cocaine enhance risk-taking behavior. These drugs are also dangerous because of the fatigue that sets in after the "high" or after a full weekend of drug-taking and dancing. Moreover, they dilate the pupils, and drivers can be blinded by the increased amount of light. Cannabis causes euphoria, somnolence, a change of visual and auditory perception, and a decrease in psychomotor abilities. The danger is markedly increased when cannabis is combined with alcohol, which is a common practice. Opiates (heroin) cause sedation, sleepiness, apathy, and pinpoint pupils. In the withdrawal phase, the subject becomes nervous, irritable, and less concentrated, which are characteristics not compatible with safe driving.

The study also reviewed the effect of medication on driving, relying on experimental and pharmaco-epidemiological studies. The most important groups are the benzodiazepines, which are used by 10–20% of the population in some countries, such as Belgium and France. Pharmaco-epidemiological studies have clearly shown that users of benzodiazepines face a two- to fivefold higher risk of being involved in an accident. This risk is even higher (8- to 10-fold) for people in the first 2 wk of treatment. Some studies have shown that the increase in crash risk is even more pronounced in young males taking long-acting benzodiazepines. Other drugs that were reviewed were antidepressants, antihistamines, neuroleptics, and opiods.

3.2. Survey of State-of-the-Art Roadside Testing Devices Available for Urine, Sweat, and Saliva Matrices

The devices that existed at the time of the study for drug testing at the roadside were inventoried *(4)*. As this information is now partially obsolete, only a brief overview of the findings will be given. A total of 19 devices were identified in the market study. Sixteen were designed for the screening of urine samples. These represented 33 brand names on the international market. Of the three devices that were developed for saliva, two were manufactured in Europe. One device could also be applied to sweat.

For urine testing, there are three kinds of test designs: a dip test (test strip or test card; the device is partially immersed in the urine for a few seconds), a pipet test (test cassette; a few drops of urine are deposited in the device with a dropper), and a cup test (the testing device is built into the side or top of a cup). Several manufacturers supplied single-parameter and multiple-parameter tests for the dip- and pipet-type devices. Most of the tests were available for the detection of amphetamines, methamphetamine, cannabinoids, cocaine, opiates, and phencyclidine. Eighty percent of the urine devices also included benzodiazepines and barbiturates in their panels. Fifty percent included methadone, and only 30% offered a test for tricyclic antidepressants.

3.3. Survey of Operational, User, and Legal Requirements Across Member States of the European Union for Roadside Testing Devices

During the initial phase of the ROSITA project, member countries collected and evaluated the specific needs and requirements of the European police forces (5). Representatives and experts for traffic safety and DUID in 21 European countries were asked to supply country-specific information by means of a structured questionnaire. Despite the fact that the majority of the European countries had not established sufficient legal conditions to fight DUID, European police forces had a rather clear picture, based on their national experiences and circumstances, of what they needed under their specific operational environment. These needs and requirements differed from country to country and sometimes even from state to state within the same country. Nevertheless, the essential requirements of roadside drug-testing devices were identified in this survey.

3.3.1. Main Target Drugs in Europe

The following classes of drugs were considered to be important enough (in decreasing order of frequency) to be included in the testing: cannabis, benzodiazepines, amphetamines, cocaine, and opiates. In Europe, cannabis is the most popular drug of abuse appearing in street traffic. This is followed by benzodiazepines, which are components of several prescribed medicines and are easily accessible. The amphetamine group also includes such "designer" drugs as methamphetamine, methylenedioxyamphetamine (MDA), and MDMA. Their use is very prevalent among people under 25 yr of age.

3.3.2. Preferred Specimen for Roadside Testing

According to European police, oral fluid was the preferred test specimen for roadside testing because of its ready availability, low level of invasiveness, and good correlation with impairment. Sweat was the second most preferred testing specimen, for similar reasons. In addition, sweat testing does not require cooperation from the drivers.

3.3.3. Test Format and Target Price

The preferred test configuration was a single-use, multi-parameter test, which was able to provide a clear, unambiguous test result on the above-mentioned groups of drugs within 5 min. The average price considered reasonable in the context of this survey for a single-parameter device was €3.9 and for a four-parameter device was €14.0.

3.4. Field Evaluation of Roadside Test Devices

3.4.1. Study Methods

In this part of the study, 11 on-site urine-test devices, 3 oral-fluid test devices, and 1 sweat-test device were tested in 2968 drivers, and positive and negative results were compared with those obtained by the reference methods as well as those in blood samples assessed by the same reference methods *(6)*. The reference methods referred to in this study are mostly gas chromatography(GC)-mass spectrometry (MS) or, in some cases, high-performance liquid chromatography with diode array detection (HPLC-DAD) or GC with electron capture detection (GC-ECD) *(see* Chapter 3). The number of subjects involved in each category and the drugs tested are given in Table 2.

Because of different legislation, the circumstances under which the tests were performed varied among the countries:

- Belgium: samples collected at the roadside were first screened by police with the Dipro Drugscreen 5 (Dipro Diagnostics) device and then by lab technicians with the other devices.
- Finland: urine was collected under police supervision in the hospital and not at the roadside. Police and laboratory staff performed the urine tests at the laboratory. Oral-fluid tests were performed at the roadside by trained police officers.
- France: on-site tests were evaluated in the laboratory.
- Germany: the tests were performed by police officers during police patrols. Oral-fluid and sweat samples were collected and tested directly at the roadside, whereas urine samples were normally collected and tested at police stations or at public lavatories. Patrols were conducted during the night, rendering reading of the results more difficult than in a police station, hospital, or laboratory.
- Italy: on-site tests were performed at the roadside by police personnel or ambulance volunteers, or in the laboratory by trained technicians. Roadside collection of blood, urine, and oral-fluid samples were made by medical personnel.
- Norway: on-site urine tests were performed by the police officers in the laboratory at the National Institute for Forensic Toxicology, in collaboration with

Table 2

Overview of the Methodological Aspects of the Roadside Testing Assessment (ROSITA) Field Tests

Countries	Number of subjects	Specimens collected	Number of on-site test devices evaluated in urine/oral fluid/sweat	Place of tests	Personnel performing tests
Belgium	180	Blood, urine, oral fluid, sweat	4/1/1	Roadside	Police, laboratory personnel
Finland	751	Blood, urine, oral fluid	11/2	Lab	Police, laboratory personnel
France	198	Blood, urine, oral fluid, sweat	3/0	Hospital	Laboratory personnel
Germany	617	Blood, urine, oral fluid, sweat	6/2/1	Roadside/ police station	Police, laboratory personnel
Italy	302	Blood, urine, oral fluid	3/1	Roadside/lab	Police, Red Cross volunteers
Norway	314	Blood, urine, oral fluid	3/2	Lab/station	Police
Spain	384	Urine, oral fluid	3/2	Roadside	Police, laboratory personnel
United Kingdom	214	Blood, urine, oral fluid	3/1	Prison/lab	Laboratory personnel

representatives from some manufacturers as assistants. The oral-fluid tests (Cozart Rapiscan [Cozart Bioscience Ltd.] and Drugwipe® [Securetec Detektions-Systeme AG]) were performed at the police station.

• Spain: on-site tests were performed by agents of the traffic police. Reading and interpretation of the results were done together by members of the Institute of Legal Medicine present during the patrol and by traffic police officers trained in the use of the devices. With one exception, the tests were performed at the roadside.

• United Kingdom: the subjects were prisoners. The on-site tests were performed by at least two members of the research team, either in the prison or in the laboratory.

The data from the evaluations in the eight countries were displayed in Microsoft Excel format. For the evaluation of opiates, specimens containing morphine, 6-acetylmorphine, or codeine were considered positives. It should be noted that other substances may cross-react and give positive results with on-site tests—for example, dihydrocodeine or pholcodine. For determination of the optimal cut-off levels in oral fluid, receiver operating characteristic (ROC) curves *(7))* were used.

Several comparisons were made between the different methods (on-site tests or reference methods) and the different matrices (blood, urine, oral fluid, or sweat). For each drug class, the following comparisons were made:

• A comparison between the reference method for blood and for the other biological fluids was made in order to assess whether findings in each matrix correspond well to those in blood. There is a general consensus that blood is the standard reference, as impairment (or recent exposure to drugs) corresponds best to the presence of drugs in blood;

• A comparison of on-site device results with those obtained from the reference methods for the same matrix;

• The validity of the roadside test for predicting blood positives by comparison with the results of blood samples assessed with a reference method.

For evaluation of the urine, oral-fluid, or sweat test devices, the accuracy, sensitivity, and specificity values have been calculated on the basis of the following definitions, where TP = true-positives, TN = true-negatives, FP = false-positives, and FN = false-negatives:

• Accuracy = percent of all samples correctly identified by the tests = (TP + TN)/(all results)

• Sensitivity = true-positives expressed as percent of all positives = TP/(TP + FN)

• Specificity = true-negatives expressed as percent of all negatives = TN/(TN + FP)

The following analytical criteria for an acceptable test were used: accuracy >95%, sensitivity >90%, specificity >90%, when compared with a reference method. Statistical analysis of the data was performed using Microsoft Excel, Medcalc (MedCalc Software), and SPSS (SPSS, Inc.).

3.4.2. Results

The study was performed on 2968 subjects. Ninety-two percent were males. Before evaluating the performance of on-site test devices, positive and negative results of a given drug class in oral-fluid, sweat, and urine samples assessed by a reference method (e.g., GC-MS) were compared with the results of blood samples assessed by the same reference method. This process allowed for the computation of the sensitivity, specificity, and accuracy of using a given reference method (e.g., GC-MS) in different fluids. In general, one can conclude that the accuracy rate of such comparisons using GC-MS ranges between 78 (cannabinoids in sweat) and 99% (cocaine in oral fluid) (Table 3). The exception is the benzodiazepine group, where the low sensitivity of the analytical methods applied in the laboratory appears to be the cause for the overall low and insufficient accuracy rate of oral fluid (29%) as a specimen for roadside screening. It is clear that there will never be a 100% correlation among the different body fluids. The results are influenced by the timing of sampling relative to the last drug intake. If a drug was taken very recently, it is possible that it can be found only in blood (and oral fluid), but not yet in urine. If a drug was taken a longer time ago, it is possible that it is no longer detectable in blood, but only in urine (and possibly in sweat).

In the next set of experiments, drug results from oral-fluid, sweat, and urine samples as assessed by various on-site testing devices were compared with those of the same fluid assessed by the reference method (i.e., GC-MS) or those of blood samples assessed by the same reference method. These results are given in Tables 4–6. The following sections provide a summary of the findings.

For amphetamines, all body fluids were appropriate for testing of this drug when GC-MS was the reference method. Both urine and oral fluid have good accuracy and predictive values (Table 3). Eighteen different on-site tests for amphetamine or methamphetamine were evaluated. If the results of amphetamines and methamphetamine were considered jointly (i.e., if one considers the test to be positive if either the amphetamine or the methamphetamine test is positive), test devices such as Rapid Drug Screen® (RDS; American Bio Medica), Dipro, and Syva® RapidTest™ (SRT; Dade Behring) satisfied the analytical criteria (accuracy >95%, sensitivity >90%, specificity >90%) (Table 4). Tests for oral fluid had much lower accuracy (80% or less in all cases; Table 5). The optimal cut-off for amphetamines in oral fluid was in the range of 70–90 ng/mL. For sweat, the low number of samples (nearly all positive) did not permit definite conclusions (Table 6), but use of sweat seemed promising.

Urine seemed to be a better fluid for detecting benzodiazepines at the roadside with the reference methods used (Table 3). Of the on-site urine test devices, Triage (Biosite Diagnostics) and RDS were the only two that met the

Table 3

Comparison of the Accuracy, Sensitivity, and Specificity of the Qualitative Results by Gas Chromatography (GC)-Mass Spectrometry (MS) in Urine, Oral Fluid, and Sweat vs GC-MS in Blood ("Gold Standard") for the Different Drugs

Analyte	Accuracy			Sensitivity			Specificity		
	Urine	Oral fluid	Sweat	Urine	Oral fluid	Sweat	Urine	Oral fluid	Sweat
Amphetamine	94%	95%	97%	97%	98%	100%	92%	91%	0%
Benzodiazepines	89%	29%		89%	21%		90%	67%	
Cannabinoids	86%	89%	78%	97%	86%	91%	81%	90%	17%
Cocaine	97%	99%	89%	95%	96%	100%	98%	99%	0%
Opiates	86%	91%	80%	97%	89%	88%	85%	91%	63%

Table 4
Number of Comparisons (*n*), Sensitivity (Se, %), Specificity (Sp, %) and Accuracy (Ac, %) of Rapid Urine Tests for Five Drug Classes

		Amphetamine + methamphetamine				Benzodiazepines				Cannabis				Cocaine				Opiates			
		n	Se	Sp	Ac	*n*	Se	Sp	Ac	*n*	Se	Sp	Ac	*n*	Se	Sp	Ac	*N*	Se	Sp	Ac
American Biomedica Rapid Drug Screen®	A + M	468	98	99	99	219	91	98	97	571	97	90	92	580	100	98	98	472	98	95	95
Cortez	A + M	186	87	93	90	189	81	84	82	369	95	95	95	393	85	98	97	387	98	95	95
Dipro Drugscreen 5 panel test	A + M	122	97 10	100	98					123	99	92	97	128	100	99	99	34	100	85	88
Frontline	A	68	0	56	68																
Mahsan Diagnostica	A	157	88	99	97					148	97	91	94	156	100	93	94	137	–	97	97
Rapitest® Multidrug panel	A	95	86	96	92	92	95	82	91	95	70	98	85	96	75	100	99	97	78	99	97
Roche TestCup 5	A	527	75	100	95					542	92	93	93	570	95	99	99	474	97	93	94
Status DS	A	92	85	96	91					92	80	100	91	92	100	99	99	94	100	97	97
Surescreen 6 Drug MultiTest	A + M	106	93 10	95	94	102	89	88	88	114	76	99	90	116	100	100	100	118	82	97	96
Syva® RapidCup™	A	52	0	100	100					88	97	92	94	90	100	98	98	85	100	96	96
Syva RapidTest™	A + M	558	97	100	100	354	98	84	86	880	93	100	97	904	96	99	99	782	95	96	96
Triage	A	395	89	99	98	394	94	99	98	396	84	99	96	396	95	100	100	396	100	99	99

The results were compared with the results obtained by gas chromatography-mass spectrometry. For amphetamines, in some cases (A + M) the combination of an amphetamine and methamphetamine test was used (*see* text).

Table 5
Accuracy, Sensitivity, and Specificity Values With Respect to the Blood Status Measured With Gas Chromatography-Mass Spectrometry for Three Oral Fluid Test Kits

Tests	Drugwipe®				Rapiscan				ORALscreen™			
Type of Drug	N	Acc. (%)	Sens. (%)	Spec. (%)	N	Acc. (%)	Sens. (%)	Spec. (%)	N	Acc. (%)	Sens. (%)	Spec. (%)
Amphetamine	142	73	90	55	111	80	87	74	0			
MDMA ("ecstasy")	130	72	90	55	61	74	67	74	0			
Benzodiazepines	0				133	56	17	90	0			
Cannabinoids	0				98	79	16	94	179	84	50	84
Cocaine	34	82	75	93	4	50	50	50	190	99	50	99
Opiates	214	81	63	83	109	81	67	83	180	86	50	87

MDMA, methylenedioxymethamphetamine.

Table 6

Accuracy, Sensitivity, and Specificity Values for Drugwipe® With Respect to the Blood and Sweat Status Measured With Gas Chromatography (GC)-Mass Spectrometry (MS)

Tests										
					Drugwipe					
		Sweat vs blood GC-MS					Sweat vs sweat GC-MS			
Type of drug	N	Acc. (%)	Sens. (%)	Spec. (%)		N	Acc. (%)	Sens. (%)	Spec. (%)
Amphetamine	38	95	100	0		37	92	94	67
MDMA ("ecstasy")	59	97	100	0		54	96	98	67
Cocaine	22	68	75	0		22	77	77	NA
Opiates	12	83	100	50		9	89	89	NA

NA, not applicable or not available; MDMA, methylenedioxymethamphetamine.

analytical criteria (Table 4). For oral fluid, the sensitivity of the on-site test devices and of some confirmation methods was very poor (Table 5). This was explained by the extremely low concentrations of benzodiazepines in oral fluid (often <1 ng/mL). This was even more so for the low levels of some benzo-diazepines, such as flunitrazepam. No on-site tests were available for sweat.

For cannabinoids, comparison of the performance of the different matri-ces showed a small advantage for oral fluid (89% accuracy; Table 3), which is not unexpected considering the much longer window of detection of cannabis metabolites in urine compared with the presence of tetrahydrocannabinol (THC) in blood. Three of 11 on-site tests for urine met the analytical criteria. These were Dipro, Cortez (Cortez Diagnostics), and SRT (Table 4). In com-parison with blood, the accuracy of the best on-site urine tests was close to 90%. For the on-site oral-fluid tests (Table 5), the sensitivity was too low (only 18 to 25% when compared with blood results). The required sensitivity of on-site oral-fluid tests was 2 ng/mL of THC. There were indications that THC may bind to the material of some sampling devices. Much higher concentra-tions of THC could be extracted from the cotton of the Salivette®, in compari-son with the THC concentrations in oral fluid. A possible explanation could be that the cotton of the Salivette absorbs the THC that has been sequestered onto teeth and gum, but this possibility needs to be confirmed. This phenome-non could be useful for increasing the sensitivity of oral-fluid analysis for THC, if a suitable extraction method can be found to release the THC trapped on the fibers of the sampling device. For testing of cannabinoids with sweat, no on-site test devices were available.

For cocaine and metabolites, both oral fluid and urine gave good correla-tion for the prediction of positive drug results in blood assessed by GC-MS (Table 3). Eight of the 11 on-site tests met the analytical criteria. These were Dipro, RDS, TesTcup (Roche Diagnostics.), Syva Rapid Cup (SRC), SRT, SureScreen™ (Surescreen Diagnostics), Status DS™ (Lifesign), and Triage (Table 4). Even when compared with blood results, four tests had an accuracy of greater than 95% and sensitivity and specificity greater than 90%: RDS, Roche TesTcup, SRT, and Triage. In oral fluid, the evaluation was hampered by the low number of positive samples (Table 5). In addition, the sensitivity of Drugwipe was too low. For sweat, the number of samples that could be evalu-ated was also small, and the evaluation was done with positive samples only. The accuracy of Drugwipe was 77% (Table 6).

When comparing the GC-MS analysis of opiates in different body fluids with the GC-MS analysis of blood samples, oral fluid had slightly better accu-racy than urine (Table 3). Six of the 11 on-site tests met the analytical criteria (Table 4): RDS, Cortez, SRC, SRT, Status DS, and Triage. With oral fluid, the on-site tests showed less accuracy than with urine tests (Table 5). The sensitivity, in particular, was too low. An ideal oral-fluid test should have a detection limit of 2–5 ng/mL for opiates.

3.4.3. Practical and Operational Aspects

When the necessary facilities were available (e.g., a sanitary van), urine could be obtained relatively easily at the roadside. When the facilities were not available, obtaining a urine sample was a problem, and it could be time-consuming if the driver had to be brought to a suitable facility. In some cases, the volume of urine obtained was low and was insufficient for certain test devices. Some countries clearly stated that sampling urine at the roadside was unacceptable. A clear majority of countries preferred oral fluid as the matrix for roadside testing, while one country favored sweat and one country favored urine. The methods for obtaining oral fluid needed further improvements. Wiping over the tongue seemed to be a well-accepted technique, but in this case the analytical detection technique needed to be very sensitive. Sampling oral fluid with dedicated devices also gave rise to the following problems:

- It was sometimes messy and uncomfortable for the subject;
- In some cases it took a long time;
- The cooperation of the subject was needed (in some cases, intentionally or not, the subject swallowed the collection device);
- Oral fluid was sometimes viscous and could not be used with some devices.

Moreover, dry mouth was a frequently encountered problem in drug users. Sampling was then even more difficult and time-consuming. However, in the present evaluation, obtaining oral fluid for testing was successful in nearly all cases. Overall, sweat and oral-fluid sampling seemed very well accepted by the subjects, much moreso than that of urine or blood.

3.4.4. Discussion

Eleven different on-site test devices for detection of illegal drugs in urine were evaluated. Most of the urine test devices only reached accuracy levels of approx 90% when correlated with the blood results. This could be a result of the discrepancy in temporal distribution of drugs in different body fluids. A much better accuracy rate is reached when the urine results of roadside test devices are correlated with urine results from GC-MS analysis. In this case, several test devices surpass the 95% accuracy rate for some drug classes. However, some limitations of the study design, which is mainly dictated by the different legal situations, must be pointed out:

- The analytical methods used in all the countries were not identical; the evaluation of the devices was done in different places—at the roadside, in the police station, or in the laboratory;

- The devices were evaluated by different persons, which made their comments on the practical and operational aspects of the study difficult to compare;
- Prevalence of drug use and the selection criteria of the subjects differed among the countries, resulting in variability in the preferential use of different specimens for different on-site test devices in different countries.

In several countries, the ROSITA evaluations were the first experience that police officers had had with roadside drug tests and, despite some problems and disappointments, police officers still liked having the tools to detect drivers under the influence of drugs. Users of on-site tests had also shown great creativity in overcoming some of the encountered problems. The oral-fluid devices available at the time of the study all had practical disadvantages, and the analytical evaluation was not satisfactory. But the need for such devices was so great that in one country, police officers preferred to perform an oral-fluid test that was imperfect, rather than no test at all. In other countries, police would rather use urine tests. Police did not have major objections to collecting specimens. A majority of the countries favored oral fluid as a test matrix. Besides the analytical evaluation discussed here, all test devices that were part of the field trials had also been evaluated by the police with respect to handling, ease of sampling, speed, and overall user-friendliness.

In the "needs and requirements" survey, most police forces in Europe expressed preferences for test devices based on oral fluid or sweat because of the ready availability of the specimen. Interestingly, sampling urine during the field-test phase was not a problem, if appropriate facilities (such as a sanitary van) were available. In other cases, drivers had to be taken to a police station or health center, which took time. In one country, when drivers were asked to give a urine sample at the roadside without suitable facilities, the refusal rate was high. Most police forces in Europe are legally not authorized to obtain a urine sample by force. Sampling oral fluid or sweat was much more acceptable to drivers. The possibility of using sweat as a testing specimen is especially of interest to the police forces.

In some cases, the volume of urine collected was not sufficient for the cup-type test devices (e.g., SRC, TesTcup, RDS). This was a problem in 3% of the cases in Germany. In that respect, RDS has the advantage that the urine can be pipetted onto the card.

In some cases, the calculation of the different analytical criteria was hampered by the skewing of the data toward one end of the positive–negative spectrum. For example, many drivers have been tested with ORALscreen, but most of the results turn out to be negative, leading to good accuracy values despite the fact that sensitivity is insufficient. The accuracy of the on-site tests for oral fluid is not satisfactory when one compares it with the reference method in the same specimen: the sensitivity is between 25% (ORALscreen cannabinoids) and 88% (Drugwipe amphetamines/MDMA). Specificity is in the range of 48% (RapiScan benzodiazepines) to 100% (RapiScan cocaine). Very high specificity values are again a result of no or very low numbers of positive samples. The performance of Drugwipe for amphetamines/MDMA and opiates in sweat seems good, but very few negative samples were analyzed. More studies will be needed to confirm these findings and to allow a proper evaluation of Drugwipe as a sweat test.

Benzodiazepines are present in oral fluids in extremely low concentrations. In a review by Kidwell *(8)*, the limits of the methods used to detect benzo-diazepines in oral fluid range from 0.05 to 5 ng/mL, with the majority being less than 0.3 ng/mL. At present, the sensitivity of the on-site test and of some confirmation methods is poor.

The sampling method for Drugwipe (wiping over the tongue) was appreciated everywhere, because of minimal discomfort and low sample-volume requirement. ORALscreen was considered "disgusting" in Germany and Scotland because of the many complications that occurred during sampling, and in nearly all cases, the fingers of the officers and researchers came into contact with oral fluid. This was certainly less acceptable to them than working with urine. Sampling with Cozart Rapiscan was also problematic. The process took a long time and was cumbersome. It was worse if drivers were able to provide only a limited volume of oral fluid, either because of low oral-fluid production or because of refusal to cooperate. The average duration of sampling with the Rapiscan was 4 min, with extremes between 1 and 12 min. Average total time for sampling plus analysis was 20 min (range was 13 to 33 min), which was considered too long for roadside use. One advantage of Cozart Rapiscan was the availability of excess (diluted) samples for performing confirmation tests in the laboratory. In the final analysis, sampling by wiping the tongue is well accepted, although this process requires a very sensitive detection method because of the low volume and the lack of sufficient sample for confirmation analysis. The other methods all have some drawbacks, and more research is needed to develop more efficient sampling methods.

In terms of practical use, none of the testing devices was fully acceptable to the police officers. In Germany, the acceptance of the oral-fluid tests was much less than any of the urine tests. Drugwipe was considered simple in terms of the training needed. The small sample volume and rapid turnaround time were appreciated; however, viewed less favorably were the availability of only single tests, the difficulty of reading of the results, and the need for water in order to perform the test. Use of the electronic reader was considered impractical in Norway, but was considered essential in all other countries. In Italy, oral fluid was considered quite easy to test at the roadside, at least through the use of Drugwipe.

With Avitar ORALscreen, problems were encountered in the transferal of oral fluid from the sampling device to the test. In Scotland, problems were encountered with the transfer of viscous oral fluid, and some samples failed to migrate to the analytical strip as a result of manufacturing faults. Some problems with reading the ORALscreen were reported. Faint lines were produced, especially for cannabinoids, resulting in difficulty in distinguishing presence or absence of drugs. The multiple pieces of equipment and the need to place them on a flat surface made the use of Cozart Rapiscan impractical for a police officer on a motorbike, and restricted its use to police officers driving a van. The equipment proved to be rather complicated to use, and the total time needed to obtain a result (sample collection, sample preparation, run time) was at least 15 min. Often, it took that long just to collect sufficient oral fluid from drivers under the influence of drugs, as they often had very dry mouth as a result of drug use. General comments from police officers were that the sample-preparation procedures (filtration, pipetting, and handling of sample tubes) were rather complicated, such that previous training in the laboratory was necessary.

3.5. Conclusions and Recommendations for Roadside Testing

The ROSITA project studied 2968 subjects and compared 11 different urine on-site drug tests and 3 on-site oral fluid tests (one of which was used on sweat as well) in eight countries. From this experience, the following conclusions can be drawn (9).

3.5.1. Role of Roadside Drug Tests in EU Traffic Safety

There is a definite need for roadside drug tests in Europe. Roadside drug tests give confidence to police officers prosecuting DUID. Without an on-site tool to confirm the suspicion, police officers are often reluctant to prosecute. Roadside drug tests save both time and money by simplifying drug law-enforcement procedures and by obviating more expensive laboratory analysis. In addition, people who are not under the influence are minimally inconvenienced and can go on their way sooner.

Most subjects are impressed by the immediate results they see, even more so if the procedures are complex or if the results are read electronically. Often, the guilty parties would confess to the crime when confronted with a positive result, sometimes even after a long and vehement denial before seeing the test results.

3.5.2. Choice of Specimens for Roadside Testing

In all countries, blood is considered the best fluid for confirmation analysis, because the presence of drugs in blood corresponds best with recent use and impairment. The ROSITA study shows that a clear majority of European countries prefer oral fluid as the matrix for roadside testing, while one country favors sweat and one country favors urine. For oral fluid, the methods of collection as well as assay sensitivity need further improvements. A drawback of urine testing is that none of the test devices score high for all the drug categories tested. There is also no clear preference for the dip- or pipet-type devices. Cup-type devices would be preferred if they did not leak and if they required a smaller sample volume.

Despite the many practical problems associated with the project, police officers still believe that the results of the study are valuable. There is general feeling that a rapid and reliable testing device will greatly simplify their work and save time. There is also a preference for multi-analyte drug tests as well as electronic readers. A reference band on the testing device is deemed necessary.

4. *ROSITA-II: Evaluation of On-Site Oral-Fluid Test in Europe and the United States*

In 2003, a follow-up project to ROSITA was started. This time, the study is being performed in collaboration with the United States. Six European partner countries of the former ROSITA project (Belgium, Finland, France, Germany, Norway, and Spain) and five states in the United States—Utah (Salt Lake City Police), Florida (Hillsborough County Sheriff's Office and Manatee County Sheriff's Office, Washington (State Patrol), Wisconsin (State Laboratory of Hygiene), and Indiana (State Department of Toxicology/Indiana State Police)—are the participants. In this study, the focus is exclusively on oral-fluid testing. In total, approx 3000 subjects will be tested in two 9-mo testing periods, separated by a 3-mo interim evaluation period. A preliminary market study identified 10 on-site test devices appropriate for testing drugs in oral fluids (Table 7). Six of the 10 have been evaluated with spiked oral-fluid samples (Table 7). Final results are expected to be published by the end of 2005.

Based on the experience with the first ROSITA project, the focus of ROSITA II will be on a more uniform protocol with identical limits of detection for the reference methods. Initial evaluations indicate that the current versions of the oral-fluid test devices have made some progress, but not as much as was hoped for in 2000. In particular, the detection of THC is still problematic. Although a detection limit of of 2 ng/mL is necessary, the best device can detect 20 ng/mL only 50% of the time (Table 8).

5. *Conclusions*

The ROSITA study has given a general boost to roadside drug testing, and laboratories, police forces, and politicians have become interested. The work of ROSITA is followed intensely by several governments considering

Table 7

Overview of Point-of-Collection Oral-Fluid Drug Tests

Manufacturer	Device	Evaluated in ROSITA-II (as of Jan 2004)
Avitar, Inc., Canton, MA 02021, USA	ORALscreen™	
Branan Medical Corporation, Irvine, CA 92618, USA	Oratect™	X
Cozart Bioscience Limited, Abingdon, Oxfordshire, UK	RapiScan	X
Dräger Safety, Lübeck, Germany	DrugTest®	
OraSure Technologies, Inc, Bethlehem, PA 18015, USA	UPlink™	X
EnviteC-Wismar GmbH, Wismar, Germany	Smartclip	
Lifepoint Inc., Ontario, CA 91761, USA	Impact® test system	
Securetec Detektions-Systeme AG, Ottobrunn, Germany	Drugwipe®II	X
Sun Biomedical Laboratories, Inc., Blackwood, NJ 08012, USA	OraLine® s.a.t. Test	
ulti med Products GmbH, Germany	Salivascreen	X
Varian Inc, Lake Forest, CA	On•Site OraLab®	X

ROSITA, Roadside Testing Assessment.

290

Table 8
Detection Limits (ng/mL) of Six Point-of-Collection Tests
in Spiked Oral-Fluid Samples *(14,15)*

	Amphetamine	Cocaine	Methamphetamine	Morphine	THC
Drugwipe®	500	200	100	20	50
Oratect™	25	40	25	20	ND
Rapiscan	25	200	100	80	50
OraLab®	500	10	500	80	100
Salivascreen	NT	40	25	20	ND
UPlink™	25	200	25	20	20

NT, not tested; ND, no tetrahydrocannabinol (THC) could be detected, even at 100 ng/mL.

legislation on drugs and driving, e.g., France, Denmark, Austria, and the Netherlands. The work of ROSITA is also cited in several high-level official documents, e.g., the Council Resolution *(2)*. The results have been presented at many scientific meetings and published in several journals *(10–13)*. Two PhD theses have been based on work in the ROSITA project. At the time of writing, the conclusions of ROSITA are still valid: oral fluid and sweat are promising specimens for roadside drug testing, but more research and development is needed. Much progress has been made in the 3 yr since the end of the project, and the dream of a reliable and practical roadside drug test is coming closer to reality. The ROSITA-II project is currently evaluating the latest generation of oral-fluid tests.

REFERENCES

1. European Commission, Energy and Transport DG. Saving 20,000 Lives on Our Roads: A Shared Responsibility, Brussels: October 2003.
2. Council of the European Union. Council Resolution on Combating the Impact of Psychoactive Substances Use on Road Accidents. CORDROGUE 73. 2003.
3. Maes V, Charlier C, Grenez O, and Verstraete AG. Drugs and medicines that are suspected to have a detrimental impact on road user performance, in ROSITA. Roadside Testing Assessment (Verstraete AG, ed), ROSITA Consortium, Gent: 2001.
4. Samyn N, Viaene B, Vandevenne L, and Verstraete AG. Inventory of state-of-the-art roadside drug testing equipment, in ROSITA. Roadside Testing Assessment (Verstraete AG, ed), ROSITA Consortium, Gent: 2001.
5. Moeller MR, Steinmeyer S, and Aberl F. Operational, user and legal requirements across EU member states for roadside drug testing equipment, in ROSITA. Roadside Testing Assessment (Verstraete AG, ed), ROSITA Consortium, Gent: 2001; pp. 103–166.

6. Verstraete AG and Puddu M. Evaluation of different roadside drug tests. In Rosita. Roadside Testing Assessment (Verstraete, A. G., ed), ROSITA Consortium, Gent: 2001; pp. 167–232.

7. Zweig MH and Campbell G. Receiver-operating characteristic (ROC) plots: a fundamental evaluation tool in clinical medicine. Clin Chem 1993;39:561–577.

8. Kidwell DA, Holland JC, and Athanaselis S. Testing for drugs of abuse in saliva and sweat. J Chromatogr B Biomed Sci Appl 1998;713:111–135.

9. Verstraete AG and Puddu M. General conclusions and recommendations, in ROSITA. Roadside Testing Assessment (Verstraete AG, ed), ROSITA Consortium, Gent: 2001; pp. 393–397.

10. Kintz P, Cirimele V, and Ludes B. Detection of cannabis in oral fluid (saliva) and forehead wipes (sweat) from impaired drivers. J Anal Toxicol 2000;24:557–561.

11. Steinmeyer S, Ohr H, Maurer HJ, et al. Practical aspects of roadside tests for administrative traffic offences in Germany. Forensic Sci Int 2001;121:33–36.

12. Gronholm M and Lillsunde P. A comparison between on-site immunoassay drug-testing devices and laboratory results. Forensic Sci Int 2001;121:37–46.

13. Samyn N, De Boeck G, and Verstraete AG. The use of oral fluid and sweat wipes for the detection of drugs of abuse in drivers. J Forensic Sci 2002;47:1380–1387.

14. Walsh JM, Flegel R, Crouch DJ, et al. An evaluation of rapid point-of-collection oral fluid drug-testing devices. J Anal Toxicol 2003;27:429–439.

15. Walsh JM. An evaluation of oral fluid point of collection testing devices phase 2, The Walsh Group, Bethesda, MD: 2003.

Chapter 18

Trends in Drug Testing
Concluding Remarks

Raphael C. Wong

1. INTRODUCTION

For the drug-testing industry, this is a time of new technologies and changes. There are various forms of lateral-flow devices making drug testing easier and providing results in matters of minutes. Test matrices other than urine are being investigated in which windows of detection can be narrowed to a few hours for detection of driving under the influence or be extended to several months to provide a long-term history of drug use. Moreover, information on drug testing is now widely available on the Internet, so that many more nonscientists are educated about drug testing. In this final chapter, we attempt to provide our personal thoughts on the industrial and scientific trends.

2. CONTINUOUS POPULARITY OF THE URINE SPECIMEN MATRIX

For the foreseeable future, urine will remain the matrix of choice. This is partly because of its abundant scientific documentation, enabling easier defensibility in court challenge. Moreover, because of its long history of use, urine tests are better understood by everyone involved than are tests with other matrices.

2.1. Increasing Utilization of On-Site Urine Screen Tests

Lateral-flow on-site devices require little training to operate, can provide results quickly, and have provided reliable results. Hence, they are gaining

From: *Forensic Science and Medicine: Drugs of Abuse: Body Fluid Testing*
Edited by R. C. Wong and H. Y. Tse © Humana Press Inc., Totowa, NJ

acceptance. Such drug screens have been widely utilized in the criminal-justice arena because of their low cost. In the workplace market segment, there is a continuous shift toward screening drugs on-site by the specimen collectors rather than sending the specimen to be tested to a reference laboratory. This practice trims down tremendously the time and cost of initial drug screens. Now a drug screen takes only minutes, with results available usually while the donors are present. Positive screen tests can still be sent to laboratories for confirmation. In light of this change, reference laboratories have been performing fewer drug screens, and competition for business among laboratories has been fierce. The end result is that there have been consolidations of laboratories, and many reference laboratories have made on-site test devices available to their customers.

3. DECREASING PRICES OF ON-SITE DEVICES AS A RESULT OF COMPETITION

With the popularity of the on-site drug screens, new manufacturers, including several from overseas, have entered the market because of the apparent low startup cost of lateral-flow technology. In order to garner market share, many of these new entrants have resorted to a low-price strategy. Although it is good news to the end-users, impacts on the US manufacturers are tremendous. In response to the lowered margin, many are forced to move manufacturing to locations in Mexico or China, while others have left the drug-testing industry altogether. Moreover, the low price also reduces funding for research and development.

4. TEST-CUP ON-SITE DEVICES GAINING POPULARITY

For urine on-site lateral-flow devices, there are basically four formats:

1. Cassette device, in which urine specimen is transferred from a collection cup to a sample hole on the cassette for testing;
2. Dipstick device, in which the lateral-flow test strip in a holder is dipped into sample in a collection cup;
3. Dipcard device, in which multiple test strips are bundled together in a card-type holder and dipped into a collection cup;
4. Test-cup device, in which test strips are incorporated into the collection cup.

Test-cup devices are preferred, because they are convenient and eliminate much of the possibility of operator exposure to urine specimens. However, as a result of the complexity and cost of manufacturing, cup devices are historically higher in price. With the decreasing prices of on-site devices, cup devices are now affordable to most users, and hence there should be a continuous increase in their use.

5. ADULTERATION REMAINS A CHALLENGE TO URINE DRUG TESTING

Addicts to abused drugs have great incentives to try to defeat drug tests, and they often use adulteration products. Because of the high profit margin, great customer demand, low cost of entry, and wide accessibility via the Internet, there are many manufacturers in this market. Not only do some of them employ innovative chemists, they also provide informative educational materials on their Web sites, which help the abusers understand how the drug-testing system works and how to defeat the tests. Although legislators in many states have banned adulterant-product sales, and guidelines for detecting their presence have been established, adulteration will remain a challenge to urine drug testing (*see* Chapters 13 and 14).

5.1. Adulteration Test Products Become a Necessity

With the spread of adulteration knowledge via the Internet, use of adulterants has increased . Hence, adulteration testing has become a necessity for guaranteeing the integrity of the drug-test process. However, laboratory-based adulterant test systems may not sufficiently detect all of the adulteration products in submitted specimens, because of the time delay involved in shipping and the quick dissemination of many newer-generation adulterants. Hence, the importance of on-site adulterant tests will increase (an example is discussed in Chapter 14). With the incorporation of adulterant test panels into lateral-flow drug test devices like the test cup, specimen integrity is established while the drug testing is being performed (an example is discussed in Chapter 12). This type of test product will become the device of choice.

6. MORE ATTENTION WILL BE PAID TO ALTERNATIVE SPECIMENS

Owing mainly to the adulteration issue and reduced obtrusiveness of the collection process, alternative specimens (*see* Chapters 2 and 7–11) have been receiving increased attention. Among them, oral fluid appears most interesting because sample collection is easiest and testing can be performed on-site for a quick result. Moreover, because drug levels in oral fluid are more closely correlated with those in blood than those in urine, oral-fluid drug tests better measure the degree to which a donor is under the influence. This potential advantage aroused the interest of many police departments, and oral-fluid test devices are being evaluated in roadside drug testing (*see* Chapter 17).

6.1. Challenges Faced in Oral-Fluid Drug Screening

Before oral-fluid drug screens can be widely accepted, additional efforts must be made to educate their users on the difference between oral-fluid tests and urine tests, emphasizing the shorter windows of detection for various drugs and the fact that the detectable molecules are parent drugs instead of metabolites for some drugs. Cut-off concentrations must be studied further to ensure that food or other ingestibles do not cause false-positive results.

For manufacturers of on-site drug screens, the challenge is to increase the sensitivity of the Δ-9-tetrahydrocannabinol so that a longer window of detection can be established. Once these challenges are met, oral-fluid drug screens can garner a substantial share of the drug-testing market.

7. GROWING ACCEPTANCE IN THE REST OF THE WORLD

Although the majority of drug testing is still being performed in the United States, acceptance of drug testing has been growing in the rest of the world. Part of this is due to the realization that there is a real correlation of decreased work performance with the use of drugs.

In Europe and Asia, moreover, there is a growing awareness of the use of adulterants. In addition, the interest in oral-fluid test devices in Europe is very high, especially in the law-enforcement sector.

8. CONCLUSIONS

The above discussion provides a glimpse of what we believe will happen in the drug-testing industry. The decreasing price of urine tests will make them more affordable. Oral-fluid tests will reduce objection to specimen collection. In the end, all of these factors should help to enable a more widespread use of drug testing. We hope that the end result will be that drug testing will contribute to the reduction or elimination of abused drug use.

Index

A

Accuracy, calculation, 278
AdultaCheck 6, adulteration detection, 228, 229, 231, 238
Adulteration,
    classification of adulterants, 220
    combined testing with drug screening, 243
    frequency, 234
    government response, 236, 237
    hair specimens, 225
    incentives, 223
    Intercept® device, 121, 126
    oral fluid specimens, 225
    prospects for testing, 295
    urine specimens,
        chemical adulterant mechanisms, 235, 236
        detection for integrity check,
        AdultaCheck 6, 228, 229, 231, 238
        glutaraldehyde, 228
        Intect® 7, 228, 229, 231, 238–243
        Multistix®, 238
        nitrite, 227
        peroxidase, 227, 228
        pyridinium chlorochromate, 226
        Urine ID™, 238
        urine properties, 226
        diluted urine, 221, 222, 235
        glutaraldehyde, 224, 225
        household chemicals, 222, 223, 234
        nitrites, 223, 224
        overview, 220, 235
        pyridinium chlorochromate, 223
        Stealth and peroxidase, 224
        substitution or synthetic urine, 220, 221, 234, 235
Alcohol, *see* Ethanol
Amphetamine,
    history of use, 218
    window of detection, 219
Amtrak Colonial accident, history of drug testing, 3
Analytical techniques, classification, 30, 31
Applications, drugs of abuse testing, 32, 33
Automation, *see* Lateral-flow assays

B

Blood specimens, advantages and limitations, 12, 13
Breast milk, specimen drug testing, 24

C

Capillary electrophoresis (CE),
    mass spectrometry coupling, 52

principles, 49, 50
Capillary isotachophoresis (CITP),
      principles, 49
Capillary zone electrophoresis (CZE),
      principles, 49
CE, *see* Capillary electrophoresis
CEDIA, *see* Cloned enzyme donor
      immunoassay
Chromatography, definition, 43
CITP, *see* Capillary isotachophoresis
Cloned enzyme donor immunoassay
      (CEDIA), principles, 38, 39
Cocaine,
      hair levels of proven users, 191–193
      history of use, 218
      window of detection, 219
Costs, drug testing devices,
      criminal justice system
            considerations, 257
      manufacturer competition and
            decreasing prices, 294
      ROSITA findings, 276
Criminal justice system,
      corrections, 6, 7, 251
      drug courts,
            administration, 250
            ancillary services, 251
            defense attorney, 249
            evaluation, 251, 252
            functional significance, 252
            judge, 248, 249
            key components, 252–254
            overview, 6, 248
            prosecutors, 249, 250
            prospects, 257, 258
      drug testing,
            importance, 254
            methodology and technology,
                  256, 257

            minimum standards, 255, 256
            volume and costs, 257
      drug treatment programs, 7, 250, 251
      drug-related crime prevalence, 258
      Europe, see European drug testing
      probation, 251
Cut-off values,
      determination, 5, 6, 33, 34
      Dräger DrugTest®, 138
      Drugwipe® device, 166–169
      Oratect® device, 147
      table of drugs, 219
CZE, *see* Capillary zone electrophoresis

D

Dräger DrugTest®,
      advantages of oral fluid testing, 133,
            134
      clinical studies and validation, 142,
            143
      cut-off values, 138
      design, 134–137
      principles, 138, 140
Drug courts, *see* Criminal justice
      system
DrugTest®, see Dräger DrugTest®
Drugwipe® device,
      amphetamine testing in sweat vs
            saliva, 171, 172
      cut-off values and ROSITA II
            confirmation, 166–169
      design, 162, 163
      methylenedioxymethamphetamine
            testing,
            saliva, 170
            sweat, 172, 173
      principles of test, 163, 164
      reader, 166

roadside study in Germany, 173–175
saliva sample collection, 165
sweat sample collection, 165, 166
technical features, 164, 165

E

Ecstasy, *see*
    Methylenedioxymethamphetamine
Efficiency, calculation, 34, 35
EIA, *see* Enzyme immunoassay
ELISA, *see* Enzyme-linked
    immunosorbent assay
Emergency medicine, drug testing, 9
EMIT, *see* Enzyme-multiplied
    immunoassay technique
Enzyme immunoassay (EIA),
    principles, 118, 119
Enzyme-enhanced chemiluminescence
    immunoassay (IMMULITE),
    principles, 40
Enzyme-linked immunosorbent assay
    (ELISA),
    Oratect® device validation, 149, 152
    principles, 36, 38
Enzyme-multiplied immunoassay
    technique (EMIT),
    historical perspective, 2
    principles, 38
eScreen® system,
    benefits of closed information
        system, 213
    development, 207–209
    laboratory service decentralization to
        point of collection, 205,
        206
    myeScreen.com portal, 213, 214
    reader, 212
    software, 211, 212

urine specimen collection, 209, 210
Ethanol,
    oral fluid specimen testing, 16
    OratectPlus™ testing, 157, 158
European drug testing,
    blood tests, 267
    devices, 266, 267
    drug targets, 262, 263
    frequency and market for testing,
        260–262
    hair tests, 268, 269
    hospitals, 265, 266
    oral fluid tests, 268
    police, 264
    prisons, 263, 264
    probation, 264
    prospects, 296
    regulation, 269
    ROSITA project, *see* ROSITA
    sweat tests, 268
    urine tests, 267
    workplace, 265

F

False-negative, definition, 34
False-positive, definition, 34
FDA, *see* Food and Drug
    Administration
Fluorescence polarization immunoassay
    (FPIA), principles, 39
Food and Drug Administration (FDA),
    regulation of drug testing
        products, 4, 5
FPIA, *see* Fluorescence polarization
    immunoassay
FRAT, *see* Free radical assay technique
Free radical assay technique (FRAT),
    historical perspective, 2

G

Gas chromatography (GC),
    carrier gas, 46, 47
    columns, 47
    computers, 48
    detectors, 47
    injector, 46
    internal standards, 46
    mass spectrometry coupling, 52–55
    principles, 44, 45
    sample preparation and
            derivatization, 45, 46
    temperature control, 47
GC, *see* Gas chromatography
Glutaraldehyde,
    adulteration of urine specimens, 224,
        225
    detection in specimens, 228

H

Hair specimens,
    adulteration, 225
    advantages, 178
    analytical techniques, 20, 170
    applications,
        criminal justice and rehabilitation,
            194
        medical applications, 195
        overview, 178
    caveats, 20, 21
    collection and handling, 179
    conferences, 19, 20
    drug incorporation mechanism, 20,
        178, 179
    drug levels in hair of proven users,
        cocaine, 191–193
        methamphetamine, 193
        opiates, 193

        tetrahydrocannabinol, 193, 194
    environmental contamination and
            washing, 184, 185
    growth and history of drug use, 19
    hair color bias studies, 185, 186
    mass spectrometry analysis,
        calibration, 188, 191
        extraction methods, 186, 187
        instrumentation, 187
        ionization, 187, 188
    preliminary screening assays for
            drugs,
        analytical goals, 180, 181
        sample preparation and matrix
                effects, 181, 183, 184
    prospects, 195, 196
    structure of hair, 178, 179
High-performance capillary
        electrophoresis (HPCE),
    principles, 49
High-performance liquid
        chromatography (HPLC),
    detectors, 48, 49
    mass spectrometry coupling, 49, 52,
        55
    principles, 48
    sample preparation, 48
Household chemicals, adulteration of
        urine specimens, 222, 223
HPCE, *see* High-performance capillary
        electrophoresis
HPLC, *see* High-performance liquid
        chromatography

I

IMMULITE, *see* Enzyme-enhanced
        chemiluminescence immunoassay
Immunoassay, *see also specific*
        immunoassays,

competitive immunoassays with
combined labels, 39, 40
heterogeneous competitive
immunoassays, 36–38
homogeneous competitive
immunoassays, 38, 39
lateral-flow assays, *see* Lateral-flow
assays
point-of-collection drugs-of-abuse
testing, 40–42
principles, 35, 36
Intect® 7
adulteration detection, 228, 229, 231,
238–243
analyses, 239–241
design, 238, 239
kinetic studies, 241–243
Intercept(r) device,
algorithm for testing, 118, 128
cross-reactivity, 121, 123–125
enzyme immunoassay principles,
118, 119
interferents and adulterants, 121, 126
limits of detection and analytical
sensitivity, 120
precision, 120–122
principles, 117, 118
urine test comparison, 128, 130
validation with gas chromatography-
mass spectrometry,
126–129
Interferents, *see also* Adulteration,
Intercept® device, 121, 126
Oratect® device,
beverages, 157
cosmetic and hygiene products, 157
ethnic meals, 155, 157
food ingredients, 157
table of compounds, 156

K

KIMS, *see* Kinetic interaction of
microparticles in solution
Kinetic interaction of microparticles in
solution (KIMS), principles, 39

L

Lateral-flow assays,
antibodies,
colloidal gold conjugation,
92–94
gold-labeled antibody application
to test strip,
pad application, 95
pad drying, 95–97
labeling approaches, 91, 92
monoclonal vs polyclonal, 90
production, 89, 90
purification, 90, 91
automation,
assembly of devices, 112, 113
design factors,
adhesives, 102
dimensioning and tolerance,
102–106
housing, 106–109
lamination of test strips,
103–106
materials selection, 100–102
high-volume manufacturing,
dispensing, 112
lamination, 112
imperatives, 113, 114
low- to moderate-volume
manufacturing,
cutting of test strips, 110, 111
dispensing, 110
lamination, 110

bar code perspective of test lines,
206, 207
detection system overview, 88, 89
immunoassays for point-of-
collection testing, 41
nitrocellulose membranes, *see*
Nitrocellulose
membranes
prospects, 97, 98
surfactants, 97
test strip design, 72, 73, 88, 99, 100
Liquid chromatography, *see* High-
performance liquid
chromatography

M

Marijuana,
history of use, 218
window of detection, 219
Mass spectrometry (MS),
computers, 52
coupling with separation techniques,
52–55
detectors, 52
hair analysis,
calibration, 188, 191
extraction methods, 186, 187
instrumentation, 187
ionization, 187, 188
ion source and ionization techniques,
50, 51
mass analyzer, 51, 52
principles, 50
tandem mass spectrometry, 55
vacuum system, 52
MDMA, *see*
Methylenedioxymethamphetamine
MECC, *see* Micellar electrokinetic
capillary chromatography

Meconium, specimen drug testing, 23
Methamphetamine, hair levels of
proven users, 193
Methylenedioxymethamphetamine
(MDMA),
Drugwipe® device testing,
saliva, 170
sweat, 172, 173
history of use, 218
window of detection, 219
Micellar electrokinetic capillary
chromatography (MECC),
principles, 49
MS, *see* Mass spectrometry
Multistix®, adulteration detection, 238

N

Nails, specimen drug testing, 24
Nitrites,
adulteration of urine specimens, 223,
224
detection in specimens, 227
Nitrocellulose membranes,
advantages in lateral-flow assays, 85
blocking agents, 83, 84
capture reagent lines,
capillary flow time effects, 81
chemical interaction effects, 81,
82
function, 79, 80
reagent application, 80
characterization,
capillary flow time, 76
overview, 75, 76
surface quality, 77
thickness, 76, 77
historical perspective, 71, 72
manufacture,
backing, 74, 75, 101, 102

casting, 74
nitrocellulose lacquers, 73, 74
nitrocellulose polymer, 73
protein-binding properties,
adsorption and retention, 78
capacity, 78
orientation, 78
reactivity, 79
signal development in lateral-flow
assays,
liquid flow uniformity, 82, 83
sensitivity, 83
test strip design, 72, 73, 88, 99, 100

O

Opiates,
gas chromatography–mass
spectrometry, 151, 153
hair levels of proven users, 193
Oral fluid specimens,
adulteration, 225
advantages, 16
analytical techniques, 17, 18
caveats, 18, 19
commercial tests, 145, 146
Dräger DrugTest®, *see* Dräger
DrugTest®
Drugwipe® test, *see* Drugwipe®
device
ethanol testing, 16
historical perspective, 15, 16
Intercept® testing, *see* Intercept®
device
limitations, 17
Oratect® testing, *see* Oratect®
device
physiology, 17, 115–117
point-of-collection testing
challenges, 146

prospects for testing, 131, 295, 296
types, 15, 116
Oratect® device,
advantages, 157, 158
cross-reactivity, 153–155
cut-off values, 147
description, 146–148
interfering substances,
beverages, 157
cosmetic and hygiene products,
157
ethnic meals, 155, 157
food ingredients, 157
table of compounds, 156
opiate detection window, 153
OratectPlus™ testing for ethanol,
157, 158
precision, 149
principles of testing, 148
test line intensity over time, 149
test procedures, 148
tetrahydrocannabinol detection over
time, 153, 155
validation,
enzyme-linked immunosorbent
assay, 149, 152
opiate gas chromatography–mass
spectrometry, 151, 153
urine gas chromatography–mass
spectrometry, 149, 151

P

PCP, *see* Phencyclidine
Peroxidase,
adulteration of urine specimens, 224
detection in specimens, 227, 228
Phencyclidine (PCP),
history of use, 218
window of detection, 219

POCT, *see* Point-of-collection testing
Point-of-collection testing (POCT), *see also specific devices*,
  bar code perspective of test lines,
      206, 207
  barriers to manual testing, 208, 209
  benefits, 202
  competitive immunoassays, 41, 42
  complications,
      accuracy concerns, 203, 204
      aliquoting of specimens, 203
      donor anonymity, 204
      transcription errors, 204, 205
  implementation, 40, 41
  laboratory service decentralization to
      point of collection, 205,
      206
  oral fluid testing challenges, 146
Pyridinium chlorochromate,
  adulteration of urine specimens, 223
  detection in specimens, 226

R

RA, *see* Receptor assay
Radioimmunoassay (RIA), principles, 36
Receptor assay (RA),
  principles, 41, 43
  radio-receptor assay, 43
RIA, *see* Radioimmunoassay
Roadside testing, *see* ROSITA
ROSITA,
  aims, 273
  device testing,
      accuracy, sensitivity, and
          specificity, 279,
          281–285
      cost comparison, 276
      study methods, 276–278
      types of devices, 274, 275

  validation, 279, 280
  difficulty of roadside testing, 286–288
  drugs and medicines affecting driver
      performance, 274
  influence on drug testing field, 289,
      291
  limitations of study, 285, 286
  official partners, 273
  practical and operational aspects of
      roadside testing, 285
  rationale for study, 272
  recommendations,
      specimen preferences, 288, 289
      traffic safety role of roadside
          testing, 288
  ROSITA II,
      detection limit findings, 289, 291
      Drugwipe® device cut-off value
          confirmation, 166–169
      overview, 289, 290
      specimen comparison, 275, 276
      target drugs, 275

S

Saliva, *see* Oral fluid specimens
SAMHSA, *see* Substance Abuse and
      Mental Health Services
      Administration
Schools, drug testing, 9, 10
Semen, specimen drug testing, 24
Sensitivity, calculation, 34, 278
Specificity, calculation, 34, 278
State regulations, drug testing, 5
Stealth,
      adulteration of urine specimens, 224
      detection in specimens, 227, 228
Substance Abuse and Mental Health
      Services Administration
      (SAMHSA),

drug testing guidelines, 4, 5, 10, 32, 33, 220
specimen validation criteria, 236, 237
Sweat specimens,
analysis, 22, 23
caveats, 23
collection, 22, 23
composition, 22
Drugwipe® test, *see* Drugwipe® device

T

Test strip, *see* Lateral-flow assays
Test-cup devices, popularity, 294
Tetrahydrocannabinol (THC),
hair levels of proven users, 193, 194
Oratect® device detection, 153, 155
THC, *see* Tetrahydrocannabinol
Thin-layer chromatography (TLC),
principles, 44
TLC, *see* Thin-layer chromatography
True-negative, definition, 34
True-positive, definition, 34
Urine ID™, adulteration detection, 238
Urine specimens,
adulteration,
chemical adulterant mechanisms, 235, 236
detection for integrity check,
AdultaCheck 6, 228, 229, 231
glutaraldehyde, 228
Intect(r) 7, 228, 229, 231
nitrite, 227
peroxidase, 227, 228

pyridinium chlorochromate, 226
urine properties, 226
diluted urine, 221, 222, 235
glutaraldehyde, 224, 225
household chemicals, 222, 223, 234
nitrites, 223, 224
overview, 220, 235
pyridinium chlorochromate, 223
Stealth and peroxidase, 224
substitution or synthetic urine, 220, 221, 234, 235
advantages, 13, 14, 293
analytical techniques, 14
caveats, 14, 15
eScreen® point-of-collection testing, *see* eScreen® system
on-site testing trends, 293, 294
US *Nimitz* accident, history of drug testing, 3

V, W

Vernix caseosa, specimen drug testing, 24
Vietnam War, history of drug testing, 2
Vitreous humor, specimen drug testing, 24
Workplace testing,
collection, 8
laboratories, 8, 9
medical review officer, 9
policy, 7
process, 7, 8
third-party administrator, 9